Seminars in the Psychiatry of Intellectual Disability

Third Edition

College Seminars Series

For details of available and forthcoming books in the College Seminars Series please visit:
www.cambridge.org/series/college-seminars-series/

Seminars in the Psychiatry of Intellectual Disability

Third Edition

Edited by
Mark Scheepers
2gether NHS Foundation Trust

Mike Kerr
Cardiff University

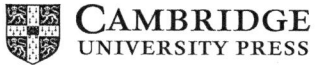

CAMBRIDGE
UNIVERSITY PRESS

University Printing House, Cambridge CB2 8BS, United Kingdom

One Liberty Plaza, 20th Floor, New York, NY 10006, USA

477 Williamstown Road, Port Melbourne, VIC 3207, Australia

314–321, 3rd Floor, Plot 3, Splendor Forum, Jasola District Centre, New Delhi – 110025, India

79 Anson Road, #06-04/06, Singapore 079906

Cambridge University Press is part of the University of Cambridge.

It furthers the University's mission by disseminating knowledge in the pursuit of education, learning, and research at the highest international levels of excellence.

www.cambridge.org
Information on this title: www.cambridge.org/9781108465069
DOI: 10.1017/9781108617444

© The Royal College of Psychiatrists 1997, 2003, 2019

This publication is in copyright. Subject to statutory exception and to the provisions of relevant collective licensing agreements, no reproduction of any part may take place without the written permission of Cambridge University Press.

This book was previously published by The Royal College of Psychiatrists.

First published 1997, The Royal College of Psychiatrists
Second edition 2003, The Royal College of Psychiatrists
This third edition published by Cambridge University Press 2019

Printed and bound in Great Britain by Clays Ltd, Elcograf S.p.A.

A catalogue record for this publication is available from the British Library.

Library of Congress Cataloging-in-Publication Data
Names: Scheepers, Mark, editor. | Kerr, Michael (Michael P.), editor.
Title: Seminars in the psychiatry of intellectual disability / edited by Mark Scheepers, Mike Kerr. Other titles: College seminars series (Cambridge, England)
Description: Third edition. | Cambridge, United Kingdom ; New York, NY : University Printing House, [2019] | Series: College seminars series | Includes bibliographical references.
Identifiers: LCCN 2018029228 | ISBN 9781108465069
Subjects: | MESH: Intellectual Disability
Classification: LCC HV3004 | NLM WM 300 | DDC 362.3–dc23
LC record available at https://lccn.loc.gov/2018029228

ISBN 978-1-108-46506-9 Paperback

Cambridge University Press has no responsibility for the persistence or accuracy of URLs for external or third-party internet websites referred to in this publication and does not guarantee that any content on such websites is, or will remain, accurate or appropriate.

....

Every effort has been made in preparing this book to provide accurate and up-to-date information that is in accord with accepted standards and practice at the time of publication. Although case histories are drawn from actual cases, every effort has been made to disguise the identities of the individuals involved. Nevertheless, the authors, editors, and publishers can make no warranties that the information contained herein is totally free from error, not least because clinical standards are constantly changing through research and regulation. The authors, editors, and publishers therefore disclaim all liability for direct or consequential damages resulting from the use of material contained in this book. Readers are strongly advised to pay careful attention to information provided by the manufacturer of any drugs or equipment that they plan to use.

Contents

List of Contributors   vii

Section 1 Understanding Intellectual Disability

1. **Epidemiology of Intellectual Disability**   1
Christine Linehan

2. **Genetics of Intellectual Disability**   12
Kate Wolfe, Andre Strydom and Nick Bass

3. **Behavioural Phenotypes**   28
Ruth Bevan and Gill Bell

4. **Communication in People with Intellectual Disability**   42
Lauren Edwards

Section 2 Co-morbidity

5. **Autism**   53
Tom Berney and Peter Carpenter

6. **Epilepsy and Intellectual Disability**   65
Mike Kerr and Lance Watkins

7. **Complex Physical Health Issues in People with Intellectual Disability**   83
Robyn A. Wallace and Mark Scheepers

8. **Mortality in People with Intellectual Disability**   102
Pauline Heslop and Matthew Hoghton

Section 3 Psychiatric and Behavioural Disorders

9. **Children with Intellectual Disabilities and Psychiatric Problems**   115
Pru Allington-Smith

10. **Adults with Intellectual Disabilities and Psychiatric Disorders**   125
Sally-Ann Cooper

11. **Management of Dementia in Intellectual Disability**   136
Vee P. Prasher and Hassan Mahmood

12. **Forensic Psychiatry and Intellectual Disability**   147
Harm Boer and Liz Beber

13. **Psychotherapy in People with Intellectual Disabilities**   158
Rajnish Attavar and Kuljit Bhogal

14. **Psychological Treatment of Common Behavioural Disorders**   165
Audrey Espie and Andrew Jahoda

15. **Challenging Behaviour and the Use of Pharmacological Interventions**   179
John Devapriam and Regi T. Alexander

Section 4 Delivering High-Quality Care

16 **History of Services for People with Disorders of Intellectual Development** 191
Peter Carpenter

17 **Inpatient Care for People with Intellectual Disability** 204
Kiran Purandare and Shaun Gravestock

18 **Legal Provisions and Restrictive Practices** 213
Kevin O'Shea

19 **Leadership and Management** 222
Paul Winterbottom

20 **Clinical Research in Intellectual Disabilities: Ethical and Methodological Challenges** 231
Niall O'Kane, Sujata Soni and Angela Hassiotis

21 **Training in Intellectual Disability Psychiatry** 245
Bernice Knight and Joanna Kingston

Index 255

Contributors

Regi T. Alexander, Consultant Psychiatrist, Hertfordshire Partnership University NHS Foundation Trust, Norwich, UK

Pru Allington-Smith, Consultant Psychiatrist in Child and Adolescent Learning Disability, Brooklands Hospital, Birmingham, UK

Rajnish Attavar, Consultant Psychiatrist in Learning Disabilities, Hertfordshire Partnership University NHS Foundation Trust, Aylesbury, UK

Nick Bass, senior lecturer/Honorary Consultant Psychiatrist, UCL Division of Psychiatry, University College London, London, UK

Liz Beber, Consultant Psychiatrist, Learning Disability Pathway, St Andrews Healthcare, Northampton, UK

Gill Bell, Consultant Forensic Adolescent Learning Disability Psychiatrist, Northumberland Tyne and Wear NHS Foundation Trust, Newcastle upon Tyne, UK

Tom Berney, Developmental Psychiatrist, Newcastle upon Tyne, UK

Ruth Bevan, Consultant in Gender Dysphoria, Northumberland Tyne and Wear NHS Foundation Trust, Newcastle upon Tyne, UK

Kuljit Bhogal, Consultant Psychiatrist in Learning Disability, Southern Health NHS Foundation Trust, Basingstoke, UK

Harm Boer, Consultant Forensic Psychiatrist for People with Learning Disability, Huntercombe Centre Birmingham, Oldbury, UK

Peter Carpenter, Honorary Consultant Psychiatrist, Avon & Wiltshire Partnership Mental Health NHS Trust, Chippenham, UK

Sally-Ann Cooper, Professor of Learning Disabilities & Honorary Consultant Psychiatrist, Institute of Health and Wellbeing, University of Glasgow, Glasgow, UK

John Devapriam, Consultant Psychiatrist and Medical Director, Worcestershire Health and Care NHS Trust, Worcester, UK

Lauren Edwards, Head of Profession for Speech and Language Therapy and Dietetics, ²gether NHS Foundation Trust, Gloucester, UK

Audrey Espie, Consultant Clinical Neuropsychologist, West Dumbarton Learning Disability Service, Glasgow, UK

Shaun Gravestock, Consultant Psychiatrist, John Howard Centre, East London Foundation NHS Trust, London, UK

Angela Hassiotis, Professor of Psychiatry of Intellectual Disability and Honorary Consultant Psychiatrist, UCL Division of Psychiatry, University College London, London, UK

Pauline Heslop, Professor of Intellectual Disabilities Research, University of Bristol, Bristol, UK

Matthew Hoghton, General Practitioner, Clevedon Medical Centre, Clevedon, UK

Andrew Jahoda, Professor of Learning Disabilities, Psychological Medicine, Gartnavel Royal Hospital, Glasgow, UK

Mike Kerr, Emeritus Professor of Learning Disability Psychiatry, Institute of Psychological Medicine and Clinical Neurosciences, Cardiff University, Cardiff, UK

Joanna Kingston, ST6 Higher Trainee in Psychiatry of Intellectual Disability, Health Education England, Bristol, UK

Bernice Knight, ST5 Higher Trainee in Psychiatry of Intellectual Disability & National Medical Director's Clinical Fellow, Health Education England, London, UK

Christine Linehan, Director UCD Centre for Disability Studies, School of Psychology, University College Dublin, Dublin, Ireland.

Hassan Mahmood, ST5 Specialist Registrar in Intellectual Disabilities, Birmingham Community Healthcare NHS Foundation Trust, Birmingham, UK

Niall O'Kane, ST6 Higher Trainee in Psychiatry of Intellectual Disability, Goodmayes Hospital, London, UK

Kevin O'Shea, Consultant Psychiatrist, Intellectual Disability (Forensic), Woodhaven Hospital, Southampton, UK

Vee P. Prasher, Consultant and Visiting Professor of Learning Disability, Birmingham Community Healthcare NHS Foundation Trust, Birmingham, UK

Kiran Purandare, Honorary Senior Clinical Lecturer, Imperial College & Consultant Psychiatrist, CNWL NHS Foundation Trust, London, UK

Mark Scheepers, Consultant Psychiatrist, Learning Disability Services, ^{2}gether NHS Foundation Trust, Gloucester, UK

Sujata Soni, Consultant Psychiatrist, Camden Learning Disability Service, London, UK

Andre Strydom, Professor of Intellectual Disabilities, Institute of Psychiatry Psychology and Neuroscience, King's College London, London, UK

Robyn A. Wallace, Clinical Associate Professor School of Medicine, University of Tasmania & Consultant Physician, SHAID (Specialised Healthcare for Adults with Intellectual Disability), Calvary Lenah Valley Hospital, Tasmania, Australia

Lance Watkins, ST6 Higher Trainee, Psychiatry of Learning Disability, Wales Deanery, Cardiff University, Cardiff, UK

Paul Winterbottom, past Medical Director & Consultant Psychiatrist, Learning Disability Services, ^{2}gether NHS Trust, Gloucester, UK

Kate Wolfe, MRC PhD student, UCL Division of Psychiatry, University College London, London, UK

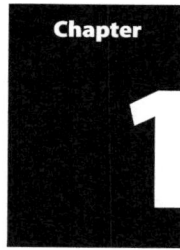

Section 1 Understanding Intellectual Disability

Chapter 1: Epidemiology of Intellectual Disability

Christine Linehan

1.1 Introduction

This chapter examines the epidemiology of intellectual disability (ID). Epidemiology is 'the study of the occurrence and distribution of health-related states or events in specified populations, including the study of the determinants influencing such states, and the application of knowledge to control the health problem' (Porta, 2008). Epidemiological research in ID is complicated not only by the stigma associated with many historical terms used to denote ID, but also by the heterogeneity of different presentations of disability represented under this single entity (Leonard & Wen, 2002). This chapter discusses first the historical and current perspectives of ID; then terminology, classification and diagnosis; prevalence and incidence; aetiology; and finally concludes with morbidity and mortality.

1.2 Perspectives of ID

A contextual approach is required when considering the epidemiology of ID. Unlike other health conditions, such as communicable disease which may more traditionally be the focus of epidemiological study, the issue of what constitutes a 'true case' of a person with an ID (caseness) has been conceptualised using various historical approaches. Schalock (2013) identifies four of these approaches:

(1) Social criterion: prior to the introduction of formal diagnostic criteria for ID, individuals were identified on the basis of their behaviour, or more specifically their 'failure' to socially adapt to their environment (Greenspan, 2003, 2006a, 2006b).
(2) Clinical criterion: 'the medical model' classified individuals with ID on the presence of specific symptoms and syndromes with a focus on heredity, organicity and pathology. The model sought to 'cure' disability and actively pursued prevention through segregation policies (Drum, 2009; Devlieger; Rusch & Pfeiffer 2003).
(3) Intellectual criterion: psychometric testing heralded the classification of individuals on the basis of intelligence as measured by the IQ test (Devlieger, 2003).
(4) Dual criterion: in 1959 the American Association on Mental Deficiency (AAMD; now AAIDD, the American Association on Intellectual and Developmental Disabilities) combined both intellectual and social criteria by defining ID as deficits originating in the developmental period in intellectual functioning with co-morbid difficulties in 'maturation, learning and social adjustment', collectively referred to as 'adaptive behaviours'.

The addition of 'adaptive behaviour' as a criterion for ID was a response to ongoing dissatisfaction with IQ as the sole indicator of ID, notably due to its failure to measure social and practical skills (Schalock et al., 2010). Originally defined as 'the effectiveness with which the individual copes with the nature and social demands of his environment' (Heber, 1959: 61), adaptive behaviour is currently conceptualised as a multidimensional concept comprising conceptual skills (e.g. linguistic and numeric skills), social skills (e.g. interpersonal skills, following rules) and practical skills (e.g. daily living and occupational skills). The addition of adaptive behaviour in the classification criteria of ID reflects efforts by the disability movement to move ID from a medical diagnostic position where ID was considered an 'absolute trait' of the individual to an ecological position where ID is influenced by the development of adaptive skills (AAIDD, 2010).

Advancing this ecological position, AAIDD developed a support needs model of disability where ID is understood as neither fixed nor dichotomised but rather as fluid and changing depending on the individual's functional limitations and the supports available within the person's environment. 'Supports' are defined as resources and strategies that promote personal development and enhance functioning, while 'support need' is identified as a psychological construct referring to both the pattern and intensity of support required for an individual with disability to participate in activities associated with 'normative human functioning' (Thompson et al., 2009). While both adaptive behaviour and support needs address typical performance on everyday tasks, they differ in focus whereby adaptive behaviour assesses the individual's level of performance or mastery on a given task, while support needs focuses on the type and intensity of support that an individual requires to successfully participate in an activity (Buntinx, 2015); 'put another way, if supports were removed, people with ID would not be able to function as successfully in typical activities and settings' (AAIDD, 2010: 113). Both adaptive behaviour and support needs are deemed relatively recent constructs which remain highly influential progressing the understanding, diagnosis and classification of ID from an intellectual limitation to an issue concerning the whole person in his or her life situation (Buntinx, 2015).

1.3 Terminology, Classification and Diagnosis

Current classification systems of ID are dominated by three systems: the fifth edition of the American Psychiatric Association's Diagnostic and Statistical Manual of Mental Disorders, known as DSM 5 (APA, 2013); the 10th edition of the World Health Organization's International Classification of Diseases, known as ICD-10 (WHO, 1992); and the 11th edition of the American Association on Intellectual and Developmental Disabilities' manual (AAIDD, 2010). Less utilised for diagnostic purposes is the World Health Organization's International Classification of Functioning, Disability and Health, known as ICF (WHO, 2001). Within the WHO family of classifications, health conditions are classified using ICD-10, while associated functioning and disability are classified using ICF (WHO, 2001). For diagnostic purposes, three criteria are common across current classification systems: deficits in intellectual functioning, deficits in adaptive behaviour, and onset during the developmental period. Deficits in intellectual functioning, typically an IQ score of 70 or less, and deficits in adaptive behaviour are objectively assessed as scoring two standard deviations below the mean on standardised psychometric tests. Intellectual functioning and adaptive behaviour are correlated but are not deemed causally associated (Tasse et al., 2016). Guidance on assessing ID is available from the British Psychological Society.[1]

---

[1] www.rcpsych.ac.uk/pdf/ID%20assessment%20guidance.pdf [accessed 11 August 2018].

Preparations for the 11th edition of WHO's ICD led to the establishment of a Working Group charged with securing international evidence-based consensus on the name, definition, subtypes and architecture of ID (Bertelli et al., 2016). The Working Group comprised various stakeholders including APA, AAIDD, the World Psychiatric Association (WPA) and the International Association for the Scientific Study of Intellectual and Developmental Disabilities (IASSIDD) (Salvador-Carulla et al., 2011). Despite ongoing debate of these definitional issues in the field (Switzky & Greenspan, 2006), the establishment of this international Working Group provided the first expert multidisciplinary discourse on the topic in forty years (Bertelli et al., 2016).

Driving much of the discussion is the apparent inconsistency among classification systems whereby ID is conceptualised as a health disorder by ICD and DSM and as a disability by ICF and AAIDD. Extreme positions in this discourse may conceptualise ID solely as a disability thereby calling for its exclusion from ICD, an action which may potentially render it invisible in many health monitoring systems. At the other extreme, conceptualising ID solely as a health condition is inconsistent with the social and biopsychosocial model of disability adopted by many jurisdictions in terms of legislation, policy and practice (Bertelli et al., 2016).

The Working Group agreed on the term 'Intellectual Developmental Disorder' (IDD) for ICD-11, which is classified within the parent category of 'Neurodevelopmental Disorder'. Intellectual Developmental Disorder is formally defined as 'a group of developmental conditions characterized by significant impairment of cognitive functions which are associated with limitations of learning, adaptive behaviour and skills' (Bertelli et al., 2016: 7). Intellectual Developmental Disorder is described as an early cognitive meta-syndrome analogous to the later-life syndrome of dementia. Conditions classified as Intellectual Developmental Disorders result from significant interference with brain development up to adolescence. Within the WHO family of classifications, Intellectual Developmental Disorder is thus coded within ICD-11, while ID is conceptualised as its functioning and disability counterpart and is coded within ICF. Reflecting this new landscape, APA replaced the term 'Mental Retardation' as used in the fourth edition of DSM (DSM IV) with the term 'Intellectual Disability (Intellectual Developmental Disorder)' (ID/IDD) when publishing the 5th edition (DSM 5) in 2013. The addition of 'Intellectual Developmental Disorder' within DSM 5 specifically aimed to harmonise DSM terminology with that proposed for ICD-11. Similarly, APA changed the classification of ID/IDD from Developmental Disorder in DSM IV to Neurodevelopmental Disorder in DSM 5, once again in order to harmonise with ICD.

Mindful of the degree of heterogeneity in limitations of intellectual functioning and adaptive behaviour among individuals with ID, both DSM and ICD employ a classification of clinical severity using four categories; mild, moderate, severe and profound. Within ICD-10 these categories are based on IQ score (IQ between 50 and 69 is classified within the mild range, 35 to 49 as moderate, 20 to 34 as severe and below 20 as profound). While DSM IV similarly used IQ scores to classify severity, DSM 5 introduces a new classification of mild, moderate, severe and profound ID based on deficits in adaptive behaviours, specifically in the areas of conceptual, social or practical skills. The rationale for employing adaptive behaviour rather than intellectual functioning is 'because it is adaptive functioning that determines the level of support required – moreover, IQ measures are less valid in the lower end of the IQ range' (APA, 2013: 33).

In addition to these four levels of severity, preparations for ICD-11 initiated a discussion of individuals with 'borderline' intellectual functioning, typically defined as individuals who score within the 70–84 IQ range. These individuals are not covered by DSM and ICD (Salvador-Carulla et al., 2011). Described as 'an invisible clinical entity', borderline intellectual functioning is defined as a heterogeneous group of specific neurodevelopmental syndromes, disorders or diseases, distinct from ID (Hassiotis, 2015), which should be prioritised for further development of definition, measurement and intervention (Salvador-Carulla et al., 2011).

1.4 Prevalence and Incidence

A meta-analysis of fifty-two worldwide studies undertaken as part of the Global Burden of Disease study (Gustavsson et al., 2011) estimated the prevalence of ID at 1% globally (95% CI 0.95–1.12), with a moderately higher prevalence among males than females (Maulik et al., 2011). Globally, higher prevalence rates are reported in low-income countries (1.64%) when compared with middle-income (1.59%) and high-income countries (0.92%). The higher prevalence observed in lower-income countries is attributed to environmental factors such as malnutrition, iron deficiency and poor-quality perinatal services (Bertelli et al., 2009).

In general, the global range of estimates is extremely wide. Of the fifty-two studies reported, the lowest prevalence estimate was 0.93 per 1,000 reported from a large screening study of 550,000 residents in Mumbai, India (Dave et al., 2005). In contrast, the highest prevalence estimate was 156.03 per 1,000 reported in one of eight developing regions in a comparative study (Stein et al., 1987). This level of disparity among prevalence estimates is, according to some commentators, 'almost certainly due to methodological flaws' (Tharper et al., 2015: 720). A number of factors are however known to influence prevalence estimates of ID: higher prevalence estimates are reported in lower-income countries; where samples are drawn from urban slums/mixed rural–urban districts; among children and adolescent populations; among population-based screening studies; and in studies where psychometric scales are employed (Maulik et al., 2011).

Epidemiological community surveys reveal the vast majority of persons with ID have 'mild' ID (85%), with only a minority having an ID within the range of 'moderate' (10%), 'severe' (4%), or 'profound' (2%) (King et al., 2009). Prevalence estimates of the severity of ID may however be hindered by a lack of available data. An extensive record linkage study of all individuals born in Western Australia from 1983 to 1992, for example, reported estimates combining mild-to-moderate ID (10.6 per 1,000) and combining severe-to-profound ID (1.4 per 1,000) as no further level of detail was available from the educational sources from which the data were obtained (Leonard et al., 2003).

Higher prevalence estimates reported among studies of child and adolescents when compared with adults are commonly observed and reflect a 'transition cliff' where the age-specific prevalence of ID ascertained from administrative databases abruptly declines during transition to adulthood. UK data, for example, reported a significant decline in prevalence from 40–50 per 1,000 for children to 6–7 per 1,000 in adulthood among individuals with ID identified through use of public services (e.g. education, social care, health services) (Emerson & Glover, 2012). This decline is observed for those with milder ID, but not among those with more severe levels of ID. The transition cliff identifies a 'hidden population' of adults with mild-to-moderate levels of ID who are essentially lost from administrative databases in the transition to adulthood. In contrast, the administrative prevalence of persons with severe or profound ID remains relatively stable from childhood through to adulthood, presumably as these individuals tend to remain in services from childhood and onward throughout adulthood (Emerson & Glover, 2012). A similar pattern is observed in an Irish national database of all persons within the state who are in receipt of, or registered as in need of ID services (Doyle & Carew, 2016). The administrative prevalence of mild ID reported nationwide for 2015 was low at 1.99 per 1,000, a reflection of the fact that many individuals with mild ID, either by choice or for eligibility reasons, are neither in receipt of nor on a waiting list for ID services. While little is known of this hidden population, they are deemed to comprise a vulnerable group who report poorer health outcomes, lower occupational prestige and greater likelihood of being involved in the criminal justice system (Emerson, 2011; Farrington et al., 2007; Wells et al., 2003).

Incidence studies of ID are scarcer than prevalence studies (McKenzie et al., 2016), largely due to the methodological challenges they present (Hatton, 2012). Most incidence studies focus on children with ID (Maulik & Harbour, 2010). A comprehensive incidence study was conducted as part of the Rochester Epidemiology Project, a pioneering record linkage study of all residents of Olmstead, Minnesota, established in 1966 (Rocca et al., 2012). Using a cohort of all children born in the region from 1976 to 1980, the cumulative incidence of ID at 8 years of age was 9 per 1,000, with little variation between boys (8.3 per 1,000) and girls (10 per 1,000). A gender difference was however noted by severity of ID; cumulative incidence for severe ID was higher in girls, while cumulative incidence for mild ID was higher in boys (Katusic et al., 1996). Incidence patterns over time were examined in Northern Finland among a cohort of individuals born in 1966 who were compared with a cohort born twenty years later. No overall difference in incidence was reported over this time period (Heikura et al., 2003). Marked differences were however observed in the incidence of ID by severity, with the incidence of mild ID increasing by 50% over the twenty years, while the incidence of moderate and severe ID decreased 55% and 34% respectively. Incidence levels for profound ID remained relatively stable (Heikura et al., 2003). The authors comment that these temporal changes are likely to reflect true differences in incidence rates resulting from a complex array of medical, social and educational changes over the twenty-year period. More recently, analysis of the Danish Civil Registration System, which provides continual medical information on all 5.6 million residents in Denmark, identified a cumulative incidence rate of ID at 50 years of 1.58% for males and 0.96% for females (Pederson et al., 2014), figures which are within the range of the 1% estimated for prevalence (Maulik et al., 2011).

1.5 Aetiology

The causal factor for ID remains unknown in almost half of all cases (Maulik et al., 2011). Where known, traditional conceptualisations propose two broad causal factors of ID: aetiology due to biological origin and aetiology due to sociocultural/familial factors (Grossman, 1983; Hatton, 2012; Ziegler, 1967). This dichotomy is deemed to reflect differing developmental pathways (Hodapp et al., 1990) with differing levels of impairment: biological causes being linked with severer levels of impairment and sociocultural/familial aetiologies being associated with milder levels of impairment (Simonoff, 2015). This 'two-group' theory is now deemed overly simplistic given the widely differing level of intellectual impairment among individuals with the same biological aetiology (e.g. Down syndrome) and among individuals with the same sociocultural/familial aetiology (e.g. social deprivation) (Simonoff, 2015).

AAIDD expanded the concept of aetiology to a multifactorial construct comprising four 'categories of risk': biomedical, social, behavioural and educational (Schalock et al., 2010). Each category of risk occurs over the lifetime of the individual, classified according to three time periods: prenatal, perinatal and postnatal. Prenatal risk factors may include chromosomal disorder (biomedical), domestic violence (social), parental alcohol use (behavioural) and lack of preparation for parenthood (educational). Of particular interest are recent biomedical advances in genetics which have led to the identification of a number of behavioural phenotypes for ID including Down syndrome, fragile X, Prader–Willi syndrome, Rett syndrome and tuberous sclerosis complex. By definition, behavioural phenotypes identify a 'heightened probability or likelihood that people with a given syndrome will exhibit certain behavioural and developmental sequelae relative to those without the syndrome' (Dykens, 1995: 523). Increased incidence of early onset dementia such as Alzheimer's disease, for example, is well evidenced among people with Down syndrome (Bush & Beail, 2004). While behavioural phenotypes are clearly useful in predicting the support needs of individuals with specific chromosomal disorders (Bertelli et al., 2009; Hatton, 2012), caution is required to avoid self-fulfilling prophecies or diagnostic overshadowing where the identification of a behavioural phenotype is equated with the inevitability of specific behaviours (Hatton 2012).

Perinatal risk factors for ID may include birth injury (biomedical), lack of access to perinatal care (social), parental abandonment (behavioural) and lack of medical referral for intervention services at discharge (educational) (Schalock et al., 2010). Postnatal aetiologies may include malnutrition (biomedical), family poverty (social), child abuse and neglect (behavioural) and delayed diagnosis (educational) (Schalock et al., 2010).

The precise impact of many risk factors for ID, however, remains poorly understood (Hatton, 2012). The relationship between socio-economic disadvantage and ID illustrates the complexity and bidirectionality of risk factors (Simonoff, 2015); poverty is a risk factor for exposure to both environmental and psychosocial hazards associated with ID (Emerson, 2012; Emerson & Hatton, 2007); having an ID is a risk factor for under- and unemployment and associated poverty (Siperstein et al., 2013); caregiving for a family member is associated with increased risk of poverty due to additional costs of transport, childcare, etc., and reduced rates of maternal employment (Parish et al., 2004; Shahtahmasedi et al., 2011). While numerous and complex, the aetiology of ID is deemed preventable in a substantial proportion of cases (Gustavsson et al., 2011).

1.6 Morbidity

ID is associated with significant health problems (Gustavsson et al., 2011) which tend to differ by severity rather than type of ID (McLaren & Bryson, 1987). A pioneering population-based Dutch study highlighting the disparity in health conditions between people with and without ID identified those with ID having on average 2.5 times more health problems than the general population, with significantly higher rates observed across a number of somatic conditions including multiple congenital abnormalities, epilepsy, musculoskeletal conditions, visual difficulties, deafness and obesity (van Schrojenstein Lantman de Valk et al., 2000).

While people with ID were traditionally reputed to necessarily have poorer physical health (Krahn et al., 2006), the observed disparity in health status with the general population is now conceptualised as resulting from a myriad of factors including genetics (e.g. thyroid problems associated with Down syndrome), social circumstances (e.g. social isolation, inadequate attention by care providers to health needs), environmental factors (e.g. exposure to contaminants, residential settings that promote inactivity), individual behaviours that contribute to co-morbidities due to inadequate access to health promotion (e.g. nutrition) and inadequate access to healthcare (Krahn et al., 2006). Disparities of access to routine healthcare are well evidenced; people with ID report lower rates of screening for cancer, blood pressure, vision, health and cholesterol (Chan et al., 1999; Iezzoni et al., 2000; Ramierz et al., 2005). These challenges of health status and access to healthcare have been reported as a 'cascade of disparities' (Krahn et al., 2006) which are deemed 'health inequities' (Havercamp & Scott, 2015) defined as 'unnecessary and avoidable but, in addition, are also considered unfair and unjust' (Whitehead, 1990: 5).

Adults with ID also experience high rates of mental ill-heath (Cooper & van der Speck, 2009). A systematic review of sixteen papers from 2003 to 2013 reported prevalence estimates of psychiatric disorders ranging from 13.9% to 74% (Buckles et al., 2013) with the authors noting that the higher end estimate may be atypical given the study identified 'psychiatric symptoms' in a population over 65 years (Strydom et al., 2005). More commonly, studies report estimates within the 30–40% range (Cooper & van der Speck, 2009; Enfield et al., 2006; Morgan et al., 2008) but observe marked variation by level of ability. A study of 113 adults with ID in residential care, for example, of whom 88% were classified within the severe and profound range, identified 83% to have a psychiatric diagnosis (Felstrom et al., 2005). A large population-based study of 1,023 adults with ID, of whom just 36% had severe-to-profound ID, used the same diagnostic measure as the study above and identified 35% of the sample as having psychiatric co-morbidity. The most common psychiatric conditions reported in this population-based study were problem behaviours (18.7%), affective disorder (5.7%) and autistic spectrum disorder (4.4%). Factors found to be associated with the presence of these conditions included having profound or severe ID, experiencing life events in the preceding twelve months, higher contact with a physician in the previous twelve months, being female, being a smoker and living with paid support. In contrast to the general population, no association was reported between these conditions and living in a deprived area, not having a daytime occupation, epilepsy and marital status (Cooper et al., 2007). The findings from this study are considered particularly robust given the use of multiple assessments, comparison of multiple criteria findings and classification of findings based on severity of ID (Buckles et al., 2013).

1.7 Mortality

Compared to the general population, people with ID have shorter life expectancy and increased risk of early death (Hollins et al., 1998; McGuigan et al., 1995). For those with mild ID, however, life expectancy is approaching that of the general population (Patja et al., 2000; Puri et al., 1995). The pattern of differing mortality by level of disability is illustrated by the survival probabilities of 8,724 individuals included on a database managed by the Disability Services Commission of Western Australia (Bittles et al., 2002); median life expectancy declined from 74.0 for persons with mild ID, to 67.6 for those with moderate ID, to 58.6 for those with severe ID.

A similar association with level of ID is observed regarding causes of mortality. A comprehensive Finnish study examining cause of death followed 2,369 individuals with

ID over a thirty-five-year period. Of the 1,095 individuals who were deceased at follow-up, the cause of death for those with milder ID mirrored that of the general population, but this trend diminished for those with more severe levels of disability (Patja et al., 2001). Across all levels of disability, vascular disease was the most common cause of death, followed by respiratory diseases and cancer.

Attempts to reduce health inequalities are required to reduce the mortality of people with ID from conditions with potentially preventable causes (Tyrer et al., 2009). This inequity was sharply placed in focus by a UK confidential inquiry into premature deaths of individuals with ID (Heslop et al., 2014). The most common underlying cause of death for 247 persons with ID was heart and circulatory disorders, followed by cancer. On examination, almost half of these deaths (48%) were deemed avoidable, defined as preventable through good-quality healthcare or public health intervention. The report concludes that 'despite numerous previous investigations and reports, many professionals are either not aware of, or do not include in their usual practice, approaches that adapt services to meet the needs of people with learning [intellectual] disabilities' (Heslop et al., 2014: 5).

1.8 Conclusion

This chapter has provided an overview of the epidemiology of ID. Two recurrent themes emerge. First, that the level of ID rather than type is a key factor impacting on individuals' somatic and psychological health, as well as influencing their life expectancy. Second, inequities pervade the literature. ID is preventable in a substantive proportion of cases; a 'cascade of disparities' is observed with regard to health status; and almost half of all deaths in a confidential inquiry were deemed avoidable. As people with ID and their advocates make strident efforts to secure their inclusion in society, it is imperative that these inequities are addressed to ensure a level playing field for all.

References

American Psychiatric Association (2013). *Diagnostic and Statistical Manual of Mental Disorders (DSM-5®)*. American Psychiatric Publishing.

Bertelli, M., Hassiotis, A., Deb, S. et al. (2009) New contributions of psychiatric research in the field of intellectual disabilities. *Advances in Psychiatry*, 3, 37–43.

Bertelli, M., Munir, K., Harris, J. et al. (2016) 'Intellectual developmental disorders': Reflections on the international consensus document for redefining 'mental retardation-intellectual disability' in ICD-11. *Advances in Mental Health and Intellectual Disabilities*, 10(1), 1–23.

Bittles, A. H., Petterson, B. A., Sullivan, S. G. et al. (2002) The influence of intellectual disability on life expectancy. *Journals of Gerontology Series A: Biological Sciences and Medical Sciences*, 57(7), M470–M472.

Buckles, J., Luckasson, R. & Keefe, E. (2013) A systematic review of the prevalence of psychiatric disorders in adults with intellectual disability 2003–2010. *Journal of Mental Health Research in Intellectual Disabilities*, 6(3), 181–207.

Buntinx, W. (2015) Adaptive behaviour and support needs. In *The Handbook of Intellectual Disability and Clinical Psychology Practice* (2nd edn) (eds. A. Carr, C. Linehan, G. O'Reilly et al.), pp. 107–35. Routledge.

Bush, A. & Beail, N. (2004) Risk factors for dementia in people with Down syndrome: Issues in assessment and diagnosis. *American Journal on Mental Retardation*, 109(2), 83–97.

Chan, L., Doctor, J. N., Maclehose, R. F. et al. (1999) Do Medicare patients with disabilities receive preventative services? A population-based study. *Archives of Physical and Medical Rehabilitation*, 80(6), 642–6.

Cooper, S. A., Smiley, E., Morrison, J., et al. (2007) Mental ill-health in adults with intellectual disabilities: Prevalence and associated factors. *British Journal of Psychiatry*, **190**(1), 27–35.

Cooper, S. A. & van der Speck, R. (2009) Epidemiology of mental ill health in adults with intellectual disabilities. *Current Opinion in Psychiatry*, 22(5), 431–6.

Dave, U., Shetty, N. & Mehta L. (2005) A community genetics approach to population screening in India for mental retardation – A model for developing countries. *Annals of human biology*, 32(2), 195–203.

Devlieger, J. P. (2003) From 'idiots' to 'person with mental retardation'. Defining differences in an effort to dissolve it. In *Rethinking Disability: The Emergence of New Definitions, Concepts and Communities* (eds. J. P. Devlieger, R. Rusch & D. Pfeiffer), pp. 169–188. Garant.

Devlieger, J. P., Rusch, F. & Pfeiffer, D. (2003) *Rethinking Disability: The Emergence of New Definition, Concepts and Communities.* Garant.

Doyle, A. & Carew, A. M. (2016) *Annual Report of the National Intellectual Disability Database Committee 2015.* Health Research Board.

Drum, C. E. (2009) Models and approaches to disability. In *Disability and Public Health* (eds. C. E. Drum, G. L. Krahn & H. Bersani), pp. 27–44. American Association on Intellectual and Developmental Disabilities.

Dykens, E. M. (1995) Measuring behavioural phenotypes: Provocations from the 'new genetics'. *American Journal on Mental Retardation*, **99**, 522–32.

Einfeld, S. L., Piccinin, A. M., Mackinnon, A. et al. (2006) Psychopathology in young people with intellectual disability. *JAMA*, **296**(16), 1981–9.

Emerson, E. (2011) Health status and health risks of the 'hidden majority' of adults with intellectual disability. *Intellectual and Developmental Disabilities*, 49, 155–65.

(2012) Deprivation, ethnicity and the prevalence of intellectual and developmental disabilities. *Journal of Epidemiology and Community Health*, 66(3), 218–24.

Emerson, E., Emerson, E. & Glover, G. (2012) The 'transition cliff' in the administrative prevalence of learning disabilities in England. *Tizard Learning Disability Review*, 17(3), 139–43.

Emerson, E. & Hatton, C. (2007) Poverty, socio-economic position, social capital and the health of children and adolescents with intellectual disabilities in Britain: A replication. *Journal of Intellectual Disability Research*, 51(11), 866–74.

Farrington, D. & Welsh, B. (2007) *Saving Children from a Life of Crime.* Oxford University Press.

Felstrom, A., Mulryan, N., Reidy, J. et al. (2005) Refining diagnoses: Applying the DC-LD to an Irish population with intellectual disability. *Journal of Intellectual Disability Research*, 49 (11), 813–19.

Greenspan, S. (2003) Mental retardation: Some issues for concern. In *What Is Mental Retardation? Ideas for an Evolving Disability* (eds. H. N. Switzky & S. Greenspan), pp. 64–74. American Association on Mental Retardation.

Greenspan, S. (2006a) Functional concepts in mental retardation: Finding the natural essence of an artificial category. *Exceptionality*, **14**, 205–24.

Greenspan, S. (2006b) Mental retardation in the real world: Why the AAMR definition is not there yet. In *What Is Mental Retardation? Ideas for an Evolving Disability* (eds. H. N. Switzky & S. Greenspan), pp. 165–83. American Association on Mental Retardation.

Grossman, H. J. (1983) *Classification in Mental Retardation* (rev. edn) American Association on Mental Deficiency.

Gustavsson, A., Svensson, M., Jacobi, F. et al. (2011) Cost of disorders of the brain in Europe 2010. *European Neuropsychopharmacology*, **21** (10), 718–79.

Hassiotis, A. (2015) Borderline intellectual functioning and neurodevelopmental disorders: Prevalence, comorbidities and treatment approaches. *Advances in Mental Health and Intellectual Disabilities*, 9(5), 275–83.

Hatton, C. (2012) Intellectual Disabilities – Classification, epidemiology and causes. In *Clinical Psychology and People with Intellectual Disabilities* (2nd edn) (eds. E. Emerson, C. Hatton, K. Dickson et al.), pp. 3–22. Wiley.

Havercamp, S. M. & Scott, H. M. (2015) National health surveillance of adults with disabilities, adults with intellectual and developmental disabilities, and adults with no disabilities. *Disability and Health Journal*, **8**(2), 165–72.

Heber, R. (1959) A manual on terminology and classification in mental retardation: *A monograph supplement to the American Journal on Mental Deficiency*, **64**.

Heikura, U., Taanila, A., Olsen, P. et al. (2003) Temporal changes in incidence and prevalence of intellectual disability between two birth cohorts in Northern Finland. *American Journal on Mental Retardation*, **108**(1), 19–31.

Heslop, P., Blair, P. S., Fleming, P. et al. (2014) The Confidential Inquiry into premature deaths of people with intellectual disabilities in the UK: A population-based study. *The Lancet*, **383** (9920), 889–95.

Hodaoom, R. M., Burack, J. A. & Zigler, E. (1990) *Issues in the Developmental Approach to Mental Retardation*. Cambridge University Press.

Hollins, S. Attard, M., van Fraunhofer, N. et al. (1998) Mortality in people with learning disability: Risks causes, and death certification findings in London. *Developmental Medicine and Child Neurology*, **40**, 50–6.

Iezzoni, L. I., McCarthy, E. P., Davis, R. B. et al. (2000) Mobility impairments and use of screening and preventative services. *American Journal of Public Health*, **90**, 955–61.

Katusic, S. K., Colligan, R. C., Beard, C. M. et al. (1996) Mental retardation in a birth cohort, 1976–1980, Rochester, Minnesota. *American Journal of Mental Retardation*, **100**(4), 335–44.

King, B. H., Toth, K. E., Hodapp, R. M. et al. (2009) Intellectual disability. In *Kaplan and Sadock's Comprehensive Textbook of Psychiatry* (eds. B. J. Sadock, V. A. Sadock, P. Ruiz), pp. 3444–74. Lippencott, Williams & Wilkins.

Krahn, G. L., Hammond, L. & Turner, A. (2006) A cascade of health disparities: Health and health care access for people with intellectual disabilities. *Mental Retardation and Developmental Disabilities Research Reviews*, **12**, 70–82.

Leonard, H., Petterson, B., Bower, C. et al. (2003) Prevalence of intellectual disability in Western Australia. *Paediatric and Perinatal Epidemiology*, **17**(1), 58–67.

Leonard, H. & Wen, X. (2002) The epidemiology of mental retardation: Challenges and opportunities in the new millennium. *Mental Retardation and Developmental Disabilities Research Reviews*, **8**(3), 117–34.

McGuidan, S. M., Hollins, S., Attard, M. (1995) Age specific standardised mortality rates in people with learning disability. *Journal of Intellectual Disability Research*, **39**, 527–31.

McKenzie, K., Milton, M., Smith, G. et al. (2016) Systematic review of the prevalence and incidence of intellectual disabilities: Current trends and issues. *Current Developmental Disorders Reports*, **3**, 104–15.

McLaren, J. & Bryson, S. E. (1987) Review of recent epidemiological studies of mental retardation: Prevalence, associated disorders, and etiology. *American Journal on Mental Retardation*, **92**, 243–54.

Maulik, P. K. & Harbour, C. K. (2010) Epidemiology of intellectual disability. In *International Encyclopedia of Rehabilitation* (eds. J. H. Stone & M. Blouin) Center for International Rehabilitation Research Information and Exchange.

Maulik, P. K., Mascarenhas, M. N., Mathers, C. D. et al. (2011) Prevalence of intellectual disability: A meta-analysis of population-based studies. *Research in Developmental Disabilities*, **32**, 419–36.

Morgan, V., Leonard, H, Bourke, J. et al. (2008) Intellectual disability co-occurring with schizophrenia and other psychiatric illness: Population-based study. *British Journal of Psychiatry*, **193**(5), 364–72.

Parish, S. L., Seltzer M. M., Greenberg, J. S. et al. (2004) Economic implications of caregiving at midlife: Comparing parents with and without children who have developmental disabilities. *Mental Retardation*, **42**(6), 413–26.

Patja, K., Iivanainen, M., Vesala, H. et al. (2000) Life expectancy of people with intellectual disability: A 35-year follow-up study. *Journal of Intellectual Disability Research*, **44**(5), 591–9.

Pedersen, C. B., Mors, O., Bertelsen, A. et al. (2014) A comprehensive nationwide study of the incidence rate and lifetime risk for treated mental disorders. *JAMA Psychiatry*, **71**(5), 573–81.

Porta, M. (ed.) (2008) *A Dictionary of Epidemiology*. Oxford University Press.

Puri, B. K., Lekh, S. K., Langa, A. et al. (1995) Mortality in a hospitalised mentally handicapped population: A 10-year survey. *Journal of Intellectual Disability Research*, **39**, 442–6.

Ramirez, A., Farmer G. C., Grant, D. et al. (2005) Disability and preventive cancer screening: Results from the 2001 California Health Interview Survey. *American Journal of Public Health*, **95**(11), 2057–64.

Rocca, W. A., Yawn, B. P., St. Sauver, J. L. et al. (2012) History of the Rochester Epidemiology Project: Half a century of medical records linkage in a US population. *Mayo Clinic Proceedings*, **87**(12), 1202–13.

Salvador-Carulla, L., García-Gutiérrez J. C., Gutiérrez-Colosía, M. R. et al. (2013) Borderline intellectual functioning: consensus and good practice guidelines. *Revista de Psiquiatría y Salud Mental (English Edition)*, **6**(3), 109–20.

Salvador-Carulla, L., Ruiz M. & Nadal, M. (2011), *Funcionamiento Intelectual Límite (FIL): Guía de Consenso y Buenas Prácticas*, Obra Social Caja Madrid.

Schalock, R. L. (2013) Introduction to the intellectual disability construct. In *The Story of Intellectual Disability: An Evolution of Meaning, Understanding, and Public Perception* (ed. M. L. Wehmeyer). Brookes.

Schalock, R. L., Borthwick-Duffy, S. A., Bradley, V. J. et al. (2010) *Intellectual Disability: Definition, Classification, and Systems of Supports*. American Association on Intellectual and Developmental Disabilities.

Shahtahmasebi, S., Emerson, E., Berridge D. et al. (2011) Child disability and the dynamics of family poverty, hardship and financial strain: Evidence from the UK. *Journal of Social Policy*, **40**(4), 653–73.

Simonoff, E. (2015) Intellectual disability. In *Rutter's Child and Adolescent Psychiatry* (6th edn) (eds. A. Thapar, D. S. Pine, J. F. Leckman et al.), pp. 719–37. Wiley-Blackwell.

Siperstein, G. N., Parker, R. C. & Drascher, M. (2013) National snapshot of adults with intellectual disabilities in the labor force. *Journal of Vocational Rehabilitation*, **39**(3), 157–65.

Stein, Z., Belmont, L. & Durkin, M. (1987) Mild mental retardation and severe mental retardation compared: Experiences in eight less developed countries. *Upsala Journal of Medical Sciences. Supplement*, **44**, 89–96.

Strydom, A., Hassiotis, A. & Livingston, G. (2005) Mental health and social care needs of older people with intellectual disabilities. *Journal of Applied Research in Intellectual Disabilities*, **18**, 229–35.

Switzky, H. N. & Greenspan, S. (2006) *What Is Mental Retardation? Ideas for an Evolving Disability in the 21st Century*. American Association of Mental Retardation.

Tassé, M. J., Luckasson, R. & Schalock, R. L. (2016) The relation between intellectual functioning and adaptive behavior in the diagnosis of intellectual disability. *Intellectual and Developmental Disabilities*, **54**(6), 381–90.

Thapar, A., Pine, D. S., Leckman, J. F. et al. (2015) *Rutter's Child and Adolescent Psychiatry*. Wiley.

Thompson, J. R., Bradley, V. J., Buntinx, W. et al. (2009) Conceptualising supports and the support needs of people with intellectual disability. *Intellectual and Developmental Disabilities*, **47**(2), 135–46.

Tyrer, F. & McGrother, C. (2009) Cause-specific mortality and death certificate reporting in adults with moderate to profound intellectual disabilities. *Journal of Intellectual Disability Research*, **53**, 898–904.

Van Schrojenstein, Lantman de Valk H., Metsemakes, J., Haveman, M. et al. (2000) Health problems in people with intellectual disability in general practice: A comparative study. *Family Practice*, **17**(5), 405–7.

Wells, T., Sandefur, G. D. & Hogan, D. P. (2003) What happens after the high school years among young persons with disabilities? *Social Forces*, **82**, 803–32.

Whitehead, M. (1990) *The Concepts and Principles of Equity in Health*. World Health Organization.

WHO (1992) *The ICD-10 Classification of Mental and Behavioural Disorders. Clinical Descriptions and Diagnostic Guidelines*. World Health Organization.

WHO (2001) *International Classification of Functioning, Disability and Health: ICF*. World Health Organization.

Ziegler, E. (1967) Familial mental retardation: A continuing dilemma. *Science*, **155**, 292–8.

Chapter 2
Genetics of Intellectual Disability

Kate Wolfe, Andre Strydom and Nick Bass

2.1 General Introduction

Intellectual disability (ID) is aetiologically heterogeneous, having a wide range of genetic and environmental origins. Its onset occurs in the developmental period with developmental delay (DD), although impaired intellectual development does not inevitability lead to ID in adulthood. This chapter will focus on the genetic causes and risk factors for ID. Technological advances in genetic investigation have led to rapid progress in our understanding of the genetics of ID over the last decade, with over 700 ID relevant genes now identified (Vissers et al., 2015). Given the breadth of the topic, we present an overview of major developments in the field – from both a research and clinical perspective – with selected examples of specific genetic aetiologies.

First, we will revisit some basic genetic principles to facilitate understanding of the chapter. Most cells in our body contain deoxyribonucleic acid (DNA), which is a two-stranded macromolecule. Each strand consists of a ribose phosphate backbone and four bases: adenine (A), thymine (T), guanine (G) and cytosine (C). These bases form base pairs with complementary bases from the other DNA strand, which are held together by hydrogen bonds to form a double helix structure. The complete genetic make-up of an individual is referred to as their genome and comprises of approximately 3 billion base pairs. Our DNA sequence is simply the sequence of bases along the DNA molecules. Although it is now clear that most of our DNA sequence is functional, only about 1% directly codes for proteins. The stretches of DNA that code for proteins are referred to as genes. There are approximately 20,000 genes in the human genome. Human DNA is packaged into structures called chromosomes, which consist of supercoiled DNA and associated proteins. We normally inherit 23 chromosome pairs; one chromosome of each pair is inherited from our mother and the other from our father. For 22 of the chromosome pairs the chromosome inherited from the mother and the father are (normally) structurally identical – these 22 chromosome pairs are known as the autosomes. The remaining pair comprises the sex chromosomes, usually females have two X chromosomes and males have an X and a Y chromosome.

Throughout this chapter, we will describe the relationship between genotype, which is the genetic makeup of an individual, and phenotype, which is the observable characteristics that arise from the interaction of the genotype with the environment. The relationship between genotype and phenotype is complex. Two important concepts in understanding genotype–phenotype correlations are penetrance and genetic pleiotropy. Penetrance is the proportion of people with a particular genotype who exhibit the phenotype associated with that genotype. A disorder is said to have reduced (or incomplete) penetrance when the aberrant genotype is present in the absence of the associated phenotype. Down syndrome (trisomy of chromosome 21) is an example of a genetic disorder with full penetrance, in that all individuals with trisomy 21 present with features of Down syndrome, including some degree of intellectual impairment. However, there is considerable variation in the extent to which some phenotypes are expressed; for example, some individuals with Down syndrome may have an IQ in the borderline ID range (IQ 70–85), while others are more severely affected with an IQ below 35 (Karmiloff-Smith et al., 2016).

Genetic pleiotropy describes the situation whereby the altered function of a gene can cause multiple phenotypic outcomes. A relatively recent observation is that there is overlap at the genetic level between seemingly distinct psychiatric phenotypes; for example, exonic deletions of the *NRXN1* gene have been identified in studies of autism spectrum disorders (ASD), schizophrenia and ID – see O'Donovan and Owen (2016), for a detailed discussion of this topic. The phenotype of ID is highly variable, both in terms of severity and the domains of intellectual functioning that are affected. Research is ongoing to identify common genetic pathways that may be associated with clinical presentations. Furthermore, ID also co-occurs with other medical and psychiatric phenotypes, such as congenital malformations, epilepsy and ASD. Historically ID has been divided into two broad categories: syndromic ID, where there is a co-occurrence of a recognisable set of clinical phenotypes, and non-syndromic ID. A large proportion of ID remains idiopathic, meaning the cause is unknown.

The chapter will broadly follow the progression of genetic discovery in ID – from syndromes and cytogenetics to idiopathic ID and next-generation sequencing (NGS). We will provide illustrative examples of genetic discoveries in ID, which are summarised in Table 2.1. In the 1950s, a technique for visualisation of the complete set of chromosomes (also known as the karyotype) under optical microscopes was developed (Tjio & Levan, 1956). This cytogenetic technique enabled the identification of abnormalities of chromosome number (aneuploidies) and large structural abnormalities. Over the past fifteen years, submicroscopic structural variations (microdeletions and microduplications) have been identified as an important class of genetic variation in neurodevelopmental disorders. These deletions and duplications are referred to as copy number variations (CNVs), and their identification has heralded a new era in the clinical investigation of idiopathic ID. CNVs typically vary in their penetrance; some CNVs have nearly 100% penetrance, such as the 22q11.2 deletion, whereas the 16p11.2 duplication has a penetrance of around 34% (see relevant sections below for more detail) (Kirov et al., 2014).

More recently the development of ultra-high-throughput NGS technologies has made it possible to rapidly sequence the whole protein-coding region of the genome (known as the exome), or even the whole genome, at a low cost. NGS is a very powerful tool for identifying pathological single-base changes in the DNA sequence, which are referred to as single-nucleotide variants (SNVs). In particular, NGS has facilitated the identification of *de novo* mutations. By definition, *de novo* mutations are not present in the parents and have arisen for the first time during egg or sperm cell formation, or in early embryonic development of the offspring. The application of these techniques to genetic research of syndromic and non-syndromic ID has proved very successful, and these techniques have now found their way into the clinical arena.

2.2 Cytogenetic Anomalies

Genetic aberrations which can be visualised by karyotype analysis include aneuploidies, and large-scale translocations, inversions and deletions or duplications. Translocations involve

Table 2.1 Overview of key genetic disorders associated with ID

	Genetic aetiology	Genetic test	Estimated prevalence (live births)	Predominant mode of transmission	Main associated psychiatric/behavioural phenotype	Reference
Down syndrome	Trisomy 21	Chromosomal analysis (Karyotyping)	1 in 400–1,500	*De novo*	Alzheimer's disease	(Wiseman et al., 2015)
Cri-du-chat syndrome	5p deletion	CMA	1 in 37,000–50,000	*De novo*	Self-injurious and aggressive behaviour	(Sigafoos et al., 2009)
Klinefelter syndrome	XXY	Chromosomal analysis (Karyotyping)	1 in 500 males	*De novo*	ADHD, anxiety, depression, psychosis	(Verri et al., 2010)
Phenylketonuria (PKU)	*PAH* gene point mutations; deletion/duplication in 1–3%	NGS, and CMA	1 in 10,000	Autosomal recessive	ADHD and ASD	(Blau et al.; Levy, 2010)
Rett syndrome	*MECP2* gene point mutations; deletion in 8%	NGS, and CMA	1 in 10,000–22,000 females	*De novo*	Self-injurious behaviour	(Neul and Zoghbi, 2004)
Fragile X syndrome	*FMR1* gene mutation	Southern blot/PCR	1 in 4,000 males, 1 in 8,000–9,000 females	X-linked dominant	ADHD and ASD	(Crawford et al., 2001)

Syndrome	Genetic cause	Method	Prevalence	Inheritance	Associated psychiatric features	Reference
Prader–Willi syndrome	Paternal 15q11–q13 deletion	CMA	1 in 10,000–30,000	*De novo*	Behavioural problems, ASD and psychosis	(Butler, 2011)
Angelman syndrome	Maternal 15q11–q13 deletion	CMA	1 in 10,000–40,000	*De novo*	ADHD and ASD	(Horsler and Oliver, 2006; Pelc et al., 2008)
22q11.2 deletion syndrome	22q11.2 deletion	CMA	1 in 2,000–4,000	*De novo*	ASD, ADHD, anxiety disorders, psychosis	(Schneider et al., 2014)
22q11.2 duplication syndrome	22q11.2 duplication	CMA	—	*De novo* and familial	ASD, protective for psychosis	(Ou et al., 2008)
16p11.2 deletion syndrome	16p11.2 deletion	CMA	1 in 2,000	*De novo* and familial	ASD	(Zufferey et al., 2012)
16p11.2 duplication syndrome	16p11.2 duplication	CMA	—	*De novo* and familial	ASD and psychosis	(D'Angelo et al., 2015)

the movement of stretches of DNA between chromosomes and can be balanced or unbalanced depending on whether there is an overall loss or gain of genetic material. Examples of syndromes arising from aneuploidies and large structural abnormalities are detailed below.

2.2.1 Down Syndrome

Down syndrome is the most prevalent genetic disorder and one of the most frequent causes of ID. The syndrome is recognisable due to characteristic facial dysmorphisms and is associated with a range of medical phenotypes, including congenital heart defects, haematopoietic disorders and gastrointestinal anomalies. Individuals with Down syndrome also have an increased risk of developing Alzheimer's disease (Wiseman et al., 2015). In 1959, cytogenetic analysis identified chromosomal aneuploidy to be the main cause of Down syndrome, due to trisomy (three copies) of chromosome 21 (Lejeune et al. 1959).

2.2.2 Sex Chromosome Aneuploidies

The sex chromosomes are particularly susceptible to aneuploidy, with Klinefelter syndrome being the most common disorder of the sex chromosomes. Klinefelter syndrome has a variable intellectual phenotype – ranging from normal intellectual functioning to specific cognitive deficits and ID. It has also been associated with a range of psychiatric phenotypes, including attention deficit hyperactivity disorder (ADHD), anxiety, depression and psychosis (Verri et al., 2010). In 1959, it was discovered that Klinefelter syndrome is caused by an extra copy of the X chromosome, which results in the karyotype 47, XXY (Jacobs & Strong, 1959). Several other sex chromosome disorders have been described, such as 48, XXYY. Typically, IQ deficits increase with the number of additional sex chromosomes (Visootsak & Graham, 2006).

2.2.3 Cri-du-Chat Syndrome

The main features of Cri-du-chat syndrome are ID, craniofacial dysmorphisms and behavioural problems, such as self-injurious and aggressive behaviour. The syndrome name stems from the distinctive cat-like cry of affected children. In 1963 a deletion of the short arm (p) of chromosome 5 was identified in individuals with cri-du-chat syndrome (Lejeune et al., 1963). While the majority of cases are caused by chromosome 5p deletions, in 10–15% of cases, the disorder arises as a result of unbalanced translocations (Sigafoos et al., 2009).

2.3 Single-Gene Disorders, Disorders of DNA Methylation and Genomic Imprinting

Mendelian disorders are disorders which exhibit a Mendelian pattern of inheritance, comprising autosomal dominant, autosomal recessive or sex-linked inheritance. Typically, Mendelian disorders are caused by mutations of bases within a single gene. For autosomal dominant disorders only one copy of the mutated gene is required to give rise to the disease phenotype, whereas in autosomal recessive conditions two abnormal copies of the gene are required. The 1970s and 1980s saw the development of molecular genetic techniques to manipulate DNA – such as the polymerase chain reaction (PCR). The PCR became a core technique in molecular genetics as it can be used to generate millions of copies of specific segments of the genome for a variety of subsequent genetic assays. With the identification of polymorphic DNA markers and application of PCR, genetic linkage analysis became a powerful tool for gene discovery in Mendelian disorders. Linkage analysis is based on the concept that polymorphic DNA markers of known chromosomal position can be used to approximately locate disease-causing genetic variation through analysis of the co-segregation of specific alleles of the markers and the disease within families. A combination of cytogenetic and linkage techniques has been instrumental in the mapping of many ID genes.

DNA methylation is an important mechanism by which genes are switched on or off, resulting in changes in gene activity. DNA methylation refers to the addition of methyl groups to regions of the DNA, which prevents gene transcription and ultimately protein production. Fragile X and Rett syndrome (see sections 2.3.2–2.3.3) are both examples of syndromic forms of ID associated with disordered DNA methylation. Normally, genes from both the maternal and paternal chromosomes are expressed, however, in a process called genomic imprinting, one of the parental genes is imprinted (epigenetically silenced by DNA methylation) and therefore only one active copy of the gene is present in the offspring. Genomic imprinting underlies the alternate phenotypes of Prader–Willi syndrome and Angelman syndrome which arise from deletion of a common region on 15q11-q13, explored in further detail below.

2.3.1 Phenylketonuria

Phenylketonuria (PKU) is an autosomal recessive disorder that can lead to the development of ID, seizures and heart problems. A range of behavioural and psychiatric phenotypes have also been observed, including ASD and ADHD (Blau et al., 2010). PKU arises due to mutations in the phenylalanine hydroxylase (*PAH*) gene. The gene encodes an enzyme that catalyses the breakdown of the amino acid phenylalanine. Mutations result in enzyme deficiency and a resultant toxic build-up of phenylalanine in the brain and body. Delineation of the inheritance pattern and metabolic pathology of PKU occurred before the *PAH* gene was mapped to chromosome 12 in the 1980s (Scriver, 2007). The enzyme deficiency can be ameliorated by implementation of a low-phenylalanine diet, preventing the development of ID and other disease pathology. Newborn screening programmes for PKU have been widely implemented and have proved to be very successful (Cederbaum, 2002).

2.3.2 Fragile X Syndrome

Fragile X syndrome is one of the most frequent causes of ID in males. It is characterised by ID, seizures and characteristic physical features, including a long narrow face, a prominent jaw and macroorchidism. From a psychiatric perspective, ASD and ADHD are common (Crawford et al., 2001). In 1991, the fragile X mental retardation 1 (*FMR1*) gene was implicated in fragile X syndrome (Pieretti et al., 1991). The disorder arises through expansion of a trinucleotide repeat sequence (CGG), which causes DNA methylation and, in turn, termination of gene transcription. Fragile X syndrome also occurs in females, but has a lower prevalence, as the presence of two X chromosomes in females buffers the effect (Rousseau et al., 2011). The FMR gene is just one of at least 102 chromosome X genes implicated in the aetiology of ID (Lubs et al., 2012).

2.3.3 Rett Syndrome

Rett syndrome is normally lethal in males and is one of the leading causes of ID in females. For the first six to eighteen months development progresses normally, but this is followed by a developmental regression. Growth slows, resulting in microcephaly, hypotonia develops and there is a gradual loss of any acquired speech/mobility. Patients tend to develop severe ID, self-injurious behaviour, seizures and characteristic hand-wringing (Chahrour & Zoghbi, 2007). Rett syndrome was first described clinically in 1966, but it was not until 1999 that the genetic aetiology was elucidated. The main gene responsible for Rett syndrome is the methyl-CpG-binding protein 2 (*MeCP2*) gene. MeCP2 is located on the X chromosome and has a major role in DNA methylation. Rett's syndrome shows an X-linked dominant pattern of inheritance, as loss of function of one copy of the gene is sufficient to rise to the phenotype (Amir et al., 1999).

2.3.4 Prader–Willi and Angelman Syndrome

The most prominent clinical feature of Prader–Willi syndrome (PWS) is childhood-onset obesity with extreme hyperphagia. Other features include mild ID, a recognisable pattern of dysmorphism, hypogonadism and growth insufficiencies. Behavioural problems, including tantrums and compulsive traits, are estimated to affect 70–90% of individuals; ASD is present in 25% of cases and psychosis in 5–10% (Cassidy and Driscoll, 2009). The genetic aetiology of PWS was established in 1981, when an interstitial deletion of the paternal chromosome was identified encompassing an imprinted region on chromosome 15q11–q13 (Ledbetter et al., 1981). A set of genes in this region are imprinted (turned off) on the maternal chromosome. Deletion of the equivalent region on the paternal chromosome results in the lack of any active copies of these genes.

Angelman syndrome (AS) presents with severe ID, virtual absence of speech, seizure disorders and mild dysmorphisms. The behavioural phenotype is particularly distinct, with hyperactivity, frequent laughter and motor stereotypies (Pelc et al., 2008). AS is the reciprocal condition to PWS, arising through a deletion of the maternal chromosome in the imprinted 15q11–q13 region. A set of genes in this region are imprinted (turned off) on the paternal chromosome, so deletion of the region from the maternal chromosome results in lack of any active copies of these genes. It is still unclear which imprinted gene(s) contribute to the PWS phenotype; however, it is known that the gene encoding ubiquitin–protein ligase E3A (*UBE3A*) explains many of the manifestations of AS and single-gene mutations can also give rise to the disorder (Van Buggenhout and Fryns, 2009).

2.4 Copy Number Variations, Chromosomal Microarray Analysis and Neuropsychiatric CNVs

For any given autosomal DNA segment, the usual copy number in an individual is two: one maternal copy and one paternal copy. Copy number variations (CNVs) are DNA segments where the copy number can vary between individuals. Variation in copy number arises through deletion or duplication of the DNA segments. Deletion results in a reduced copy number (usually to one) and duplication in an increased copy number (usually to three). Dosage changes in one or multiple genes can lead to changes in gene expression and protein function. However, it must be emphasised that not all CNVs have a deleterious effect on human health. Studies of healthy control populations have revealed that CNVs are common across the human genome (Iafrate et al., 2004; Sebat et al., 2004). Approximately 12% of the human genome is thought to exhibit CNVs (Redon et al., 2006). Curation of CNVs in control populations across the world is ongoing; the largest online resource is the Database of Genomic Variants (DGV) (MacDonald et al., 2014).

2.4.1 DNA Microarrays and Chromosomal Microarray Analysis

DNA microarrays, also known as nucleic acid arrays, are small slides to which thousands of nucleic acid probes are bound. This enables hundreds of thousands of genotyping reactions to be carried out simultaneously. Currently there are two main types of microarray used for chromosomal microarray analysis (CMA): microarray-based comparative genomic hybridisation (array CGH) and single-nucleotide polymorphism (SNP) microarrays. In array CGH, DNA from the patient and a reference control are differentially fluorescently labelled and changes in genomic copy number, using probes at varying intervals, are made visible by differences in florescence levels (Carter, 2007). SNP platforms were primarily developed to detect changes to single bases of the DNA sequence. However, it is also possible to determine genomic copy number using SNP arrays by detecting changes in the intensity information of segments of DNA (LaFramboise, 2009).

CMA has had a major impact on the clinical investigation of DD and ID. In 2010, a consensus statement from the International Standard Cytogenomic Array (ISCA) Consortium identified CMA as one of the recommended first-line tests, replacing karyotyping, for postnatal investigation of idiopathic DD/ID, multiple congenital abnormalities and ASD. A review of 33 studies, including 21,698 patients with ID and congenital abnormalities, suggested an average diagnostic yield of 15–20% (Miller et al., 2010).

To date, the investigation of CNVs in large cohorts with DD/ID has predominantly occurred in paediatric patients. One of the first large analyses of pathogenic CNVs in children with DD/ID and congenital defects was undertaken in 2011 on 15,767 cases and 8,329 controls. It was estimated that approximately 14.2% of CNVs >400 kb were responsible for disease in the case group (Cooper et al., 2011). A refined CNV morbidity map, comprising data from 29,085 children (some of which were included in the previous sample), has subsequently been generated allowing the identification of 70 CNV regions significantly associated with DD/ID (Coe et al., 2014). Through this mechanism of integrating data from large datasets, new CNV syndromes are being identified and characterised.

2.4.2 CNVs in ID and Psychiatric Disorders

There is an increased prevalence of psychiatric disorders in adults with ID compared to the general population. For example, the point prevalence of psychosis has been estimated as 10 times higher in ID (Cooper et al. 2007). Large-scale studies of CNVs in DD/ID and psychiatric disorder patient groups have revealed that many CNVs are strong risk factors for more than one disorder. Investigation of *de novo* CNVs in simplex families with ASD, in which there is only one affected family member, has confirmed six main risk loci for ASD (1q21.1, 3q29, 7q11.23, 16p11.2, 15q11.2–q13 and 22q11.2). All of these CNVs have also been shown to confer risk for ID (Sanders et al. 2015).

Similarly, all CNVs that have been shown to increase risk for developing schizophrenia have also been implicated in risk for ID. An analysis of 51 ID risk CNVs in a large cohort of patients with schizophrenia and healthy controls found a significant enrichment of ID

CNVs in the schizophrenia cohort. For a detailed description of these CNVs and population rates in cases versus controls, see Rees et al. (2016). Thus, it appears that these CNVs are better conceptualised as generic risk factors for abnormal neurodevelopment, rather than disorder-specific risk factors, which further challenges traditional categorical diagnostic classifications. It has been hypothesised that psychiatric disorders lie on a neurodevelopmental continuum, of which ID is the most severe brain insult, followed by ASD and schizophrenia (Doherty & Owen, 2014).

Historically, clinical genetic screening has not been a routine part of the assessment of adults with ID who present to psychiatric services (de Villiers & Porteous, 2012). In order to assess the rate of undiagnosed CNVs in this patient group, a recent UK study recruited adults with idiopathic ID and challenging behaviours and/or co-morbid psychiatric diagnoses from ID psychiatry services. This study indicated that 11% of adults with ID and co-morbid psychiatric phenotypes have undiagnosed likely pathogenic CNVs (Wolfe, Strydom et al., 2017). We will now consider two specific examples of CNVs with shared psychiatric risk.

2.4.3 22q11.2 Deletions and Duplications

The clinical presentation of 22q11.2 deletion syndrome (also known as velocardiofacial syndrome or DiGeorge syndrome) is highly variable, with more than 180 clinical features described (Shprintzen, 2008). Congenital cardiac malformations, immune deficiencies, palate defects and ID occur in approximately 70% of cases. Minor facial dysmorphisms, renal abnormalities and hearing impairments are among other common features (Habel et al., 2014). The 22q11.2 deletion syndrome is the strongest known risk factor for psychotic disorders, with prevalence estimates as high as 30% (Monks et al., 2014). Other behavioural and psychiatric phenotypes are also common. It has been estimated that up to 60% of children meet the criteria for at least one psychiatric diagnosis, notably ADHD and anxiety disorders (Hooper et al., 2013). Initially, these variable phenotypes were thought to be the result of different syndromes; however, cytogenetic analysis, followed by molecular analysis, identified a common deletion at the 22q11.2 locus typically spanning 30 to 40 genes (Shprintzen, 2008).

The 22q11.2 duplication syndrome shares some features with the reciprocal deletion, such as heart defects, congenital abnormalities, ID and mild dysmorphic features (Portnoï, 2009). While the phenotype is again variable, it is generally mild in comparison with the deletion syndrome and familial transmission is frequently observed (Ou et al., 2008). Psychiatric and behavioural problems include ASD, which occurs in approximately 14–25% of carriers. Interestingly, psychosis is infrequently observed and the 22q11.2 duplication has been proposed as a protective mutation for schizophrenia (Rees et al., 2014).

2.4.4 16p11.2 Deletions and Duplications

Deletions and reciprocal duplications at 16p11.2 were initially found to confer risk for DD and ASD, accounting for approximately 1% of cases (Weiss et al., 2008). The 16p11.2 deletion syndrome is commonly associated with ID, macrocephaly, seizures and obesity. IQ testing in a cohort of 16p11.2 deletion carriers found that their full-scale IQ is typically two standard deviations lower than non-carrier relatives. It has been estimated that around 80% of 16p11.2 deletion carriers exhibit psychiatric disorders, of which 15% of children present with ASD (Zufferey et al., 2012).

The clinical features of the 16p11.2 duplication syndrome exhibit a mirror phenotype to the deletion; for example, it has been associated with microcephaly and a reduced body mass index. IQ testing in the duplication carriers has revealed a higher variance than in deletion carriers (D'Angelo et al., 2015), and penetrance is incomplete, with some individuals (even in the same family) presenting with mild or absent features. A meta-analysis of 16p11.2 duplication studies found that the disorder confers a fourteen-fold increased risk of psychosis and a sixteen-fold increased risk of schizophrenia (Giaroli et al., 2014).

2.5 The Human Genome Project and Next-Generation Sequencing

The Human Genome Initiative, more commonly known as the Human Genome Project (HGP), was conceived in 1986 and set out to sequence all 3 billion base pairs of the human genome. This ambitious international collaborative effort started in 1990 and was completed in 2003. The project has conveyed us into the era of genomic medicine. The sequence was made publicly available and has enabled the development of bioinformatic resources, which provide powerful tools for genetic investigation and clinical genetics (Lehner et al., 2014). One of these tools is the University of California Santa Cruz (UCSC) genome browser, which was the first graphical user interface for viewing the draft genome sequence (http://genome-euro.ucsc.edu). The sequence continues to be revised and new assemblies (also known as builds) of the genome are released regularly. Furthermore, the HGP provided the driving force behind the development of NGS. NGS has been applied to the study of ID with great success in terms of identification of causative SNVs. Initially, targeted NGS was used, focusing on the protein-coding regions of the genome (exons), which are more likely to harbour causative variants. It is now feasible to undertake large-scale sequencing studies of the whole genome, although this creates an enormous amount of data, and methodology to interpret this at scale is still in development.

2.5.1 Exome Sequencing in ID

Exome sequencing has been applied to rare syndromes with unexplained aetiology, sporadic ID and non-syndromic forms of ID. Aneuploidies and large structural abnormalities usually arise *de novo* in the affected individual. Until the advent of NGS, it was very difficult to test whether *de novo* SNVs contribute to sporadic ID. It is estimated that each newborn acquires 50–100 *de novo* mutations in his or her genome, of which 0.86, on average, are novel, amino acid-altering mutations (Lynch, 2010). NGS has demonstrated that the *de novo* SNV paradigm is particularly important in the aetiology of sporadic ID of moderate–severe severity. The first exome sequencing study to explore the *de novo* paradigm analysed ten patient–parent trios and identified an average of five candidate non-synonymous *de novo* mutations per affected individual (Vissers et al., 2010). Non-synonymous exonic mutations alter the normal amino acid sequence, which can result in changes in protein configuration and gene function.

Exome sequencing has also been applied to large cohorts with DD/ID. For example, the Deciphering Developmental Disorders (DDD) study sequenced the exomes of individuals with severe idiopathic developmental disorders and their families ($N=4{,}293$) and found 42% of cases carried pathogenic damaging *de novo* mutations (DNMs). They estimated that DNMs have a prevalence of 1 in 213 to 1 in 448 births, depending on parental age

(McRae et al., 2017). The data from this study and others has been made publicly available on one of the largest, anonymised data-sharing platforms for DD/ID (https://decipher.sanger.ac.uk/browser). Exome sequencing has also proved successful in the study of autosomal recessive ID. A study of consanguineous families identified plausible pathogenic mutations in single genes in 78 out of the 136 families that were investigated. This comprised 23 genes that were previously implicated in ID, or related neurological disorders, and 50 novel candidate genes (Najmabadi et al., 2011).

2.5.2 Genome Sequencing Studies

Whole-genome sequencing (WGS) is now being applied to the study of ID. The first major WGS study comprised patient–parent trios in a cohort of fifty patients with severe idiopathic ID. The cohort had previously undergone extensive genetic testing, including single-gene testing, CMA and exome sequencing analysis. The diagnostic yield for WGS was 42%, in comparison with an average diagnostic yield of 12% for CMA and 27% for whole exome sequencing. Interestingly, the variants identified were all in the coding regions of the genome and had been missed using the other technologies, which highlights that intragenic variant interpretation remains challenging (Gilissen et al., 2014).

2.5.3 Genetic Testing in the Clinic

If a syndromic form of ID is suspected, then a specific genetic test may be indicated (see Table 2.1 for details of genetic tests for specific forms of ID). CMA is one of the first-line clinical genetic investigations for idiopathic DD/ID. However, many CNVs are extremely rare, which presents challenges for variant categorisation. Factors that influence pathogenicity classifications include the inheritance status, size and genetic content of the CNV. Interpretation of CNV findings remains in a state of flux. For example, one study reinterpreted CNV results from 67 individuals with idiopathic ID two years after the initial analysis and found a statistically significant increase in potentially pathogenic CNVs (Palmer et al., 2014). Furthermore, it is assumed that gene–gene and gene–environment interactions affect the penetrance and pleiotropic effects of CNVs but, to date, little empirical data has been generated. These issues of reduced penetrance and pleiotropic effects pose a particular challenge for genetic counselling.

Most adults with ID will not have had genetic investigation using new technologies, such as CMA or NGS. Therefore, it may be appropriate to offer adults with idiopathic ID genetic testing, particularly if they present with co-morbid psychiatric conditions, dysmorphic features, a family history of ID or physical disorders such as epilepsy or a history of congenital heart disease. Close liaison with regional clinical genetics services pre and post testing is recommended. A recent survey of Royal College of Psychiatrists' child and adolescent and ID psychiatrists identified differences in existing views and practices in relation to genetic testing. Increased training and collaboration with clinical genetic services were identified as key areas for improvement of clinical practices (Wolfe, Stueber et al., 2017).

Confirmation of a genetic diagnosis can facilitate screening for associated medical and psychiatric disorders. Information leaflets with clinical guidelines are available for an increasing number of rare genetic syndromes (e.g. www.rarechromo.co.uk/html/Disorder Guides.asp, www.orpha.net/consor/cgi-bin/Disease.php). A genetic diagnosis can also enable access to disorder-specific or general support groups, such as the Unique chromosomal disorder support group. Furthermore, a genetic diagnosis may have broader implications for the family and indicate genetic counselling and cascade testing via regional clinical genetics services.

2.6 Future Directions

Exome sequencing is beginning to be used regularly in the clinical arena, and research has indicated that this will increase diagnostic yields for the genetic investigation of ID. The interpretation of results, patient feedback and strategies for dealing with incidental findings, however, pose clinical challenges (Gilissen et al., 2014). In 2015, the 100,000 genomes project was launched (www.genomicsengland.co.uk). This project is the first large-scale clinical application of WGS for patients with rare diseases, including patients with DD/ID. WGS is likely to be the next step for clinical diagnostics in ID, as both exonic and intronic causative variants can be identified. Pipelines for identifying CNVs from WGS data are also improving, which should make WGS the most comprehensive single genome screen to date.

There are, however, other mechanisms that give rise to ID, which are not captured by current technologies. Thus far, the aberrations we have described relate to those found in the germline of the individual, which means that these mutations are present in all cells of the body and can be passed onto offspring. Somatic mutations, on the other hand, arise during cell replication and are only present in particular cell lines of the body (e.g. neuronal cells). Given that patient DNA samples are typically derived from blood or saliva, it is not always possible to detect all somatic mutations, also known as somatic mosaicisms. Targeted sequencing of individuals with brain malformations has identified that of the 17% of causal variants identified in participants, 30% of these mutations were found to be mosaic (Jamuar et al., 2014). Novel methods for the detection of somatic variation could also be an important development for comprehensive genetic screening in DD/ID.

Understanding the genetic aetiologies of ID is only the starting point as the ultimate goal is to use this aetiological information to personalise therapeutic interventions and so improve patient outcomes. Some progress has been made in pharmacological development for Rett syndrome and fragile X syndrome. In 2007, the Rett syndrome like neurological phenotype in *MECP2* deficient mice was shown to be reversed by delayed restoration of the gene (Guy et al., 2007). This has led to clinical trials of several drugs, with recombinant human insulin-like growth factor 1 (IGF-1) being a particularly promising agent (Khwaja et al., 2014). In fragile X syndrome, methylation of the *FMR1* gene prevents expression of the fragile X mental retardation protein (FMRP). One downstream effect of this is increased metabotropic glutamate receptor 5 (mGluR5) activity. As mGluR5 has an important role in synaptic transmission, clinical trials have focused on mGluR5 antagonists. However, despite these advances there are currently few examples of successful therapeutic interventions or pharmacological treatments.

2.7   Summary

In this chapter we have seen how genetic discovery has moved from gene mapping of syndromes with characteristic phenotypes to a genotype-first approach, whereby genome-wide screening defines causative variants and the range of associated phenotypes enlarges as different patient cohorts are investigated. Not only do the same phenotypes arise from different genetic variants, but the same genetic variant can confer risk for multiple disorders. Study of the complex trajectory from genotype to phenotype, taking into account environmental interactions, will be key to bridging the current gaps in our understanding and achieving the goal of personalised medicine.

In conclusion there has been a vast expansion in the number of genetic variants known to cause (or act as strong risk factors for) ID in recent years. However, this continues to be a highly active field of research and discovery of further ID relevant variants is expected. From a clinical perspective, genetic investigation of DD/ID has moved from karyotyping and specific genetics tests for suspected syndromes to comprehensive genome wide screening for CNVs and SNVs. The genetics of ID is likely to become increasingly relevant to the practice of ID psychiatry, in terms of ordering of genetic investigations, clinical management of associated medical/psychiatric problems, and communicating with patients, carers and other professionals around genetic diagnoses. However, interpretation of genetic findings is often complex and closer links with clinical genetics services will be necessary.

References

Amir, R. E. et al. (1999) Rett syndrome is caused by mutations in X-linked MECP2, encoding methyl-CpG-binding protein 2. *Nature Genetics*, 23, 185–8. doi: 10.1038/13810

Blau, N., Van Spronsen, F. J. & Levy, H. L. (2010) Phenylketonuria. *The Lancet*, 376(9750), 1417–27. doi: 10.1016/S0140-6736(10)60961-0

Butler, M. G. (2011) Prader–Willi syndrome: Obesity due to genomic imprinting, *Current Genomics*, 12(3), 204–15, doi: 10.2174/138920211795677877

Carter, N. (2007) Methods and strategies for analyzing copy number variation using DNA microarrays. *Nature Genetics*, 39, S16–S21. doi: 10.1038/ng2028.Methods

Cassidy, S. B. & Driscoll, D. J. (2009) Prader–Willi syndrome. *European Journal of Human Genetics*, 17(1), 3–13. doi: 10.1038/ejhg.2008.165

Cederbaum, S. (2002) Phenylketonuria: An update. *Current Opinion in Pediatrics*, 14(6), 702–6.

Chahrour, M. & Zoghbi, H. Y. (2007) The story of Rett syndrome: From clinic to neurobiology. *Neuron*, 56(3), 422–37. doi: 10.1016/j.neuron.2007.10.001

Coe, B. P. et al. (2014) Refining analyses of copy number variation identifies specific genes associated with developmental delay. *Nature Genetics*, 46(10). doi: 10.1038/ng.3092

Cooper, G. M. et al. (2011) A copy number variation morbidity map of developmental delay. *Nature Genetics*, 43(9), 838–46. doi: 10.1038/ng.909

Crawford, D. C., Acuña, J. M. & Sherman, S. L. (2001) FMR1 and the fragile X syndrome: human genome epidemiology review. *Genetics in Medicine: Official Journal of the American College of Medical Genetics*, 3(5), 359–71. doi: 10.1097/00125817-200109000-00006

D'Angelo, D. et al. (2015) Defining the effect of the 16p11.2 duplication on cognition, behavior, and medical comorbidities. *JAMA Psychiatry*, 10032, 1. doi: 10.1001/jamapsychiatry.2015.2123

Doherty, J. L. & Owen, M. J. (2014) Genomic insights into the overlap between psychiatric disorders: Implications for research and clinical practice. *Genome Medicine*, 6(4), 29. doi: 10.1186/gm546

Giaroli, G. et al. (2014) Does rare matter? Copy number variants at 16p11.2 and the risk of psychosis: A systematic review of literature and meta-analysis. *Schizophrenia research*, 159(2–3), 340–6. doi: 10.1016/j.schres.2014.09.025

Gilissen, C. et al. (2014) Genome sequencing identifies major causes of severe intellectual disability. *Nature*, 511(7509), 344–7. doi: 10.1038/nature13394

Guy, J. et al. (2007) Reversal of neurological defects in a mouse model of Rett syndrome. *Science*, 315(5815), 1143–7. doi: 10.1126/science.1138389

Habel, A. et al. (2014) Towards a safety net for management of 22q11.2 deletion syndrome:

Guidelines for our times. *European Journal of Pediatrics*, 173(6), 757–65. doi: 10.1007/s00431-013-2240-z

Hooper, S. R. et al. (2013) A longitudinal examination of the psychoeducational, neurocognitive, and psychiatric functioning in children with 22q11.2 deletion syndrome. *Research in Developmental Disabilities*, 34(5), 1758–69. doi: 10.1016/j.ridd.2012.12.003

Horsler, K. & Oliver, C. (2006) The behavioural phenotype of Angelman syndrome. *Journal of Intellectual Disability Research*, 50(1), 33–53. doi: 10.1111/j.1365-2788.2005.00730.x

Iafrate, A. J. et al. (2004) Detection of large-scale variation in the human genome. *Nature Genetics*, 36(9), 949–51. doi: 10.1038/ng1416

Jacobs, P. A. & Strong, J. A. (1959) A case of human intersexuality having a possible XXY sex-determining mechanism. *Nature*, 183 (4657), 302–3. Available at: www.ncbi.nlm.nih.gov/pubmed/13632697

Jamuar, S. S. et al. (2014) Somatic mutations in cerebral cortical malformations. *New England Journal of Medicine*, 371(8), 733–43. doi: 10.1056/NEJMoa1314432

Karmiloff-Smith, A. et al. (2016) The importance of understanding individual differences in Down syndrome. *F1000Research*, 5, 389. doi: 10.12688/f1000research.7506.1

Khwaja, O. S. et al. (2014) Safety, pharmacokinetics, and preliminary assessment of efficacy of mecasermin (recombinant human IGF-1) for the treatment of Rett syndrome. *Proceedings of the National Academy of Sciences of the United States of America*, 111(12), 4596–601. doi: 10.1073/pnas.1311141111

Kirov, G. et al. (2014) The penetrance of copy number variations for schizophrenia and developmental delay. *Biological Psychiatry*, 75 (5), 378–85. doi: 10.1016/j.biopsych.2013.07.022

LaFramboise, T. (2009) Single nucleotide polymorphism arrays: A decade of biological, computational and technological advances. *Nucleic Acids Research*, 37(13), 4181–93. doi: 10.1093/nar/gkp552

Ledbetter, D. H. et al. (1981) Deletions of chromosome 15 as a cause of the Prader–Willi syndrome. *New England Journal of Medicine*, 304(6), 325–9. doi: 10.1056/NEJM198102053040604

Lehner, T., Senthil, G. & Addington, A. M. (2014) Convergence of advances in genomics, team science, and repositories as drivers of progress in psychiatric genomics. *Biological Psychiatry*, 77(1), 6–14. doi: 10.1016/j.biopsych.2014.01.003

Lejeune, J. et al. (1959) Les chromosomes humains en culture de tissus. *Comptes rendus hebdomadaires des séances de l'Académie des sciences*, (248), 602–3.

Lejeune, J. et al. (1963) Ségrégation familiale d'une translocation 5–13 déterminant une monosomie et une trisomie partielles du bras court du chromosome 5: Maladie du 'cri du chat' et sa 'réciproque'. *Comptes rendus hebdomadaires des séances de l'Académie des sciences*, 257, 3098–102. Available at: www.ncbi.nlm.nih.gov/pubmed/14095841

Lubs, H. A., Stevenson, R. E. & Schwartz, C. E. (2012) Fragile X and X-linked intellectual disability: Four decades of discovery. *American Journal of Human Genetics*, 90(4), 579–90. doi: 10.1016/j.ajhg.2012.02.018

Lynch, M. (2010) Rate, molecular spectrum, and consequences of human mutation. *Proceedings of the National Academy of Sciences*, 107(3), 961–8. doi: 10.1073/pnas.0912629107

MacDonald, J. R. et al. (2014) The Database of Genomic Variants: A curated collection of structural variation in the human genome. *Nucleic Acids Research*, 42, D986–92. doi: 10.1093/nar/gkt958

McRae, J. F. et al. (2017) Prevalence and architecture of de novo mutations in developmental disorders. *Nature*, 542(7642), 433–8. doi: 10.1038/nature21062

Miller, D. T. et al. (2010) Consensus statement: Chromosomal microarray is a first-tier clinical diagnostic test for individuals with developmental disabilities or congenital anomalies. *American Journal of Human Genetics*, 86(5), 749–64. doi: 10.1016/j.ajhg.2010.04.006

Monks, S. et al. (2014) Further evidence for high rates of schizophrenia in 22q11.2 deletion syndrome. *Schizophrenia Research*, 153(1–3), 231–6. doi: 10.1016/j.schres.2014.01.020

Najmabadi, H. et al. (2011) Deep sequencing reveals 50 novel genes for recessive cognitive disorders. *Nature*, **478**(7367), 57–63. doi: 10.1038/nature10423

Neul, J. L. & Zoghbi, H. Y. (2004) Rett Syndrome: A prototypical neurodevelopmental disorder. *Neuroscientist*, **10**(2), 118–28. doi: 10.1177/1073858403260995

O'Donovan, M. C. & Owen, M. J. (2016) The implications of the shared genetics of psychiatric disorders. *Nature Medicine*, **22**(11). doi: 10.1038/nm.4196

Ou, Z. et al. (2008) Microduplications of 22q11.2 are frequently inherited and are associated with variable phenotypes. *Genetics in Medicine: Official Journal of the American College of Medical Genetics*, **10**(4), 267–77. doi: 10.1097/GIM.0b013e31816b64c2

Palmer, E. et al. (2014) Changing interpretation of chromosomal microarray over time in a community cohort with intellectual disability. *American Journal of Medical Genetics. Part A*, **164A**(2), 377–85. doi: 10.1002/ajmg.a.36279

Pelc, K., Cheron, G. & Dan, B. (2008) Behavior and neuropsychiatry manifestations in Angelman syndrome. *Neuropsychiatric Disease and Treatment*, **4**(3), 577–84. doi: 10.2147/NDT.S2749

Pieretti, M. et al. (1991) Absence of expression of the FMR-1 gene in fragile X syndrome. *Cell*, **66**(4), 817–22. Available at: www.ncbi.nlm.nih.gov/pubmed/1878973

Portnoï, M. F. (2009) Microduplication 22q11.2: A new chromosomal syndrome. *European Journal of Medical Genetics. Elsevier Masson SAS*, **52**(2–3), 88–93. doi: 10.1016/j.ejmg.2009.02.008

Redon, R. et al. (2006) Global variation in copy number in the human genome. *Nature*, **444**(7118), 444–54. doi: 10.1038/nature05329

Rees, E. et al. (2014) Evidence that duplications of 22q11.2 protect against schizophrenia. *Molecular Psychiatry*, **19**(1), 37–40. doi: 10.1038/mp.2013.156

Rees, E. et al. (2016) Analysis of intellectual disability copy number variants for association with schizophrenia. *JAMA Psychiatry*, **73**(9), 963–9. doi: 10.1001/jamapsychiatry.2016.1831

Rousseau, F. et al. (2011) The fragile X mental retardation syndrome 20 years after the FMR1 gene discovery: an expanding universe of knowledge. *Clinical Biochemist. Reviews*, **32**(3), 135–62. Available at: www.ncbi.nlm.nih.gov/pubmed/21912443

Schneider, M. et al. (2014) Psychiatric disorders from childhood to adulthood in 22q11.2 deletion syndrome: Results from the International Consortium on Brain and Behavior in 22q11.2 Deletion Syndrome. *American Journal of Psychiatry*, **171**(6), 627–39. doi: 10.1176/appi.ajp.2013.13070864

Scriver, C. R. (2007) The PAH gene, phenylketonuria, and a paradigm shift. *Human Mutation*, **28**(9), 831–45. doi: 10.1002/humu.20526

Sebat, J. et al. (2004) Large-scale copy number polymorphism in the human genome. *Science*, **305**(5683), 525–8. doi: 10.1126/science.1098918

Shprintzen, R. J. (2008) Velo-Cardio-Facial Syndrome: 30 years of study. *Developmental Disabilities Research Reviews*, **14**(1), 3–10. doi: 10.1002/ddrr.2.Velo-Cardio-Facial

Sigafoos, J., O'Reilly, M. F. & Lancioni, G. E. (2009) Cri-du-chat. *Developmental Neurorehabilitation*, **12**(3), 119–21. doi: 10.1080/17518420902975720

Tjio, J. H. & Levan, A. (1956) The chromosome number of man. *Hereditas*, **42**, 1–6. doi: 10.1111/j.1601-5223.1956.tb03010.x

Van Buggenhout, G. & Fryns, J.-P. (2009) Angelman syndrome (AS, MIM 105830). *European Journal of Human Genetics*, **17**(11), 1367–73. doi: 10.1038/ejhg.2009.67

Verri, A. et al. (2010) Klinefelter's syndrome and psychoneurologic function. *Molecular Human Reproduction*, **16**(6), 425–33. doi: 10.1093/molehr/gaq018

de Villiers, J. & Porteous, M. (2012) Genetic testing of adults with intellectual disability. *Psychiatrist*, **36**(11), 409–13. doi: 10.1192/pb.bp.111.038216

Visootsak, J. & Graham, J. M. (2006) Klinefelter syndrome and other sex chromosomal aneuploidies. *Orphanet Journal of Rare Diseases*, **1**, 42. doi: 10.1186/1750-1172-1-42

Vissers, L. E. et al. (2010) A *de novo* paradigm for mental retardation. 42(12), 1109–12. doi: 10.1038/ng.712

Vissers, L. E. L. M., Gilissen, C. & Veltman, J. A. (2015) Genetic studies in intellectual disability and related disorders. *Nature Reviews Genetics*, **17**(1), 9–18. doi: 10.1038/nrg3999

Weiss, L. A. et al. (2008) Association between microdeletion and microduplication at 16p11.2 and autism. *New England Journal of Medicine*, **358**(7), 667–75. doi: 10.1056/NEJMoa075974

Wiseman, F. K. et al. (2015) A genetic cause of Alzheimer disease: Mechanistic insights from Down syndrome. *Nature Reviews Neuroscience*, **16**(9), 564–74. doi: 10.1038/nrn3983

Wolfe, K., Strydom, A. et al. (2017) Chromosomal microarray testing in adults with intellectual disability presenting with comorbid psychiatric disorders. *European Journal of Human Genetics: EJHG*, **25**(1), 66–72. doi: 10.1038/ejhg.2016.107

Wolfe, K., Stueber, K. et al. (2017) Genetic testing in intellectual disability psychiatry: Opinions and practices of UK child and intellectual disability psychiatrists. *Journal of Applied Research in Intellectual Disabilities*, **23**, 1–12. doi: 10.1111/jar.12391

Zufferey, F. et al. (2012) A 600 kb deletion syndrome at 16p11.2 leads to energy imbalance and neuropsychiatric disorders. *Journal of Medical Genetics*, **49**(10), 660–8. doi: 10.1136/jmedgenet-2012-101203

Chapter 3
Behavioural Phenotypes

Ruth Bevan and Gill Bell

3.1 Introduction

In this chapter we talk about the behavioural phenotype, being the expression of underlying genotype or neurobiological disorder, with an awareness that this changes across the developmental stages.

We will focus on the psychosocial and behavioural components of the phenotype and use a number of syndromes as exemplars. One must be mindful of the pervasive nature of these conditions, affecting multiple organs and systems. Further information about this can be found in textbooks such as *The A–Z Reference Book of Syndromes and Inherited Disorders* (Gilbert, 2013).

A definition of behavioural phenotype is given by O'Brien (2002: 1–2) as: 'a characteristic pattern of motor, cognitive, linguistic and social observations that is consistently associated with a biological disorder. In some cases, the behavioural phenotype may constitute a psychiatric disorder; in others, behaviours which are not usually regarded as symptoms of psychiatric diagnoses may occur.'

It is understandable that parents and carers of individuals with a syndrome will have questions about what lies ahead for their child or loved one. They may ask professionals to make predictions about the future. Their concern may be around level of intellect, behaviour, social function or illness, both physical and psychiatric. Of course, the relationship between genotype and phenotype is complex, influenced by many factors. However, the study of behavioural phenotypes has given us clues as to what the future may hold. This can be helpful in planning for future education, occupation and care.

Using the framework of a behavioural phenotype is not without its problems. There is an argument that it may reinforce stereotypes and stigma. Making negative predictions about the future may become a 'self-fulfilling prophecy' and encourage therapeutic nihilism. In the case of the sex aneuploidy, XYY, early research indicated an association between this genotype and aggressive, violent and criminal behaviour. However, the sample population was drawn from psychiatric and penal institutions resulting in a selection bias. The increased incidence of antisocial behaviour seen in this cohort could be explained by other factors, such as large stature, intellectual disability (ID) and impulsivity. Interpretations from generalisations must, therefore, first and foremost bear in mind the individual, their strengths, vulnerabilities and needs. The key to assessing a suspected behavioural phenotype, whether or not the individual has a diagnosed disorder, is to look for a constellation of features and behaviours. There are assessment tools which can aid this. O'Brien et al. (2001) provide a review of such assessment schedules.

It should be borne in mind that there are limits to the validity and usefulness of these tools. Many disorders are rare, and research findings are hampered by small case numbers and an inability to produce statistically significant results. The origins of our awareness and understanding of the behavioural phenotype have, in part, come from anecdotal reports given by families and carers.

3.2 Physical Health

Physical health is an important consideration in the assessment of individuals with a syndromal disorder. For multiple reasons, many are associated with higher rates of physical illness. Epilepsy is common and will influence the behavioural phenotype. Frequently, sensory deficits, such as hearing and visual problems, exacerbate difficulties in development, speech and social communication. Certain illnesses may be a particular feature of the syndrome, such as hypothyroidism in Down syndrome, or are a direct consequence of the underlying disability, for example, the effects of obesity in Prader–Willi syndrome. It must be remembered that illness can be iatrogenic, such as arising from the effects of medications. Socio-economic status, accessibility to appropriate healthcare and financial hardship are additional factors which disproportionately affect this group.

The following provides a summary of the behavioural phenotypes of individual syndromes. Where possible, information has been broken down into specific areas of functioning: cognition, communication, behaviour, social functioning and propensity for psychiatric illnesses.

3.3 Down Syndrome

Down syndrome, arising in most cases from trisomy 21, is the most common chromosomal cause of ID. In a minority it arises from an unbalanced translocation or mosaicism.

Most have between a mild and moderate ID. Strengths lie in visual special tasks and visual memories (Fletcher et al., 2007). Weaknesses include working memory and planning with a cognitively avoidant learning style (Daunhauer & Fidler, 2011).

Receptive language skills and comprehension often outperform expressive capabilities. Relatively strong non-verbal communication facilitates social interaction. While there is a general perception that those with Down syndrome, and in particular children, are highly sociable and have good 'people' skills, there is evidence to suggest that subtle social cognitive difficulties exist (Cebula et al., 2010).

The behavioural phenotype is further characterised by inattention, impulsivity and disobedience (Fletcher et al., 2007). Hyperactivity is less likely to feature but obsessive slowness and repetitive behaviour are more commonly seen.

An increasing incidence of individuals diagnosed with Down syndrome and co-morbid autism spectrum disorder (ASD) has been reported. Some studies suggest 5–10% meet the criteria for ASD (Daunhauer & Fidler, 2011). These figures are still below what is expected in individuals with non-specific ID (Ghazziuddin et al., 1992). There is a higher incidence of depressive disorder, anxiety and obsessive–compulsive disorder as well as an atypical and often transient psychotic disorder which tends to affect young adults (Fletcher et al., 2007). Down syndrome is referred to as a 'syndrome of precocious ageing' which in part refers to the high rates of early onset Alzheimer's dementia. Personality change, depression and loss of existing skills are early indicators of dementia of the Alzheimer's type.

3.4 Angelman Syndrome

Angelman syndrome arises from the deletion of region 15q11.2-q13 occurring on the maternally derived chromosome. Additional mechanisms have, however, been identified, all causing disruption of the *UBE3A* gene. Although there are some differences, the overarching clinical and behavioural features of the syndrome are consistent across the genetic mechanisms.

Those affected have severe ID, a movement or balance disorder, such as ataxia and tremulousness, and severe speech delay. Associated features include seizures, feeding difficulties and sleep disturbance.

A unique behavioural phenotype is characterised by an apparent happy disposition, paroxysmal laughter, which can also occur in response to apparent unpleasant events, prosocial behaviours, attraction to water, repetitive hand flapping and mouthing.

In those with a more profound ID, severe seizure disorder and unstable family or out-of-home placement may be less likely to exhibit an apparent happy demeanour (Williams, 2010).

Restlessness, hyperactivity and short attention span are reported in childhood and may abate in adulthood (Clayton-Smith, 2001).

Some children demonstrate features of ASD, such as problems with social reciprocity, language impairment and motor stereotypies. Such features are more likely in those with maternal deletion (Williams, 2010). Anxiety is commonly reported in adults.

3.5 Prader–Willi Syndrome

Prader–Willi syndrome results from a number of genetic mechanisms affecting chromosome 15's long arm. These include parental deletion (70%), maternal disomy (25%) and unbalanced translocations and mutations of the imprinting centre (5%) (Holland et al., 2003).

The behavioural profile varies according to the underlying genetic defect. However, there is no difference between the subtypes in full-scale intelligence quotient (IQ) (Zarcone et al., 2007). Level of ID is variable, but most individuals function in the mild-to-moderate ID range. Strengths lie in reading, long-term memory and visuospatial functioning (Fletcher et al., 2007). A talent for jigsaws has been reported (Rosner et al., 2004), as has excessive talking in childhood (Sinnema et al., 2011).

Characteristic of Prader–Willi syndrome is neonatal hypotonia with feeding problems, in early infancy failure to thrive, followed by food seeking, hyperphagia and insatiability during childhood, leading to potential obesity and associated health problems such as respiratory compromise, diabetes mellitus and arthritis in adolescence and adulthood. Other characteristic behaviours displayed are tantrums, aggression, skin picking and compulsive behaviours such as hoarding, orderliness and exactness (Holland et al., 2003). Unusual water intake is described with some individuals consuming excessive amounts which may be clinically significant, particularly if also taking neuroleptic medication (Akefeldt, 2009). Behavioural problems are described as increasing in adolescents and young adults but then subside in older adults although not all studies support this view (Sinnema et al., 2011). Maintenance of lower body mass index (BMI) may result in stress which could impact on behaviour (Sinnema et al., 2011).

Adaptive skills often fall below IQ expectations (Holland et al., 2003), and interpersonal relationships tend to be poor. Social competence may not improve with age (Rosner et al., 2004).

Regarding psychiatric symptoms, mood fluctuations and irritability are reported (Holland et al., 2003) and depression and major anxiety are common (Fletcher et al., 2007). Repetitive and ritualistic behaviour and rigidity are similar to that seen in ASD and many also meet the criteria for obsessive–compulsive disorder.

High rates of atypical psychosis and affective disorder are seen in Prader–Willi syndrome, which is linked to the maternal uniparental disomy subtype (Fletcher et al., 2007; Sinnema et al., 2011).

3.6 Cornelia de Lange Syndrome

Cornelia de Lange syndrome (CdLS) arises from a number of genetic defects, affecting chromosomes 5, 10 and X, producing a variety of physical and behavioural abnormalities. The condition commonly results in a moderate-to-profound ID and expressive language deficits (Wulffaert et al., 2009). Partial epilepsy, with favourable prognosis, is the most common type of epilepsy (Parisi et al., 2015).

Behavioural features of CdLS are self-injury, compulsive, repetitive and impulsive behaviours, hyperactivity and aggression. Behavioural difficulties may be linked to environmental factors or physical symptoms such as pain from gastro-oesophageal reflux (a common physical health problem associated with the condition).

Rates of ASD are comparatively high in those with CdLS. However, the profile and developmental trajectory of ASD characteristics are potentially different to those observed in idiopathic ASD. Attention deficit and hyperactivity disorder (ADHD), depression, obsessive–compulsive behaviours and social anxiety, particularly in adolescence, are also described, and often worsen with age (Parisi et al., 2015).

3.7 Foetal Valproate Syndrome

The physical effects of exposure to sodium valproate on the developing foetus are well known. There is clear evidence to suggest that exposure to sodium valproate in utero has adverse cognitive, emotional and behavioural consequences (Vinten et al., 2008).

In such cases there are numerous genetic and environmental confounders such as maternal seizures, co-morbidity and socio-economic circumstances (Tomson & Battino, 2008).

Exposure to sodium valproate in utero has been associated with language delay, reduced IQ scores and an increase in special educational needs (Baker et al., 2015 Moore et al., 2000). Studies have reported evidence of a sodium valproate dose–response relationship (Baker et al., 2014).

The behavioural phenotype includes hyperactivity, lack of concentration, behavioural disturbance and poor social skills (Vinten et al., 2008).

Higher rates of ASD are also reported (Christensen et al., 2013).

3.8 Foetal Alcohol Syndrome

The teratogenic effects of alcohol during pregnancy are widely reported. One of the most serious outcomes is foetal alcohol syndrome (FAS), now better understood as part of a spectrum disorder (FASD). The pathognomonic facial features associated with FASD are absent in the majority of those affected, leading to this disorder being frequently overlooked (Koren et al., 2014).

Individuals exhibit difficulties with communication: pronunciation, fluency (stuttering), auditory processing, language comprehension, storytelling and sequencing, and social communication skills (Ganthous et al., 2015; Wyper & Rasmussen, 2011).

In FASD the range of deficits is wide and nonspecific. They include reduced IQ, difficulties with communication and mild-to-severe behavioural disturbance. Features of the behavioural phenotype include hyperactivity, inattention and oppositional defiance.

It may be difficult to disentangle the effects of prenatal alcohol exposure from other risk factors which may co-occur, such as social deprivation, maternal smoking, drug use and maternal history of mental illness and/or abuse and neglect (Koren et al., 2014).

ADHD occurs in as many as 70% of those with FASD. Oppositional defiant and conduct disorder are the next most common diagnosable disorders (Koren et al., 2014). Anxiety and emotional problems are also reported (Steinhausen et al., 2003).

3.9 Fragile X Syndrome

Fragile X syndrome (FXS) is one of a group of FMR1 mutation-related disorders, termed fragile X-associated disorders (FXD) (Boyle & Kaufmann, 2010). It is the most common identifiable cause of inherited ID. It results from a trinucleotide repeat expansion (CGG) towards the tip of the X chromosome's long arm, at position Xq27.3. The defective gene results in a reduction in a protein, Fragile X mental retardation protein (FMRP), leading to abnormal brain development. Several factors influence the severity of phenotype, including, crucially, the length of gene expansion, degree of mosaicism and extent of gene methylation. Because it is X-linked, males and females are differentially affected.

Males with the full mutation (>200 CGG repeats) often have mild-to-moderate ID and females a borderline ID (Fletcher et al., 2007). Seizures affect approximately 20% during childhood. These are usually generalised tonic–clonic or benign rolandic seizures, and usually improve or disappear with age (Howlin & Udwin, 2002). Memory is a particular strength; however, working memory deficits are common. Studies suggest reduced rates of acquisition of new skills which can manifest as cognitive decline over time (Boyle & Kaufmann, 2010). From middle age onwards, a substantial proportion of fragile X pre-mutation (55–200 CGG repeats) carriers develop an insidious and progressive tremor-ataxia syndrome with associated cognitive decline.

Language is commonly delayed, with expressive language more impaired than receptive. Deficits include perseverative speech, echolalia, self-talking and cluttering (Fletcher et al., 2007). However, individuals with FXS tend to have better verbal than non-verbal skills (Boyle & Kaufmann, 2010).

The behavioural phenotype is characterised by inattention, hyperarousal, hyperactivity and impulsivity, tendency to aggression, tactile defensiveness, hand biting and stereotypic movements including hand flapping. Hyperactivity and impulsivity may improve with age although inattention and problems with inhibitory control persist (Cornish et al., 2008). Females display a milder version of the behavioural phenotype.

Interactions with others are adversely affected by social anxiety and gaze avoidance, although there is not thought to be a pervasive lack of interest in social contact (Fletcher et al., 2007). Areas of strength are a sense of humour, imitation skills and adaptive living skills (Howlin & Udin, 2002). This means that many are able, with support, to engage in occupational activities.

Unsurprisingly, many meet the criteria for a diagnosis of ADHD, features of which are reported in up to 84% of males and 67% of females (Boyle & Kaufmann, 2010). There are also high rates of ASD, with FXS reported to be one of the principal genetic causes of ASD. Prevalence rates vary between studies ranging from 15% to 60% in males (Budimirovic & Kaufmann, 2011). Higher rates of ASD are also reported in females. There has been uncertainty regarding whether ASD in individuals with FXS is qualitatively similar or different to idiopathic autism (Smith et al., 2012). An example of a difference is seen in social deficits. In FSX, gaze avoidance is postulated to arise from social anxiety and hyperarousal rather than a lack of understanding or interest in others (Cornish et al., 2008). There is support for a spectrum view with variable autistic manifestations in premutation/full mutation individuals (Clifford et al., 2007). Other more common psychiatric symptoms are mood instability and anxiety.

3.10 Rett Syndrome

Rett syndrome is a progressive neurological disorder arising, in the majority of cases, from a spontaneous mutation on the long arm of the X chromosome. In males, who have only one X chromosome, it is thought to be incompatible with life.

The natural history of Rett syndrome is one of normal development to the age of six to eighteen months, followed by decelerated head growth, global developmental regression, loss of verbal ability, ataxia and abnormal gait. The resultant ID is within the severe to profound range.

Behaviours frequently described are repetitive hand stereotypies, rocking, breath-holding or hyperventilation. Facial grimacing and repetitive mouth and tongue movements are also reported.

Psychiatric symptoms include mood variability, anxiety and a strong association with ASD.

3.11 Lesch–Nyhan Syndrome

Lesch–Nyhan is an X-linked recessive syndrome caused by deficiency of the activity of the enzyme hypoxanthine guanine phosphoribosyltransferase (HPRT). It almost exclusively affects males, with one-third of cases arising *de novo*. There are a variety of clinical phenotypes of HPRT deficiency, with Lesch–Nyhan syndrome being the most severe.

The majority have mild or moderate ID. Developmental delays usually become apparent during the first year of life alongside a motor disorder which may give a clinical picture similar to cerebral palsy. Initial hypotonia gives way to dystonia, spasticity and occasionally choreoathetosis and seizures.

Self-injury is a prominent feature of this behavioural phenotype and emerges between two and four years of age. It appears to be compulsive in nature and frequently involves biting of the fingers or lips or self-hitting. Other features include aggression, impulsivity, spitting or use of socially unacceptable language (Torres et al., 2012).

Due to the varied effects of hyperuricemia, even with effective treatment, life expectancy is shortened with most individuals only surviving into the second or third decade of life.

3.12 Sex Aneuploidy

Sex aneuploidy is the presence of an abnormal number of sex chromosomes. Examples are Turner syndrome (45, XO), Klinefelter syndrome (47, XXY) and other trisomies of the sex chromosomes (47, XXX and 47, XYY).

While there is significant inter-individual variation, Klinefelter syndrome confers an increased risk of developmental delay, language-based difficulties, speech delay and executive dysfunction with poor adaptive functioning. Reports describe normally distributed cognitive scores but with the mean score shifted to the left compared to the general population (Bender et al., 1986). The vast majority of those affected will not have significant problems. Reported behaviours include social difficulties such as shyness and withdrawal. There are higher rates of anxiety, depression, ADHD (predominantly inattentive) and ASD (Tartaglia et al., 2010).

The syndrome is also characterised by hypogonadism, androgen deficiency and infertility. There is some evidence that early androgen therapy can have positive effects on the behavioural phenotype (Samango-Sprouse et al., 2015).

Similarities in the features of XYY and Klinefelter syndrome include cognitive ability, speech delay, inattention and ADHD. Boys with XYY have normal pubertal development and testosterone levels.

The XYY syndrome is reported to be associated with impulsivity, behavioural problems and increased risk of ASD comparative to Klinefelter syndrome (Ross et al., 2012).

Trisomy X commonly goes undetected; therefore it is difficult to make generalisations about its effects. Reports suggest that those affected may be less well adapted, experience communication and social difficulties such as shyness, avoidance and social immaturity. It may also be associated with traits of ASD (van Rijn et al., 2014).

The physical features of Turner syndrome are well described. Most have normal intelligence but may demonstrate immaturity, hyperactivity, problems concentrating, nervousness, poor peer relations, academic difficulties and social adjustment problems (Rovet & Ireland, 1994). The behavioural phenotype may differ depending on the parentage of the X chromosome, with maternally derived X chromosome resulting in greater social deficits (Skuse et al., 1997).

3.13 Smith–Magenis Syndrome

Smith–Magenis syndrome results from deletion on chromosome 17 (17p11.2). ID is most commonly within the moderate range. Affected individuals have higher rates of seizures.

Speech is delayed and the voice is notably hoarse and deep.

The behavioural phenotype includes sleep disorder, hyperactivity, attention deficits, self-harm and aggression/disruptive behaviour. Many individuals demonstrate a preference for adult contact and an eagerness to please. Challenging behaviour may be a response to environmental events, most notably, decreased levels of adult attention (Taylor & Oliver, 2008). Certain behaviours are described as 'unique' to Smith–Magenis syndrome. These include self-hugging, hand squeezing, hand licking and page flipping.

Co-morbidities of ADHD and ASD are common in individuals with Smith–Magenis syndrome. Mood fluctuations are also described.

3.14 Tuberous Sclerosis Complex

Tuberous sclerosis complex (TSC) is an autosomal dominant genetic disorder affecting multiple organ systems, including the brain. TSC arises from mutations in *TSC1*, the gene on chromosome 9q34, and in *TSC2*, the gene on chromosome 16p13. About two-thirds of all cases of TSC are sporadic. This disease is characterised by the widespread development of hamartias, or non-growing lesions, and hamartomas, benign tumours that rarely progress to malignancy.

The cognitive profile and behavioural phenotype is highly variable and likely dependent upon distribution of the lesions, in particular within the brain. Individuals with *TSC2* mutations appear to have greater difficulties than those with *TSC1*.

There are high rates of seizures (86% in TS1 and 99% in TS2). The age of onset and type of seizure disorder and degree of seizure control will impact the clinical picture. ID is reported in between 46% and 72% with moderate-to-severe ID in 14% to 46%. Social withdrawal and/or language abnormalities are reported in up to one-third of cases (Curatolo et al., 2008).

Other features of the behavioural phenotype include hyperactivity, sleep disorders, peer problems, emotional problems, aggression and self-injury.

ASD is diagnosed in around 50% and there are high rates of ADHD and conduct disorder. Adults are at risk of anxiety disorder and depression (de Vries et al., 2005).

3.15 William Syndrome

William syndrome (WS) is a multisystem genomic disorder caused by a sporadic deletion of twenty-six to twenty-eight genes including the elastin gene on chromosome 7q11.23, which results in connective tissue abnormalities.

William syndrome has a well-recognised behavioural phenotype. It is characterised by global developmental delay, difficulties with motor control, abnormalities of visual processing and hyperacusis. There are a wide range of cognitive abilities, although most are within the mild ID range.

Although delayed, language is a relative strength. Individuals with William syndrome demonstrate comparatively good concrete receptive and expressive language and fluency. This may lead others to overestimate their abilities. There are difficulties with the pragmatics of language. Individuals show an interest in social engagement with hyper-sociability and demonstrate empathy. However, there are deficits in emotional recognition, social judgements, misinterpretation of cues and disinhibition. These features can result in poor peer relationships and vulnerability. Children and adults with WS have weaknesses in adaptive living skills, and adults have difficulty coping with demands of employment (Rosner et al., 2004).

ADHD and anxiety, including specific phobias, are recognised as common diagnoses in WS (Morris, 2010).

3.16 Phenylketonuria and Congenital Hypothyroidism

The behavioural phenotypes of phenylketonuria (PKU) and congenital hypothyroidism are well recognised. Due to neonatal screening and effective treatments, both of these conditions are now extremely rare in countries with well-developed healthcare systems.

PKU is an inherited, autosomal recessive condition, affecting the phenylalanine hydroxylase gene and leading to a build-up of toxic levels of phenylalanine. There is a spectrum of presentations; however, the classic form results in microcephaly, developmental delay, typically a severe ID, seizures and hyperactivity. An association with autism is reported (Baieli et al., 2003).

Congenital hypothyroidism is an endocrine disorder of newborns arising from early insufficiency of thyroid hormone, necessary for normal brain development. Again, there is a spectrum of clinical presentations which include ID ranging from mild-to-severe and variable neurological impairments. Even with treatment some individuals may show subtle persistent neurocognitive deficits (Triantafyllou et al., 2015).

Table 3.1 Common syndromes and their associations

Syndrome	Aetiology	Degree of ID	Common physical features	Notable features of behavioural phenotype	Common psychiatric features
Down syndrome	Trisomy 21 (commonly)	Mild to moderate	Includes congenital heart disease & hypothyroidism	Inattention Apparent sociability	Depression Anxiety Alzheimer dementia
Angelman syndrome	Deletion of region 15q11.2-q13	Severe	Movement disorder Seizures	Apparent happy disposition Repetitive hand flapping and mouthing	Hyperactivity, anxiety and ASD features
Prader–Willi syndrome	Defects of chromosome 15's long arm	Mild to moderate	Neonatal hypotonia Hyperphagia Obesity	Aggression Skin picking	Mood disorders Atypical psychosis OCD ASD
Cornelia de Lange syndrome	Defects affecting chromosomes 5, 10 and X	Moderate to profound	Gastro-oesophageal reflux Epilepsy	Self-injury Compulsive & repetitive behaviour	ADHD ASD features Mood disorder
Foetal valproate syndrome	Intrauterine exposure	Variable	Include neural tube defects and craniofacial abnormalities	Hyperactivity & poor concentration Behavioural disturbance Poor social skills	ASD
Foetal alcohol syndrome	Intrauterine exposure	Reduced IQ	May not be present	Behavioural disturbance Disobedience	ADHD Oppositional defiant disorder Conduct disorder

Syndrome	Cause	Intellectual disability	Physical characteristics	Behavioural characteristics	Mental health
Fragile X syndrome	Trinucleotide repeat of the X chromosome	Mild to moderate	Seizures Tremor-ataxia syndrome	Inattention & hyperactivity Stereotypic movements Social anxiety & gaze avoidance	Anxiety ADHD ASD
Rett syndrome	Mutation of the X chromosome	Severe to profound	Normal development followed by regression of skills Ataxia & abnormal gait	Repetitive hand stereotypies & mouth movements Breath-holding/hyperventilation	Mood disorder ASD
Lesch–Nyhan syndrome	X-linked deficiency of HPRT	Mild or moderate	Hyperuricemia Motor disorder Seizures	Self-injury Aggression	Impulsivity
Sex aneuploidy	Abnormal number of sex chromosomes	None or mild	Hypogonadism (Klinefelter) Infertility (Klinefelter & Turner)	Social difficulties (Klinefelter, XXX & Turner) Behavioural problems (XYY)	ADHD & ASD (Klinefelter, XYY & possibly XXX) Mood disorder (Klinefelter)
Smith–Magenis syndrome	Deletion on chromosome 17p11.2	Moderate	Seizures Deep/hoarse voice	Sleep disorder Self-harm Aggression/disruptive behaviour Self-hugging/hand squeezing Hand licking and page flipping	ADHD ASD
Tuberous sclerosis complex	Mutations in genes TSC1 or TSC2 resulting in	Highly variable	Highly variable Include seizures	Social difficulties Aggression Self-injury	ADHD ASD Mood disorder

Table 3.1 (cont.)

Syndrome	Aetiology	Degree of ID	Common physical features	Notable features of behavioural phenotype	Common psychiatric features
	development of hamartias & hamartomas				
William syndrome	Deletion on chromosome 7	Mild	Poor motor control Visual processing difficulties Hyperacusis	Hyper-sociability Problems in social judgements Disinhibition	ADHD Anxiety
Phenylketonuria	Abnormalities in the phenylalanine hydroxylase gene	Severe	Microcephaly Seizures	Variable Hyperactivity	ASD
Congenital hypothyroidism	Early insufficiency of thyroid hormone	Mild to severe	Variable neurological impairments	Variable	

3.17 Conclusion

Alongside our knowledge about genetic disorders, our knowledge about behavioural phenotypes has grown. As individuals with an ID continue to live longer, we gain a greater understanding of changes across the developmental stages.

In this brief overview we have provided a definition of behavioural phenotype and described several examples. Table 3.1 provides a summary.

It is important to remember that even within a syndrome, the behavioural phenotype is highly variable and dynamic, across the developmental trajectory. Influential factors include the underlying genetic mechanism, physical health, the environment and co-morbid disorders such as ASD.

Awareness of behavioural phenotypes may be particularly helpful in identifying underlying causes of behaviour and impairment in syndromes when dysmorphic features or typical physical characteristics are less obvious or absent, such as in FASD.

Knowledge of behavioural phenotypes helps us to consider differential diagnoses, what may be expected within a given disorder or what may be out of the ordinary. It may help us to avoid over-pathologising. Behavioural phenotypes should not be used to make rigid individual predictions and doing so can be unhelpful. There is also a risk that we may be overinclusive in ascribing a feature as part of the behavioural phenotype, thereby neglecting to address a problem that may be more easily remedied.

There is evidence that through our understanding, adaptations to the environment and appropriate support, behavioural phenotypes can be positively influenced. Further research in this area may allow us to design targeted interventions.

Features of ASD are commonly described within the behavioural phenotype of most syndromes. It is important to compare rates of this and other co-morbid disorders with rates in those with equivalent levels of non-syndromal ID.

The Society for the Study of Behavioural Phenotypes, set up in 1987, promotes awareness, research and treatment. Further information can be found on their website (www.ssbp.org.uk/index.html). More specialist texts which expand on this subject are also available, such as O'Brien (2002).

References

Akefeldt, A. (2009) Water intake and risk of hyponatraemia in Prader–Willi syndrome. *Journal of Intellectual Disability Research*, 53, 521–8.

Baieli, S., Pavone, L., Meli, C. et al. (2003) Autism and phenylketonuria. *Journal of Autism and Developmental Disorders*, 33(2), 201–4.

Baker, G. A., Bromley, R. L., Briggs, M. et al. (2015) IQ at 6 years after in utero exposure to antiepileptic drugs: A controlled cohort study. *Neurology*, 84(4), 382–90.

Bender, B. G., Puck, M. H., Salbenblatt, J. A. et al. (1986) Dyslexia in 47, XXXY boys identified at birth. *Behavior genetics*, 16(3), 343–54.

Boyle, L. & Kaufmann, W. E. (2010) The behavioral phenotype of FMR1 mutations. *American Journal of Medical Genetics Part C Seminars in Medical Genetics*, 154C, 469–76.

Budimirovic, D. B. & Kaufmann, W. E. (2011) What can we learn about Autism from studying fragile X syndrome? *Developmental Neuroscience*, 33, 379–94.

Cebula, K. R., Moore, D. G. & Wishart, J. G. (2010) Social cognition in children with Down's syndrome: Challenges to research and theory building. *Journal of Intellectual Disability Research*, 54(2), 113–34.

Christensen, J., Grønborg, T. K., Sørensen, M. J. et al. (2013) Prenatal valproate exposure and risk of autism spectrum disorders and childhood autism. *Jama*, 309(16), 1696–1703.

Clayton-Smith, J. (2001) Angelman syndrome: Evolution of the phenotype in adolescents and adults. *Developmental Medicine and Child Neurology*, **43**, 476–80.

Clifford, S., Dissanayake, C., Bui, Q. et al. (2007) Autism spectrum phenotype in males and females with fragile X full mutation and permutation. *Journal of Autism Development Disorders*, **37**, 738–47.

Cornish, K., Turk, J. & Hagerman, R. (2008) The fragile X continuum: New advances and perspectives. *Journal of Intellectual Disability Research*, **52**(6), 469–82.

Curatolo, P., D'Argenzio, L., Pinci, M. et al. (2008) Behavioural and cognitive phenotypes in tuberous sclerosis complex. *European Journal of Paediatric Neurology*, **12**(suppl. 1), S4.

Daunhauer, L. & Fidler, D. (2011) The Down syndrome behavioural phenotype: Implications for practice and research in occupational therapy. *Occupational Therapy in Health Care*, **25**(1), 7–25.

de Vries, P. Humphrey, A., McCartney, D. et al. (2005) Consensus clinical guidelines for the assessment of cognitive and behavioural problems in tuberous sclerosis. *European Child and Adolescent Psychiatry*, **14** (4) 183–90.

Fletcher, R, Loschen, E., Stavrakaki, C. et al. (2007) *Diagnostic Manual – Intellectual Disability: A Textbook of Diagnosis of Mental Disorders in Persons with Intellectual Disability.* Nadd Press.

Ganthous, G. and Rossi, N. F. & Giacheti, G. (2015) Language in fetal alcohol spectrum disorder: A review. *Revista CEFAC*, **17**(1), 253–63.

Ghazziuddin, M., Tsai, L. Y. & Ghazziuddin, N. (1992) Autism in Down's syndrome: Presentation and diagnosis. *Journal of Intellectual Disability Research*, **36**, 449–56.

Gilbert, P. (2013) *The A–Z Reference Book of Syndromes and Inherited Disorders.* Springer.

Holland, A. J., Whittington, J. E., Butler, J. et al. (2003) Behavioural phenotypes associated with specific genetic disorders: Evidence from a population-based study of people with Prader–Willi syndrome. *Psychological Medicine*, **33**, 141–53.

Howlin, P. & Udwin, O. (eds.) (2002), *Outcomes in Neurodevelopmental and Genetic Disorders.* Cambridge University Press.

Koren, G., Zelner, I., Nash, K. et al. (2014) Foetal alcohol spectrum disorder. *Current Opinion in Psychiatry*, **27**(2), 98.

Moore, S., Turnpenny, P, Quinn, A. et al. (2000). A clinical study of 57 children with fetal anticonvulsant syndromes. *Journal of Medical Genetics*, **37**(7), 489–97.

Morris, C. A. (2010) The behavioural phenotype of Williams syndrome: A recognizable pattern of neurodevelopment. *American Journal of Medical Genetics Part C Seminars in Medical Genetics*, **154C**, 427–31.

O'Brien, G. (2002) *Behavioural Phenotypes in Clinical Practice. No. 157.* Cambridge University Press.

O'Brien, G., Pearson, J., Berney, T. et al. (2001) Measuring behaviour in developmental disability: A review of existing schedules. *Developmental Medicine & Child Neurology*, **43** (suppl. 87), 1–70

Parisi, L., Di Filippo, T. & Roccella, M. (2015) Behavioural phenotype and autism spectrum disorders in Cornelia de Lange syndrome. *Mental illness*, **7**(2), 5988.

Rosner, B., Hodapp, R., Fidler, D. et al. (2004) Social competence in persons with Prader–Willi, Williams and Down's syndromes. *Journal of Applied Research in Intellectual Disabilities*, **17**, 209–17.

Ross, J. L., Roeltgen, D. P., Kushner, H. et al. (2012) Behavioral and social phenotypes in boys with 47, XYY syndrome or 47, XXY Klinefelter syndrome. *Pediatrics*, **129**(4), 769–78.

Rovet, J. & Ireland, L. (1994) Behavioral phenotype in children with Turner syndrome. *Journal of Pediatric Psychology*, **19**(6), 779–90.

Samango-Sprouse, C., Stapleton, E. J., Lawson, P. et al. (2015). Positive effects of early androgen therapy on the behavioral phenotype of boys with 47, XXY. *American Journal of Medical Genetics Part C Seminars in Medical Genetics*, **169**(2), 150–7.

Sinnema, M., Einfeld, S. L., Schrander-Stumpel, C. T. R. M. et al. (2011) Behavioural phenotype in adults with Prader–Willi syndrome. *Research in Developmental Disabilities*, **32**, 604–12.

Skuse, D. H., James, R. S., Bishop, D. V. et al. (1997). Evidence from Turner's syndrome of an imprinted X-linked locus affecting cognitive function. *Nature*, 387, 705–8.

Smith, L. E., Barker, E. T., Mailick Seltzer, M. et al. (2012) Behavioral phenotype of fragile X syndrome in adolescence and adulthood. *American Journal on Intellectual and Developmental Disabilities*, 117, 1–17.

Steinhausen, H. C., Willms, J., Winkler, C. et al. (2003) Behavioural phenotype in foetal alcohol syndrome and foetal alcohol effects. *Developmental Medicine & Child Neurology*, 45 179–82.

Tartaglia, N., Cordeiro, L., Howell, S. et al. (2010) The spectrum of the behavioral phenotype in boys and adolescents 47, XXY (Klinefelter syndrome). *Pediatric Endocrinology Reviews*, 8(01), 151.

Taylor, L. & Oliver, C. (2008) The behavioural phenotype of Smith–Magenis syndrome: Evidence for a gene–environment interaction. *Journal of Intellectual Disability Research*, 52 (10), 830–41.

Tomson, T. & Battino, D. (2008) Teratogenic effects of antiepileptic drugs. *Seizure*, 17(2), 166–71.

Torres, R. J., Puig, J. G. & Jinnah, H. A. (2012) Update on the phenotypic spectrum of Lesch–Nyhan disease and its attenuated variants. *Current Rheumatology Reports*, 14(2), 189–94.

Triantafyllou, P., Katzos, G., Rousso, I. et al. (2015) Neurophysiologic evaluation of infants with congenital hypothyroidism before and after treatment. *Acta Neurologica Belgica*, 115(2), 129–36.

van Rijn, S., Stockmann, L., Borghgraef, M. et al. (2014) The social behavioral phenotype in boys and girls with an extra X chromosome (Klinefelter syndrome and trisomy X): A comparison with autism spectrum disorder. *Journal of Autism and Developmental Disorders*, 44(2), 310–20.

Vinten, J., Bromley, R. L., Taylor, J. et al. (2008) The behavioral consequences of exposure to antiepileptic drug in utero. *Epilepsy & Behavior*, 14(1), 197–201.

Williams, C. A. (2010) The behavioural phenotype of the Angelman syndrome. *American Journal of Medical Genetics Part C Seminars in Medical Genetics*, 154C, 432–7.

Wulffaert, J., Berckelaer-Onnes, I., Kroonenberg, P. et al. (2009) Simultaneous analysis of the behavioural phenotype, physical factors, and parenting stress in people with Cornelia de Lange syndrome. *Journal of Intellectual Disability Research*, 53, 604–19.

Wyper, K. R. & Rasmussen, C. R. (2011) Language impairments in children with fetal alcohol spectrum disorders. *Journal of Population Therapeutics and Clinical Pharmacology*, 18(2), e364–e376.

Zarcone, J., Napolitano, D., Peterson, C. et al. (2007) The relationship between compulsive behaviour and academic achievement across the three genetic subtypes of Prader–Willi syndrome. *Journal of Intellectual Disability Research*, 51, 478–87.

Chapter 4

Communication in People with Intellectual Disability

Lauren Edwards

4.1 Introduction

Effective communication is key to indicating choice and consent, building relationships, expressing feelings and preferences, and to living as independently as possible. It is core to education, work and fulfilling a meaningful role in society. Communication is a complex and multifaceted skill that allows us to share our personality with others and to participate in everyday life.

Up to 90% of people with intellectual disability (ID) experience difficulties with communication, with half having significant additional needs in this area (Royal College of Speech and Language Therapists, 2010). Communication strengths and difficulties vary significantly between individuals and so basic proficiency across a range of communication modalities is helpful in order to achieve an effective relationship and level of engagement during consultations.

This chapter provides some simple definitions which will be helpful when considering and describing the communication abilities of an individual. It goes on to provide some guidance on how to effectively engage with people experiencing communication difficulties, particularly those with ID.

4.2 Communication

In its broadest terms, communication can be categorised as 'speech' or 'language'.

4.2.1 Speech

Speech is the range of speech sounds that are combined in order to form spoken output. The range of sounds used varies between languages and dialects. Speech difficulties may take the form of single sounds that are produced incorrectly (as is often seen in childhood) or imprecisely/weakly (a common problem with neurological impairments). There is a developmental pattern in which speech sounds are typically acquired and deviation from this may take the form of a speech delay (sounds are not acquired age-appropriately) or a speech disorder (speech sound errors are atypical or so significantly delayed that they are categorised as being disordered). A mild difficulty can make speech a little difficult for an unfamiliar listener to understand whereas a severe problem can render the words completely unintelligible. Table 4.1 summarises the developmental pattern of speech sound acquisition.

Speech sound problems are more common in children with ID compared to those without, frequently due to a combination of developmental and physical needs. People with Down syndrome are particularly likely to exhibit speech sound difficulties due to low muscle tone impacting on the accuracy and strength of articulatory placement. Hearing loss

Table 4.1 The developmental norms for speech sound acquisition (English)

2 years	p, b, t, d, m, n, w
3 years	f, s, k, g, y
4 years	Most speech sounds are in use
	Emerging sounds: ch, j, sh, v, l, z

(taken from an I CAN fact sheet, 2016)

is a feature of certain syndromes associated with ID, and impaired auditory function will affect speech sound acquisition.

4.2.2 Language

Language is the content of the message that is conveyed during an interaction. It can be divided into two categories: receptive and expressive. Expressive language is the means by which an individual conveys their message (i.e. their output). This can take many forms, ranging from spoken or written words to expressing a choice through eye-pointing. Receptive language refers to the ability to effectively receive a message. Examples include understanding speech, the ability to read for meaning, or correctly interpreting someone's behaviour, facial expression or gesture.

Typical language acquisition follows a developmental pattern (see Table 4.2). For example, linking two words together can be expected by 2-year-olds, and the use of prepositions (in, on, under) usually precedes the use of plurals.

Table 4.2 Average order for the acquisition of grammar

Present progressive	Run*ning*; eat*ing*
Prepositions	*In; on;*
Plurals	Book*s*; plate*s*
Irregular past tense	*Took; ate; fell*
Articles	*The* floor; *a* pan
Possessive	Sarah*'s* chair; Tom*'s* cup
3rd person present tense irregular	Jo *has* a new car
Copula contractible	I*'m* going; you *are* singing
Regular past tense	Jump*ed*; watch*ed*
3rd person present tense regular	She eat*s*; he cook*s*
Copula uncontractible	This *is* your brush
Auxiliary contractible	Will*'s* going later; We *will* watch
Auxiliary uncontractible	He *was* running away; *do* you want more?

(see de Villiers & de Villiers, 1973)

Early vocabulary development sees many of the same words acquired across individuals. These words vary between cultures and there are some that are specific to the person and their environment, but certain vocabulary is seen within the first fifty words with high frequency.

Specialist language assessments can be completed by a speech and language therapist in order to determine the precise level of language functioning of an individual. Targeted input may be indicated if expressive and receptive language skills are assessed as being at significantly disparate levels. For example, someone may have better receptive language (understanding) compared to expressive language (output). This could be due to an insufficient vocabulary to allow them to effectively convey their message.

4.3 Expressive language

Adults with ID may use one or several methods to communicate their message. The most common methods of communication are outlined below, starting with the most complex to acquire.

4.3.1 Spoken Output

Complexity of spoken language can vary significantly. Someone may be functioning at a single word level, where their output is characterised by the use of one key word to convey a very basic message; for example, they may say 'car' to communicate that they wish to go out. An individual communicating in single words is unlikely to have a broad vocabulary and so the range of messages that can be conveyed will be very limited. The opposite end of the scale of difficulty would be someone with an ability to produce grammatically complex sentences in order to convey detailed messages and abstract concepts.

Many individuals with ID have spoken output at a level somewhere in between the above two extremes. Many people use short, simple sentences that contain high-frequency words with very few grammatical markers. Such sentences can be used effectively to indicate choice, share information and establish relationships. These simplified sentences often contain nouns and high-frequency verbs but connecting words and tenses are frequently omitted, for example 'John walk shop' or 'Sarah watch TV bedroom'.

Spoken output is the most complex form of expressive language due to its lack of permanence (i.e. as soon as a word is spoken it is gone, leaving the listener with nothing to refer to if they require increased processing time) and the fact that a combination of sounds bears no clear link to the objects or concepts to which it relates.

4.3.2 Written Language

Like speech, written output is a difficult form of language to master due to its abstract nature (i.e. the shapes that form letters and words have no obvious correlation to the sounds or objects that they represent). However, the permanence of written words increases the time that an individual has to recognise the words and process the meaning.

The complexity of written output varies significantly. Some individuals may write single words or short phrases whereas others have the ability to write reams in order to express their thoughts or worries. It is unusual for writing to be the main form of communication for an individual with ID, but clearly this should be facilitated if it is their preference.

4.3.3 Signing

Various formal signing systems are used by people with communication difficulties. Makaton and Signalong are the two systems most frequently used by people with ID in the UK. They are both based heavily on natural gesture, but increased complexity can be introduced as required. A benefit of being gesture-based is that people with no formal training are likely to understand and use many of the signs, increasing opportunities for social interactions in the wider community.

The programme for the teaching of signs tends to shadow the pattern of spoken language acquisition (i.e. a vocabulary of single signs, followed by encouragement of linking of two signs together, production of simple phrases). Early sign vocabulary is chosen according to the individual's needs and the words most commonly acquired developmentally. Some family and carers may express concerns that the introduction of signing may discourage the use of speech, but research shows that signing in fact supports spoken language development rather than hinders it.

Some individuals will use natural gesture rather than a formal signing system. The gestures may be transparent and readily understood by strangers, or the person may have developed their own vocabulary of signs that are only understood by people who know them well. It is common to see adults adding their own 'accent' to formally recognised signs. They may have been introduced to a formal signing system in childhood, but the accuracy has reduced over the years and may bear only a loose resemblance to the original. Effective recording and sharing of an individual's communication style and preferences (often called a communication passport) is therefore an essential role of anyone supporting them.

As with speech, signs and gestures lack permanence and this can pose a challenge for those who require additional time to decipher a message. Signs that are gesture-based are easier to understand than those which bear no tangible link to the target word (i.e. the sign for drink comprises making the hand-to-mouth movement required to drink from a cup).

4.3.4 Symbols, Pictures and Photographs

It is most common for symbols/pictures to be available in a printed format. An individual may choose a symbol/picture (e.g. a cup of coffee) and indicate their choice via pointing or handing over the picture to the person with whom they are communicating. They may also demonstrate their selection (by a nod, vocalisation or gesture) as their conversation partner shows them each of the symbol options. Teaching of symbol use follows the natural order in which spoken output would be acquired. High-frequency words are encouraged initially, followed by combining two symbols to make a short phrase.

Various formal symbol systems are available, and these range from very simple line drawings to those with more detail. They tend to be easily understood by people who are unfamiliar with the symbol system and often have the written word underneath, increasing communication opportunities for the person with ID. For individuals who require the vocabulary to produce more complex phrases, abstract symbols can be introduced to represent words such as 'to', 'finished' or 'where'.

The drawing of simple pictures can be used to express a basic message but variability in interpretation across individuals can cause confusion. The use of photographs can be helpful when talking about a particular person, place or object but thought should be given to the complexity of the background, as the focus may be unclear. Consideration should also be given to an individual's ability to generalise; they may struggle to grasp the

Table 4.3 PECS® phases

Phase I	HOW TO COMMUNICATE	
	Exchanging single pictures for items/activities that they really want.	
Phase II	DISTANCE AND PERSISTENCE	
	Generalising the use of single pictures by using in different places, with different people and across distances. They are becoming more persistent communicators.	
Phase III	PICTURE DISCRIMINATION	
	Selecting from 2 or more pictures to request favourite things. The pictures are in a communication book (ring binder with Velcro strips allowing pictures to be stored and easily removed for communication)	
Phase IV	SENTENCE STRUCTURE	
	Constructing simple sentences on a detachable strip using an 'I want' picture followed by the item being requested.	
Attributes and language expansion	ATTRIBUTES AND LANGUAGE EXPANSION	
	Expanding sentences by adding adjectives, verbs, prepositions, etc.	
Phase V	ANSWERING QUESTIONS	
	Answering the question 'What do you want?'	
Phase VI	COMMENTING	
	Commenting in response to questions like 'What do you see?', 'What is it?'. Using sentences starting with 'I see', 'It is a', etc.	

(with permission of Pyramid Educational Consultants (www.pecs.com). All rights reserved (Pyramid Educational Consultants, 2016))

idea that a photograph of a bed they have not seen before is referring to the bed in their own room.

The Picture Exchange Communication System® (PECS®) is a widely used structured system for the use of pictures or symbols to communicate. Individuals can use this system at a variety of levels of complexity (see Table 4.3).

4.3.5 Real Objects

Real objects can be used to effectively convey basic messages. This might be picking up a mug to ask if someone would like a drink or holding up their coat to convey that they are going out. Introduction of an 'objects of reference' system supports an individual to effectively communicate messages using a range of objects which have certain meanings attached to them (Ockelford, 1994). Such a system was originally used with blind people but is now often used with people with profound and multiple ID. The use of real objects as a communication system is the most basic level to which communication can be reduced.

Table 4.4 Complexity of choice for Objects of Reference system

Complexity	Type of object	Example
Low	A real object that will actually be used in the task	A wooden spoon that will be used during the cookery session
↓	A real object that represents the task	A toilet roll to represent going to the toilet
	Part of a real object	A square of bath towel to represent having a shower
	Miniature version of an object	A toy car to represent going out in the car
High	Abstract objects	A silk scarf to represent a particular person

(see Ockelford, 1994)

Objects provide information through touch, are a permanent point of reference, thus allowing increased processing time, and are concrete objects, so are easier to interpret compared to symbolic communication methods such as speech or written words. There is, however, a scale of complexity that it is helpful to consider, as outlined in Table 4.4.

4.4 Receptive Language

Receptive language is an individual's ability to understand a message. This may be comprehension of spoken words, signs or gestures, objects, symbols or pictures, or the ability to read. A referral to a speech and language therapist can be made in order to gain a clear picture of an individual's ability to understand messages presented in a range of formats. Following assessment, guidelines can be provided which outline the most effective ways to engage with the person. This will help support clinicians to tailor the way they communicate with the individual in order to increase the likelihood of being understood and maximise the level of engagement.

4.4.1 Auditory Memory

Auditory memory refers to a person's ability to retain information that is presented verbally. It can change considerably dependent on context, for example it is likely to be reduced in environments with many distractions or when an individual is feeling stressed or anxious. Having an understanding of levels of auditory memory function is key to ensuring that spoken information is 'chunked' into appropriately sized pieces for the individual.

Testing forward digit span is a crude yet quick way to gauge the level of someone's auditory memory functioning. This is done by asking the person to repeat back a gradually increasing list of random numbers (e.g. 'Copy me: 1, 5, 9, 2'). The ability to follow spoken instructions containing an increasing number of key words will also provide information about auditory memory. Key words are those which are essential for the message to be correctly understood. For example, 'put the pen under the book' tests the ability to follow three key words and 'stand up and tap the wall twice' tests recall of four key words. If an auditory memory difficulty is identified, then the provision written or drawn/symbolic material may support processing of information.

4.5 Inclusive Communication

Inclusive communication and total communication (often used interchangeably) are terms used to describe a holistic approach to communication. Instead of using a single method of communication this approach values and responds to all methods of communication (speech; facial expression; gesture; body language; signing; objects of reference; photographs; drawings; symbols with written words; multisensory channels; communication aids). The approach places equal importance on the environment, method and the message itself. It encourages communication partners to model the use of a combination of communication methods. This could be using basic gesture or a Makaton signs when verbally asking if someone wants to watch TV, supporting spoken menu choices with symbols or using facial expression and pointing when asking if someone's stomach hurts. The use of a combination of communication methods provides an individual with the best possible chance of understanding a message. By consistently modelling a range of communication methods, individuals may gradually begin to adopt some of what they see.

An inclusive communication approach is essential when considering the capacity of an individual. One of the five key principles of the Mental Capacity Act 2005 is that all practicable steps are taken to support a person to make an informed decision. The use of inclusive communication helps to ensure that an appropriate combination of methods has been used to maximise the individual's ability to make a decision.

4.6 Easy Read information

Since July 2016 all organisations providing NHS or adult social care in England have been required to adhere to the Accessible Information Standard (NHS England, 2015). The aim is to ensure that people have access to information that they can understand and are supported to express themselves, regardless of their communication needs or disability. The Standard requires professionals to enquire about and record communication needs and preferences and to take steps to ensure that these needs are met.

The provision of Easy Read information is a key way to make information more accessible. It is characterised by the provision of key information using short, simple sentences (no more than twelve words per sentence) that are supported by relevant simple pictures. National guidance is available regarding how to make good-quality Easy Read documents and there is much content freely available online, particularly in relation to specific health conditions and wider health and social care issues. The quality of online information can vary considerably, so all documents should be reviewed prior to being shared with patients.

4.7 Basic Neurology of Speech and Language

4.7.1 Language

The majority of the population has their language functions represented in the left hemisphere of the brain, although the right hemisphere is involved in some aspects of language processing, for example the recognition of tone of voice (Berko Gleason, 1997). Damage to the language areas of the brain results in aphasia, a language disorder with highly variable presentation dependent on the location of the damage. Damage to the brain resulting from epilepsy may impact significantly on communicative function. Speech and/or language can be affected, and the effects can be transient or chronic.

There are two main language areas in the brain: Broca's area and Wernicke's area. Broca's area is found in the third frontal gyrus of the dominant hemisphere (usually the left). Damage to this area tends to result in good receptive language but poor expressive language. There is often difficulty with grammatical structures and output tends to be telegraphic, containing incomplete sentences with only key words, for example, 'John shop Saturday' rather than 'John wants to go shopping on Saturday'. Broca's area plays a key role in motor speech programming, and damage to this region can result in apraxia of speech. Wernicke's area is located in the posterior left temporal lobe, and damage to this area can result in fluent sentences that contain non-words (nonsense words) or strings of words that make no sense together. Receptive language (understanding) is impaired if there is damage to Wernicke's area and self-awareness of communication difficulties can be minimal. The temporal lobe also contains the cortical centre for understanding sound (Heschl's gyrus), and damage to this area may result in difficulties with auditory processing.

It is worth noting that damage to the limbic lobe can result in altered prosody (stress and intonation used in speech) or pragmatic language impairment (difficulty with the social aspects of language, following conversational rules, etc.).

4.7.2 Speech and the Brain

The precentral gyrus, also known as the primary motor cortex, lies immediately in front of the central sulcus and controls the voluntary movement of muscles on the opposite side of the body. The neurons for motor movement of the face and neck are closest to the lateral fissure. There are vast numbers of neurons committed to the movement of the small muscles of the face, jaw, tongue, palate and larynx. The premotor and supplementary motor areas are found anterior to the precentral gyrus. Their function is to receive information from other areas of the brain in order to plan or programme motor speech production.

The basal ganglia control voluntary motor movements and interpret sensory information to guide motor behaviour. The cerebellum does not initiate motor movements but helps to coordinate skilled, voluntary muscle movements produced elsewhere. The brainstem contains the medulla oblongata, pons, midbrain, thalamus and hypothalamus. The medulla and pons both have nuclei for the cranial nerves and connections to the cortex that are involved during speech production. The midbrain contains the substantia nigra, responsible for the production of dopamine, which helps in motor control and muscle tone. The thalamus relays sensory information to and from the sensory regions of the cortex, linking it to motor speech systems.

4.7.3 Motor System for Speech

The motor pathways for speech involve all levels of the nervous system and comprise the pyramidal and extrapyramidal system. The corticobulbar tract is within the pyramidal system and controls the skilled voluntary movements of speech musculature. The tract begins in the motor cortex and descends to the motor nuclei of the cranial nerves within the pons and medulla. The indirect activation pathway and the control circuit areas are the two main constituents of the extrapyramidal system. The indirect activation pathway is influenced by the basal ganglia and cerebellar control circuits. It comprises several short pathways that start in the cerebral cortex and end in the spinal cord and cranial nerves. The pathway has many tracts with an inhibitive function, as it helps to moderate reflexes. The control circuits provide information and sensory feedback to the pyramidal system and indirect activation pathways regarding the posture, tone and the environment in which coordinated muscle movement will take place. A problem with the basal ganglia control circuit often results in dyskinesia, whereas issues with the cerebellar control circuits can present as hypotonia and incoordination.

Upper motor neuron (UMN) pathways serve to activate the lower motor neuron (LMN). Spastic paralysis can occur if there is damage to the UMN. This can present as hyperreflexia, hypertonia, lack of atrophy and absence of fasciculations and may be described as a spastic dysarthria. The LMN comprises thirty-one pairs of spinal nerves and twelve pairs of cranial nerves. Once activated by the UMN, the LMN sends impulses to the muscles to stimulate movement. Damage to the LMN can present as hyporeflexia, hypotonia, muscle atrophy and fasciculations and may be described as flaccid dysarthria.

The cranial nerves, their main functions and impact on speech are outlined in Table 4.5.

Table 4.5 Cranial nerves

Cranial nerve	Function	Impact on speech
I. Olfactory	Sensory: smell	
II. Optic	Sensory: vision	
III. Oculomotor	Motor: eye movement	
IV. Trochlear	Motor: eye movement	
V. Trigeminal	Sensory: jaw, lips, face, tongue	Articulation and prosody
	Motor: jaw	
VI. Abducens	Motor: eye movement	
VII. Facial	Sensory: tongue, soft palate, nasopharynx	Articulation, prosody, facial expression
	Motor: face, lips, stapedius (middle ear)	
VIII. Vestibulocochlear	Sensory: vestibular (balance), cochlear (hearing)	Articulation, prosody, loudness
IX. Glossopharyngeal	Sensory: tongue, pharynx	Phonation, resonance
	Motor: pharynx, larynx	
X. Vagus	Sensory: larynx, pharynx, soft palate, thoracic and abdominal viscera	Phonation, resonance, articulation, prosody
	Motor: larynx, pharynx, soft palate	
XI. Spinal accessory	Motor: spinal (neck, shoulder), cranial (soft palate, pharynx, larynx)	Phonation, resonance
XII. Hypoglossal	Sensory: tongue	Articulation, prosody
	Motor: tongue	

4.8 Communication during a Clinical Appointment

The Royal College of Speech and Language Therapists have published the Five Good Communication Standards that people with a learning disability can expect from specialist hospital and residential care settings (Royal College of Speech and Language Therapists, 2013). The Five Good Standards are listed in Table 4.6. If an individual has communication difficulties, then the people supporting them to attend clinic appointments should be able to advise on their preferred style and level of communication.

The following pointers can help to maximise an individual's ability to understand a message:

- Try to gain eye contact with the person and maintain this when you are speaking with them. This helps them to realise that you are talking to them and also allows you to read their facial expression/non-verbal reactions for signs that they have or have not understood. If the person has autism, then it may not be possible to obtain eye contact.
- Use short sentences with simple grammar and high-frequency words.
- Support your speech with basic gesture, appropriate facial expression, tone of voice and real objects or pictures. Drawing pictures or writing words may be helpful to the individual.
- Asking open questions may be more challenging for the person to respond to but provides them with a greater opportunity to express their opinion, compared to closed (yes/no) questions.
- Allow extra time for the individual to respond. They may require additional time to process what has been said or to formulate their response. Do not make them feel rushed.
- Be an active listener. Keep eye contact when the person is communicating with you. This shows that you are listening and value their view, as well as allowing you to pick up on any non-verbal cues that may support their message.
- Encourage and support them to use all their communication tools, for example any communication aids, drawing or signing/gesture. Acknowledging and responding to their range of communication methods shows that you value all their communication attempts and provides the best opportunity for them to effectively convey their message.

Table 4.6 Five Good Communication Standards

1. There is a detailed description of how best to communicate with individuals.
2. Services demonstrate how they support individuals with communication needs to be involved with decisions about their care and their services.
3. Staff value and use competently the best approaches to communication with each individual they support.
4. Services create opportunities, relationships and environments that make individuals want to communicate.
5. Individuals are supported to understand and express their needs in relation to their health and wellbeing.

(Royal College of Speech and Language Therapists (2013), reproduced with permission)

- Be watchful for any patterns in the individual's responses. When offered a choice do they always opt for the first or last item because it is the only thing that they can recall?
- Check with the person that you have correctly understood what it is they are saying.
- If communication is proving difficult, involve the family or carers. They know the person best and will be able to support your conversation.

References

Berko Gleason, J. (1997) *The Development of Language* (4th edn). Allyn & Bacon.

de Villiers, J. & de Villiers, P. (1973) A cross-sectional study of the acquisition of grammatical morphemes in child speech. *Journal of Psycholinguistic Research*, 2(3), 267–78.

I CAN (2016) Speech sounds factsheet. Available at: www.ican.org.uk/~/media/Ican2/What%20We%20Do/Enquiry%20Service/Speech%20Sounds%20factsheet.ashx [accessed 2 January 2017]

NHS England (2015) Accessible Information Standard. Available at: www.england.nhs.uk/ourwork/accessibleinfo [accessed 30 September 2016].

Ockelford, A. (1994) *Objects of Reference*. RNIB.

Pyramid Educational Consultants (2016) Picture Exchange Communication System. Available at: www.pecs-unitedkingdom.com/pecs.php [accessed 5 December 2016].

Royal College of Speech and Language Therapists (2010) Adults with learning disabilities: Position paper. Available at: www.rcslt.org/members/publications/ald_position_paper [accessed 01 December 2017].

Royal College of Speech and Language Therapists (2013a) *Five Good Communication Standards*. RCSLT.

Royal College of Speech and Language Therapists (2013b) *Five Good Communication Standards: Reasonable Adjustments that Individuals with Learning Disability and/or Autism Should Expect in Specialist Hospital and Residential Settings*, RCSLT.

Further Reading

Bondy, A. and Frost, L. (1994) The Picture Exchange Communication System. *Focus on Autistic Behaviour*, 9(3), 1–19.

Department of Health (2009) *Basic Guidelines for People Who Commission Easy Read Information*. Department of Health.

Gloucestershire Total Communication (2005) Total communication. Available at: www.totalcommunication.org.uk [accessed 10 December 2016].

Halpern, H. and Goldfarb, R. (2012) *Language and Motor Speech Disorders in Adults* (3rd edn). Jones and Bartlett Learning.

Makaton (2017) About Makaton. Available at: www.makaton.org [accessed 10 December 2016].

Royal College of Speech and Language Therapists (2016) Inclusive communication and the role of speech and language therapy. Available at: www.rcslt.org/cq_live/resources_a_z/docs/inclusive/ICposition_paper [accessed 10 December 2016].

Signalong Group (2017) Signalong. Available at: www.signalong.org.uk [accessed 11 December 2016].

Section 2 Co-morbidity

Chapter 5

Autism

Tom Berney and Peter Carpenter

5.1 Evolving Concepts

Autism is a relatively modern concept which emerged from two case series, published independently in 1943/4, by Leo Kanner in Baltimore and Hans Asperger in Austria (Silberman, 2015), and which set in chain two parallel concepts. Kanner emphasised the social isolation, need for sameness and its innate and characteristic developmental quality. Calling it infantile autism, he then identified it as the early presentation of a unitary psychosis, childhood schizophrenia, a concept widely viewed through a psychoanalytic lens. As such, it appeared in DSM II in 1952 and a London committee set out criteria, very like those of today (Creak's nine points) in 1964. It was only towards the end of the 1960s that Kolvin and Rutter identified autism as a neurodevelopmental disorder (an innate, genetically based disorder moulded by development). Their view, formalised as childhood autism in ICD-9 (1977) and DSM III (1980), encouraged a more biological perception and an educational/behavioural approach to its management.

Asperger saw his cases as a form of personality disorder, as did Sukhareva describing a similar group in Moscow in 1925 and as would Sula Wolff in Edinburgh in the 1970s who drew on Kretschmer's category of schizoid personality disorder (suggestive of a prodromal association with schizophrenia). Reviewing this, Lorna Wing cemented the relationship of Asperger syndrome to autism, noting that they differed in the former having good, syntactical speech and greater ability (1981). Since then, biological psychiatry has intensified the search for a reconciliation with schizophrenia with the emergence of a more complex relationship based in shared aetiological factors.

The effort to distinguish Asperger syndrome from high-functioning autism (Tantam, 1988) led to formal criteria being posted in ICD-10 in 1992 and DSM IV in 1994 (Gillberg, 1998). By the time DSM-5 was published, the consensus was that Asperger syndrome was not a separate disorder but one of several points within autism's diagnostic cluster, all to be subsumed under the overarching diagnosis of autism spectrum disorder (ASD). However, the term is likely to keep its social currency as a summary explanation for a range of disability and unusual behaviour.

These shifts in diagnostic definition may reduce estimates of the prevalence of autism. Derived from earlier concepts of 'semantic pragmatic disorder' and 'pragmatic language impairment', DSM-5 introduces a new category, social communication disorder (SCD), which is effectively ASD without the second domain of restricted, repetitive patterns of behaviour. ICD-11's snappy equivalent looks to be 'developmental language disorder with impairment of mainly pragmatic language'. It is unclear how commonly this occurs, but it seems that it might embrace a number of people who previously would have been identified as having atypical autism (ICD-10) or PDD-NOS (DSM IV) (Wilson et al., 2013).

> **Box 5.1 Autism**
>
> Autism is a syndrome characterised by impaired social interaction and a need for sameness. The descriptions in DSM and ICD are evolving but they require abnormality in both domains during childhood. While 'social interaction' includes a combination of empathic and non-verbal skills, the 'need for sameness' may manifest as a mental rigidity, restricted and repetitive behaviours, focal interests and has been linked with unusual sensory sensitivities.
>
> As such, autism is a behavioural phenotype which is secondary to a variety of medical disorders. It also can be a primary condition, a neurodevelopmental disorder arising from a mix of genetic predisposition and environmental influence.

'Pathological demand avoidance' (PDA) identifies a group of people characterised by their extreme need to avoid everyday demands and expectations; appearing driven by anxiety, they have to be in control. The syndrome, identified by Elizabeth Newson in 1980, is arguably part of the spectrum but with its characteristics overlaid by a social understanding and an ability to role play and fantasise rather better than might be expected in autism (O'Nions et al., 2014). Its management demands an approach so substantially different, being less direct and more negotiated, as to suggest that PDA might be managed as a disorder in its own right (Eaton et al., 2012; Newson et al., 2003).

The very varied presentation has led to a vigorous debate as to whether autism is a disorder, a disability or a condition, terms which carry connotations of health care (and treatment), social care (with its emphasis on support and reasonable adjustment to the setting), or social acceptance and celebration (Box 5.1). Discussion becomes polarised, focusing on autism's part in defining someone's identity while ignoring its dimensional nature and disabling qualities. However, something so varied in its form and circumstances requires flexibility rather than a monolithic uniformity (Kenny et al., 2016).

Autism is a *continuum* in which Kanner's florid syndrome fades into the subtler personality traits found in the general population. The diagnostic cut-off, a clinical judgement, marks the point at which these traits coalesce into something that interferes with everyday functioning.

The intensities of these individual elements vary so much relative to each other as to give the presentation a kaleidoscopic quality, Lorna Wing's *spectrum*, analogous to light's constituent colours. This presentational diversity now looks as if it might be the result of lumping together a variety of specific developmental disabilities. The scientific concept of autism is fragmenting (Waterhouse et al., 2016), while, at the same time, its social identity is strengthening. This was fuelled in England by the 2009 Autism Act, followed by a series of directives and guidance to improve its management, with similar strategies under way in the other UK administrations.

5.2 The Identification of Autism: Screening and Diagnosis

5.2.1 The Criteria

Overall, the various criteria proposed by different researchers have given way to the consensus set out in DSM-5 and ICD-11 (Box 5.2). Condensing three domains to two, they require impairment of both, 'social communication and social interaction' (which emphasises non-verbal as well as verbal communication) and 'restricted, repetitive patterns

> **Box 5.2 DSM 5 and ICD-11**
>
> Although their account of autism is essentially the same, these two international classifications serve different audiences and therefore have different functions:
>
> ICD provides a descriptive prototype to guide clinicians and is freely available on the internet. Publication of ICD-11 is likely to be in 2018 but there is a beta draft at http://apps.who.int/classifications/icd11/browse/f/en. It is to be an updated, more systematic revision of the Clinical Descriptions and Diagnostic Guidelines (set out in the 'Blue Book') but there are no plans to update the Research Diagnostic Criteria (the 'Green Book').
>
> DSM-5, published in 2013, provides diagnostic criteria which must be satisfied. It is available for purchase from the American Psychiatric Association.

of behaviour, interests or activities' (RRBI). The latter now includes an unusual response to, or awareness of, sensory stimuli. This puts an emphasis on the broader symptom, RRBI, to distinguish autism from other disorders involving impaired socialising.

Both classifications give a vivid picture of autism, but it is important to appreciate that they focus on the symptoms necessary for diagnosis and omit less discriminative symptoms, even though they are frequently present.

While the diagnosis requires the onset of autism to be in the early developmental period, its symptoms may pass unnoticed until later when they emerge in response to the increasing demands that come with school or moving into a less supportive peer group. Conversely, symptoms need not be current; their historical presence is sufficient to support a diagnosis.

However autism is defined, the diagnosis, its methodology and threshold will be shaped by its purpose. A research diagnosis is likely to be stringent and made by rigid rules, often expressed in an algorithm. On the other hand, clinical diagnosis will include a wider range of cases for whom it will be a gateway to services as well as the basis of their management programme. The range and complexity of symptomatology require a diagnostician's interpretation: algorithms are inappropriate.

5.2.2 Instruments

Autism's variegated nature means that there are many instruments to elicit and record relevant information for different circumstances (Charman et al., 2013); CR191 summarises those specific to adults (Royal College of Psychiatrists, 2014). Designed for completion by either the patient or an informant (a parent, carer or someone who knows the patient well), they take two main forms – questionnaires or interview schedules.

5.2.2.1 Questionnaires

Some are freely available on the internet, while others must be bought; they provide an opening for self-diagnosis, survey and to select people for further assessment. Some instruments focus on associated characteristics, such as the ability to identify emotions from facial expression or the appearance of the eyes. Their validity will depend on the size and nature of the population on which they have been tested, but they are not diagnostic and they cannot exclude autism, a more difficult task than making a positive diagnosis.

5.2.2.2 Interviews

Interviews range from brief, survey or screening interviews through to those lasting several hours, particularly for an especially complex or marginal patient. A diagnostician has to take into account the patient's overall ability, level of communication and mental health; facets which may need separate assessments as well as those of physical health and motor control. A diagnostic interview, simply determining the presence or absence of autism and its associated disorders, falls far short of the full assessment recommended by official guidelines (National Institute for Health & Care Excellence, 2011, 2012).

The diagnostic process is at its most straightforward in the school-going child when the informants are parents and teachers and, besides interviewing the child, the clinician can observe their behaviour with others in the unsupported setting of a playground. In adulthood, circumstances may require a different methodology. Innate maturation and learned, compensatory skills may combine with a less demanding environment to minimise symptoms. Leaving the structure of school to move into isolation in a community or the support or stress of marriage and employment may conceal or reveal symptomatology. All that is certain is that the intensity and character of a patient's presentation will change with age and circumstance, and this must be explored in a diagnostic interview.

Although a degree of gender bias may be innate to autism, the range of variation of 2–16 males to one female suggests that the diagnostic process often overlooks women (Rutherford et al., 2016). For example, social difficulties in women may be masked by greater attention to playing a role. At the same time an intense interest in dolls, jewellery, clothes or other people's habits may not seem too unusual, let alone qualify as an RRBI.

Intellectual disability (ID), closely associated with autism, further complicates diagnosis as it is easy to misattribute symptoms such as unresponsiveness in deafness or 'immature' behaviour in ID. Because delayed or absent behaviour goes with intellectual delay, it puts more emphasis on positive, deviant behaviours: for example, on repetitive activity, motor stereotypies, echolalia and a lack of social interest. It also means making a broader assessment of someone's functional abilities seeking a revealing discrepancy between, say, their social, communication and daily living skills.

5.3 Aetiology

The efforts to understand autism's aetiology have exposed its heterogeneity which goes some way to explaining the lack of success of research programmes that treats it as a single, categorical entity (Brunsdon et al., 2014; Waterhouse et al., 2016). The search moves on to find endophenotypes that might align with the syndrome's components: impairments in theory of mind, central coherence and executive function have produced inconsistent results, possibly because each one is itself a mix of simpler elements (Brunsdon et al., 2014). Other markers, anatomical, physiological and biochemical, have also resulted in mirage-like associations that fail to come to fruition. The MMR controversy and its resulting impact on immunisation rates highlight the possible explosive consequences of how conclusions are publicised.

Autism is associated with ID, and the greater the degree of disability, the more likely it is to appear. Even making allowance for this, certain conditions are disproportionately prone to autism, notably neurofibromatosis, Smith–Lemli–Opitz and fragile X syndromes. In tuberous sclerosis and phenylketonuria, the link appears to be with early seizures rather than directly with their genetic basis. Dysmorphic features generally identify this group with secondary, syndromic autism, categorised as 'complex autism' by geneticists (Miles et al., 2005).

This contrasts with primary, idiosyncratic or 'essential' autism which is a highly heritable condition with a monozygotic twin concordance of 60–90% as against a dizygotic concordance of 0–20% and frequent autistic traits in close relatives (the broader autism phenotype). While research has shown that copy number variations (CNVs) are frequent and that certain chromosomal sites are affected more frequently, there is no consistent genetic mechanism to explain autism's strong familial course.

The current thinking is that this syndrome, with its great range of intensity and presentation, might be a final common pathway for the interaction between a pleiotropic genetic predisposition and environmental modifiers. This mechanism, like that of many other psychiatric disorders, affects genes involved in neuronal growth, synaptogenesis and pruning.

The identification of a rare form of childhood obsessive–compulsive disorder (paediatric autoimmune neuropsychiatric disorders associated with streptococcal infections, PANDAS) and the recognition that familial autoimmune disorder and maternal infection during pregnancy can be contributory to autism have led to a renewed focus on autoimmune causes (Meltzer et al., 2017). Recent animal studies are linking in such disparate elements as maternal diet, the microbiome and oxytocin, all combining to affect sociability (Buffington et al., 2016).

5.4 Epidemiology

5.4.1 Prevalence

Two methods are used to identify ASD in the general population: surveillance and survey. Surveys use a screening instrument to select a sample for more detailed assessment so that there is a consistency in the instruments and researchers across the study. These have given prevalence figures of 1.16% (95% CI = 9.0–14.2) for 9- to 10-year-old children (Baird et al., 2006) and of 1.1% (95% CI = 0.3–1.9) for adults (Brugha et al., 2016).

Surveillance relies on diagnosed cases for its data which will depend on how and why people were identified. For example, the USA's Center for Disease Control and Prevention found the prevalence in 8-year-olds to rank from 0.57 to 2.19% across 11 sites. Besides the geographical disparity, there was ethnic and socio-economic status variation, all of which probably reflected differences in diagnostic fashion and services (Center for Disease Control and Prevention, 2014).

A progressive increase led to claims of an autism epidemic and a search for an explanation in environmental factors. However, increased public awareness, better services and autism's positive image in comparison to that of ID as well as clinician subjectivity and changes in diagnostic criteria were sufficient to explain the change.

An important question is how the prevalence is affected by age, ability and gender which, as noted above, affect the diagnostic process. In a study of 9- to 10-year-old children, 45% of those with ASD had an IQ>70, 15% had an IQ<50 and 40% had an IQ of 50–70. The last group is likely to stand out in the educational system but to disappear after leaving school (Baird et al., 2006).

Clinic surveys are subject to the bias that comes from referral's selection pressure. Consequently, a general adult mental health clinic might find ASD in 3–5% of its patients, nearly all with the coexistent psychiatric disorder which led to referral. On the other hand, while it is only to be expected that most of those attending a specialist diagnostic clinic for ASD will have ASD, relatively few will have coexistent psychiatric disorder.

This leads to the question as to whether ASD predisposes to psychiatric disorder and, if so, to which. There is a strong suggestion that ASD is associated with high levels of anxiety and an increased frequency of affective disorder and psychosis. However, referral bias and active recruitment will both distort the composition of the clinic population.

5.4.2 Co-morbidity

Neurodevelopmental disorders frequently occur together. As none of its rich mix of symptoms are unique to autism, their allocation can be unclear. For instance, although symptoms such as prosopagnosia, alexithymia (inability to identify/describe one's emotions) (Milosavljevic et al., 2015) and unusually heightened or diminished sensory awareness are frequent in autism, they also occur with a variety of other disorders in the absence of autism. This leaves categorical diagnosis in a dither between a hierarchical approach and the recognition of coexistent disorder. The categories produced by clustering specific disabilities will be distorted by the initial selection of symptoms and cases: someone actively seeking autism, will find it. However, as a descriptive catalogue of traits and symptoms is too unwieldy for clinical practice, we must remain with our ever-evolving, categorical concepts.

Epilepsy is associated with autism, the lifetime expectancy being about 8% (in the absence of ID) while the prevalence in siblings, at about 2%, is double that of the normal population (Christensen et al., 2016; Spence et al., 2009)

Attention deficit hyperactivity disorder (ADHD) occurs in up to 50% of those with autism in clinic populations. Here the innate, stimulant responsive, distractibility and hyperactivity of ADHD must be distinguished from autism's inattentiveness which can come from a failure to comprehend what's being said or to recognise communicative intent, an over rigid focus on, or distraction by, a specific sensory stimulus, or an unawareness of the social cues that might direct the individual's attention. DSM-IV and ICD-10 resolved this by prohibiting the diagnosis of ADHD in the presence of autism; the new editions recognise their co-occurrence.

Similarly, clumsiness, once proposed as a characteristic of Asperger syndrome, is now seen as symptomatic of coexistent developmental coordination disorder. However, its diagnostic boundaries have become stretched by the inclusion of other non-motor symptoms (such as the ability to plan and organise) with the risk of engulfing ADHD.

Autism's relationship to personality disorder is problematic. First, there is the suggestion that Asperger syndrome itself might be a form of personality disorder. Next, within its characteristics, it is possible to discern a number of personality traits (notably schizoid, paranoid and narcissistic) which are accepted indiscriminately by the existing personality measures. Finally, should there be a coexistent disorder, its symptoms might well be ascribed to autism, depending on the intensity of its presentation and the level of cognitive ability. Consequently, the diagnosis of personality disorder in a patient with autism should be based on symptoms which have been observed and recorded rather than just on overall judgement. Thus, for psychopathic personality disorder, it should be clear that there is a lack of concern for others rather than simply a lack of awareness of the impact of their behaviour.

Autism must be considered as an alternative possibility where an emotionally unstable personality disorder or an attachment disorder is suspected, especially if RRBI have been thought to be present. However, given the widespread occurrence of anxiety in autism, these are rarely justified as additional, coexistent diagnoses.

Anxiety and depression are frequent symptoms in adolescence. They are often based on a skewed emotional development in which limited communication and social ineptness are barriers to informal learning from childhood. Bullying, rejection and victimisation in adolescence encourage a poor self-image and sense of being inexplicably different. The more able leave school with a sense of low achievement, low expectations and limited self-help skills. Alexithymia, present in 40–65% of adults with ASD, appears to compound these difficulties, being correlated with the pathological anxiety present in 40–80% (Milosavljevic et al., 2015)

Anxiety can trigger obsessive–compulsive disorders although they may be difficult to disentangle from autism as the distinction depends on the patient's subjective response. Here, the repetitive mannerisms and rituals that are part of the criteria for autism (and are typically used for pleasure, relaxation or stimulation) have to be separated from obsessional routines or thoughts, maintained by anxiety and which are egodystonic even if not resisted.

Mood disorders are more common than in the general population: both a general mood instability, especially in the more intellectually disabled, and formal depression, which often presents as a masked depression (although this may reflect alexithymia). Suicide is more frequent, but it is unclear how far this is due to depression, a lack of insight or a failure to appreciate death as an outcome.

Autism probably predisposes to later psychosis although contradictory results (Taylor et al., 2015) underline the need to qualify a complex relationship in which:

- the boundary between autism and prodromal schizophrenia (in the form of schizoid and schizotypal personality disorders) is ill-defined;
- the categorisation of psychosis is unclear, particularly the relationship between brief psychotic disorder (acute or transient psychotic disorder) and schizophrenia, as well as the significance of catatonia;
- it is unclear whether the relationship is confined to autism and schizophrenia (Palmen et al., 2012) or is a broader one between neurodevelopmental disorder and psychosis. Interestingly, the association appears stronger with diminished RRBI (Larson et al., 2016);
- the symptoms of autism can be mistaken for those occurring in schizophrenia. Although neither are RRBI a feature of schizophrenia nor hallucinations of autism, the interests and beliefs of someone with autism can sound delusional if taken at face value.

More specific associations have been found between autism and the following:

- Brief psychotic disorder – a sudden, acute state, usually in response to severe emotional arousal and lasting less than a month and without the longer-term functional detriment of schizophrenia.
- Schizophrenia, which typically has its onset in adolescence and young adulthood (Palmen et al., 2012; Selten et al., 2015), but there is an even closer link with childhood-onset schizophrenia. There is pre-existing autism in 30–50% of cases of this very unusual and malignant form of psychosis (Rapoport et al., 2009).
- Catatonic symptoms which occur in up to 20% of patients. Only infrequently do these come to dominate the presentation with a global deterioration in psychomotor function,

speech and responsiveness that can become crippling and chronic. Effective treatment is based on general measures to alleviate autism (a structured and predictable environment), benzodiazepines and, if necessary, ECT (Dhossche, 2014).
- Bipolar disorder is substantially more frequent, not only in the individuals themselves, but also to a lesser extent in their families (Selten et al., 2015).

Several studies have concluded that the presence of autism is associated with a reduced life expectancy although their methodology is limited by sampling bias and a failure to control for ID and their conclusions distorted by the politics of disability. Closer examination suggests that, where there is premature mortality it is likely to be the consequence of coexistent disorder; notably epilepsy and, in the more able, suicide (Hirvikoski et al., 2016).

5.5 Management

5.5.1 Management of Autism

Given the profound impact on an individual and their family, it is unsurprising that there should be a wide variety of interventions and therapies. Research Autism (http://researchautism.net/autism-interventions) maintains an up-to-date review of these and of their supporting evidence. While no 'cure' has been found, any intervention that improves the individual's comfort and well-being will reduce autism's symptoms. Thus, the treatment of co-morbidity, ranging from toothache to anxiety, will improve their autism.

The management of autism itself centres on:
- Improving communication by teaching not only the individual but also the family and carers to use communication at an appropriate level and with various methods (often with visual cues). Facilitated communication had a brief vogue until it became clear that the voices of the individual and the facilitator were inextricably entangled.
- Education and training that provides formal tuition to offset the difficulties with informal learning, as well as compensatory skills and strategies to cope with the world.
- Finding employment and then support to maintain it. In the UK, there is an onus on the employer to make reasonable adaptations to offset disability, an example being the predicament of a doctor with autism (Berney, 2014).
- Psychological interventions: the current fashion is for applied behavioural analysis (ABA) – based on the work of Ivar Lovaas from 1970 – a programme of intensive individual training by certified therapists, typically for forty hours per week. Although this approach is supported by what is probably the strongest evidence (in an area where it is difficult to enrol subjects for trials), it is also criticised fiercely as imposing a robotic conformity. There are many offshoots including positive behavioural support and pivotal response training. Counselling and problem-solving work can help people accommodate these changes.
- The support and education of family and carers.
- Making a more 'autism-friendly' environment. Broadly this means reducing anything that might cause discomfort, distraction and unpredictability. These elements become more tolerable if they are under the individual's control as, for example, being in a crowd as long as there is a ready escape.

For those seeking cure, underneath the smoke there smoulders a range of anomalous results, as disparate as unusual levels of amino acids, inflammatory proteins or abnormal bowel physiology or proteins. Their significance is unclear, but they fuel the continuing search (and funding) for a breakthrough treatment.

There is an ongoing debate as to the extent to which people with autism should access standard services or require specialist provision. What happens will depend on national policy, what already exists locally and fashion, the whole being nudged by a succession of guidance papers (National Institute for Health & Care Excellence, 2011, 2012, 2013, 2014; NHS England, 2015; Royal College of Psychiatrists, 2014).

5.5.2 Management of Co-morbid Disorders

Most co-morbid conditions can be treated successfully using conventional treatments. Medication should be used cautiously as the person's level of tolerance may be abnormally low or high and adverse effects more frequent and unusual.

Psychotherapy can be effective but may need adaptation to accommodate sensory needs and to ensure clarity and predictability within the sessions. CBT and other behavioural techniques are often used, augmented with visual reinforcements and simplified, to give more concrete descriptions and targets. Implicit assumptions usually need to be made explicit.

5.6 Legal Issues

5.6.1 Offending Behaviour

Overall, there is little evidence linking autism to criminality other than, perhaps, through a common association with co-morbid disorders (notably ADHD) (Maras et al., 2015). The nature and frequency of violence in autism is controversial and, where there is additional ID, it is usually labelled challenging behaviour and never enters offending statistics.

Prosecution of those who are more able is for arson, harassment, sexual offences, computer and terrorist crimes, but this may reflect policies rather than a propensity for these offences. For example, stalking or sexual harassment might be expected to be more common in autism given it is dependent on the person's ability to judge the social interest of others and to understand that 'no' means 'no'. Coupled with a tendency to focal obsession, it is easy to see why this might take someone into the realm of offending and, with increased public sensitivity, likely prosecution.

At this point, the presence of autism may mean that, needing a tailored, specialist provision, many are effectively excluded from standard forensic services (Pearce et al., 2016).

5.6.2 The Ability to Testify

In the UK, vulnerable people are required to have an appropriate adult present when interviewed by the police. People with autism respond poorly to the standard cognitive interview but are helped using visual aids such as drawing and by being allowed to tell their story in their own fashion.

Although there is not usually any difficulty with recalling events, there may be difficulties in remembering their temporal relationship, something which can be helped by constructing a visual time line.

Although autism may result in increased compliance, it is not linked to suggestibility. An individual can prove an effective witness but may require adaptations to reduce stimuli (e.g. a video link), a clear, timetabled role and regular checks that they understand questions and their implications – in England, they can be helped by a court intermediary (Maras et al., 2014).

5.6.3 Decision-making and Mental Capacity

Autism is a recognised mental impairment, so its diagnosis opens to question an individual's capacity to make decisions. Any assessment has to seek optimal understanding and communication with the help of those who know the person well. This may include using the person's eclectic communication method (such as a picture symbol system), images, diagrams and written summaries of what is being discussed, or even prior reading or visits to the places concerned. For major decisions, a formal communication assessment is often useful to clarify the level of comprehension.

The usual key is deciding what it is that needs to be understood or weighed up for that specific decision, but there is case law on such matters as care needs, residence and sexual intercourse. The individual should be asked what he thinks is important to the decision. Frequently problematic is the ability to understand future consequences (including those that come from not making a decision or haven't been experienced) and to think clearly about the future, present and past.

If communication about the topic is difficult, it is often useful to determine what the person is able to understand and choose in their everyday activities such as selecting clothes, meals and activities (especially with novel items) and to understand and manage their time and money.

A common trap is to assume that fluent speech, repetition of a learned phrase or recital of what has been read indicate understanding. The individual needs to be asked what is meant to check understanding. Sentences usually need to be shorter and more concrete and visual aids can help, although the assessor must be clear that they are not leading the decision process, especially in weighing information.

Finally, the clinician must determine whether any deficit in capacity is due to the autism. This is a clinical assumption, and often relies on the process of deciding how a person of the same age and ability but without autism would tackle the problem.

5.7 Conclusion

Whether autism is seen as a variant on personality or a more pronounced disorder, people with autism are at a profound disadvantage in a world that expects a team player with empathic social skills. Although it brings its assets, the psychiatrist will be seeing people who have not been able to cope, and will need to negotiate either their autism or a co-morbid disorder that has not readily responded to standard remedies.

Whatever its underlying basis, it is a condition that can be helped immeasurably by its recognition and, where necessary, the involvement of a wide range specialised services and forms of support.

References

Baird, G., Simonoff, E., Pickles, A. et al. (2006) Prevalence of disorders of the autism spectrum in a population cohort of children in South Thames: The Special Needs and Autism Project (SNAP). *The Lancet*, **368**, 210–15.

Berney, T. (2014) Doctors with autism spectrum disorder (ASD): Is there a problem? *Newsletter of the Faculty of Intellectual Disability Psychiatry*, **16**.

Brugha, T. S., Spiers, N, Bankart, J. et al. (2016) Epidemiology of autism in adults across age groups and ability levels. *British Journal of Psychiatry*, **209**, 498–503.

Brunsdon, V. E. & Happé, F. (2014) Exploring the 'fractionation' of autism at the cognitive level. *Autism*, **18**, 17–30.

Buffington, S. A., Di Prisco, G. V., Auchtung, T. A. et al. (2016) Microbial reconstitution reverses maternal diet-induced social and synaptic deficits in offspring. *Cell*, **165**, 1762–75.

Center for Disease Control and Prevention (2014) Prevalence of autism spectrum disorder among children aged 8 years – Autism and Developmental Disabilities Monitoring Network, 11 sites, United States, 2010. *Morbidity and Mortality Weekly Report (MMWR)*, **63**, 1–21.

Charman, T. & Gotham, K. (2013) Screening and diagnostic instruments for autism spectrum disorders: Lessons from research and practice. *Child and Adolescent Mental Health*, **18**, 52–63.

Christensen, J., Overgaard, M., Parner, E. T. et al. (2016) Risk of epilepsy and autism in full and half siblings – A population-based cohort study. *Epilepsia*, **57**, 2011–18.

Dhossche, D. M. (2014) Decalogue of catatonia in autism spectrum disorders. *Frontiers in Psychiatry*, **5**, 157.

Eaton, J. & Banting, R. (2012) Adult diagnosis of pathological demand avoidance – Subsequent care planning. *Journal of Learning Disabilities and Offending Behaviour*, **3**, 150–7.

Gillberg, C. (1998) Asperger syndrome and high-functioning autism. *British Journal of Psychiatry*, **172**, 200–9.

Hirvikoski, T., Mittendorfer-Rutz, E., Boman, M. et al. (2016) Premature mortality in autism spectrum disorder. *British Journal of Psychiatry*, **208**, 232–8.

Kenny, L., Hattersley, C., Molins, B. et al. (2016) Which terms should be used to describe autism? Perspectives from the UK autism community. *Autism*, **20**, 442–62.

Larson, F. V., Wagner, A. P., Jones, P. B. et al. (2016) Psychosis in autism: Comparison of the features of both conditions in a dually affected cohort. *British Journal of Psychiatry*, 1–7.

Maras, K. L. & Bowler, D. M. (2014) Eyewitness testimony in autism spectrum disorder: A review. *Journal of Autism and Developmental Disorders*, **44**, 2682–97.

Maras, K., Mulcahy S, Crane L (2015) Is autism linked to criminality? *Autism*, **19**, 515–16.

Meltzer, A. & Van de Water, J. (2017) The role of the immune system in autism spectrum disorder. *Neuropsychopharmacology*, **42**(1), 284–98.

Miles, J. H., Takahashi, T. N., Bagby, S. et al. (2005) Essential versus complex autism: Definition of fundamental prognostic subtypes. *American Journal of Medical Genetics. Part A*, **135**, 171–80.

Milosavljevic, B., Carter Leno, V., Simonoff, E. et al. (2015) Alexithymia in adolescents with autism spectrum disorder: Its relationship to internalising difficulties, sensory modulation and social cognition. *Journal of Autism and Developmental Disorders*, **46**, 1354–67.

National Institute for Health & Care Excellence (2011) Autism diagnosis in children and young people: Recognition, referral and diagnosis of children and young people on the autism spectrum CG128. National Collaborating Centre for Women's and Children's Health.

National Institute for Health & Care Excellence (2012) Autism: recognition, referral, diagnosis and management of adults on the autism spectrum. CG142. National Collaborating Centre for Mental Health.

National Institute for Health & Care Excellence (2013) Autism: The management and support of children and young people on the autism spectrum (CG170). National Collaborating Centre for Mental Health.

National Institute for Health & Care Excellence (2014) Quality Standard for Autism. QS51. National Collaborating Centre for Mental Health.

Newson, E., Le Marechal, K. & David, C. (2003) Pathological demand avoidance syndrome: A necessary distinction within the pervasive developmental disorders. *Archives of Disease in Childhood*, **88**, 595–600.

NHS England (2015) Transforming care. Department of Health. Available at: www.engΩland.nhs.uk/wp-content/uploads/2015/01/transΩform-care-nxt-stps.pdf [accessed 10 August 2018].

O'Nions, E., Christie, P., Gould, J. et al. (2014) Development of the 'Extreme Demand Avoidance Questionnaire' (EDA-Q): Preliminary observations on a trait measure for pathological demand avoidance. *Journal of Child Psychology and Psychiatry*, **55**, 758–68.

Palmen, S. & van Engeland, H. (2012) The relationship between autism and schizophrenia: A reappraisal. In *Brain, Mind, and Developmental Psychopathology in Childhood* (eds. E. Garralda & J.-P. Raynaud), pp. 123–44. Jason Aronson.

Pearce, H. & Berney, T. (2016) Autism and offending behaviour: Needs and services. *Advances in Autism*, **2**, 172–8.

Rapoport, J., Chavez, A., Greenstein, D. et al. (2009) Autism spectrum disorders and childhood-onset schizophrenia: Clinical and biological contributions to a relation revisited. *Journal of the American Academy of Child and Adolescent Psychiatry*, **48**, 10–18.

Royal College of Psychiatrists (2014) *Good Practice in the Management of Autism (Including Asperger Syndrome) in Adults*. Royal College of Psychiatrists.

Rutherford, M., McKenzie, K., Johnson, T. et al. (2016) Gender ratio in a clinical population sample, age of diagnosis and duration of assessment in children and adults with autism spectrum disorder. *Autism*, **20**, 628–34.

Selten, J., Lundberg, M., Rai, D. et al. (2015) Risks for nonaffective psychotic disorder and bipolar disorder in young people with autism spectrum disorder: A population-based study. *JAMA Psychiatry*, **72**, 483–9.

Silberman, S. (2015) *Neurotribes: The Legacy of Autism and the Future of Neurodiversity*. Penguin.

Spence, S. J. & Schneider, M. T. (2009) The role of epilepsy and epileptiform EEGs in autism spectrum disorders. *Pediatric Research*, **65**, 599–606.

Tantam, D. (1988) Asperger's syndrome. *Journal of Child Psychology and Psychiatry and Allied Disciplines*, **29**, 245–55.

Taylor, M. J., Robinson, E. B., Happé, F. et al. (2015) A longitudinal twin study of the association between childhood autistic traits and psychotic experiences in adolescence. *Molecular Autism*, **6**, 44.

Waterhouse, L., London, E. & Gillberg, C. (2016) ASD Validity. *Review Journal of Autism and Developmental Disorders*, **3**, 302–20.

Wilson, C. E., Gillan, N., Spain, D. et al. (2013) Comparison of ICD-10R, DSM-IV-TR and DSM-5 in an Adult Autism Spectrum Disorder Diagnostic Clinic. *Journal of Autism and Developmental Disorders*, 1–11.

Wing, L. (1981) Asperger's syndrome: A clinical account. *Psychological Medicine*, **11**, 115–29.

Chapter 6
Epilepsy and Intellectual Disability

Mike Kerr and Lance Watkins

Epilepsy is associated with significant morbidity and an increased risk of premature mortality. There is a strong relationship between epilepsy and intellectual disability (ID), therefore insight into the key themes of assessment and management are essential to clinical practice in the psychiatry of ID. A good understanding of (1) the impact of epilepsy, (2) risk reduction and (3) personalising treatment are key competencies when working with people with ID.

6.1 Epidemiology

There is limited comprehensive research into the epidemiology of epilepsy in the ID population. Any epidemiological research into defined populations poses significant methodological challenges (Sander & Shorvon, 1987). These challenges include case ascertainment, and standardising diagnostic criteria – which has improved following the development of the International League Against Epilepsy guidelines (Berg et al., 2010). Cohort effects, due to year of birth, are also important in defining prevalence in both ID (Fryers, 1987) and epilepsy (Cockrell et al., 1995). Large variations in prevalence have been observed in different contexts, for example between community samples and institutional samples (Bowley & Kerr, 2000). The vast majority of epidemiological studies have investigated the prevalence of ID and epilepsy in samples of children. Therefore, it may be difficult to draw comparisons with the adult population (McGrother et al., 2006). The result of the varying epidemiological methods and lack of standardisation is that consideration is required when interpreting how representative findings are of the true relationship between ID and epilepsy.

The estimated prevalence of epilepsy in the general population is between 0.4 and 1% (Chadwick, 1994). The prevalence of epilepsy in the ID population is far higher, anywhere from 14% to 44% depending upon the sample (Table 6.1). A recent meta-analysis has reported a pooled estimate of 22% (Robertson et al., 2015). We also know that up to 41% of the epilepsy population has an ID (Steffenburg et al., 1995). A direct proportional relationship between the severity of ID and the prevalence of epilepsy has been established (Richardson et al., 1981; Steffenburg et al., 1995). However, there is also evidence that the aetiological factors leading to an ID are important when considering the risk of co-morbid epilepsy in an individual. The burden of the disease in this population is therefore considerable, and associated with increased morbidity and mortality (Bowley & Kerr, 2000).

Table 6.1 Epidemiological surveys of the prevalence of epilepsy in people with ID

Study	Sample	Prevalence (%)
Corbett et al. (1975)	community children under age 14 severe ID	20
Richardson et al. (1981)	community children followed up to age 22	24
	– mild ID	44
	– severe ID	
Mariani et al. (1993)	institution	
	all levels ID	32
Steffenburg et al. (1995)	children age 6–13 community	
	– mild ID	14
	– severe ID	24
Welsh Office (1995)	community adults	
	all levels ID	22.1
Morgan et al. (2003)	institution and community	
	all levels ID	16.1
McGrother et al. (2006)	community adults	
	all levels ID	25.9
Matthews et al. (2007)	community age 17 and over	
	all levels ID	18

6.2 Aetiology

Advances in genomics are helping us gain a greater understanding of specific genetic causes of both ID and epilepsy. The clinical importance of gaining insight into the aetiology of epilepsy and ID is that we will be able to work towards providing more personalised medicine. Treatment plans could be tailored to individual needs considering gender, seizure profile, epilepsy phenotype and risk.

Both ID and epilepsy may result from a wide range of pathological processes that influence varying stages of neurological development. However, the relationship between ID and epilepsy is not always straightforward. The nature of the ID may have a direct impact upon seizure type and prognosis (Bowley & Kerr, 2000). Conversely, the level of ID may also be directly affected by specific epilepsy syndromes (Forsgren et al., 1990). Evidence consistently demonstrates that additional neurological deficits increase the risk of epilepsy in the ID population. There is a particularly strong relationship between cerebral palsy, ID and epilepsy (Airaksinen et al., 2000; Forsgren et al., 1990; Steffenburg et al., 1995). Similar correlations have also been found with autism (McDermott et al., 2005).

The cause of both the ID and epilepsy may well be one and the same. An insult upon neurological development may occur at any stage – prenatal, perinatal, postnatal or in combination. Unfortunately, at present a cause is often not identified. There is considerable genetic heterogeneity between genetic abnormalities associated with all neurodevelopmental disorders. Single-gene disorders have been identified for rare epilepsy syndromes (Bate & Gardiner, 1999) and for ID (Morgan et al., 2012). Unfortunately, there is often no single candidate gene, but a wide array of pleiotropic common genetic risk alleles (Owen, 2014).

6.2.1 Epilepsy Phenotypes

There are a number of epilepsy phenotypes that are of particular clinical relevance in this population. This is a rapidly expanding area of clinical understanding. Down syndrome and tuberous sclerosis provide good examples of the clinical utility of understanding the epilepsy phenotype.

The nature of epilepsy in Down's syndrome has been well characterised. There are two peak incidences, in the first year of life and the third decade (Pueschel et al., 1991). The latter peak is associated with the neuropathological process of Alzheimer's disease (Stafstrom, 1993). Seizures can be the presenting feature of the Alzheimer's dementia; these are usually generalised myoclonic seizures, at times these are of great severity and frequency. Unusually for a late-onset epilepsy, treatment should be focused on antiepileptic drugs (AEDs) for generalised seizures.

At least 69% of individuals with tuberous sclerosis will have a diagnosis of epilepsy (Webb et al., 1991). The onset of seizures is usually in infancy and up to 30% may present with infantile spasms (Curatolo et al., 2002). Tuberous sclerosis is the most common cause of infantile spasms, and they tend to have an early onset at around four to six months. Infantile spasms have a typical hypsarrhythmia electroencephalogram (EEG) pattern (Saxena & Sampson, 2015). In later childhood this may progress to the specific seizure pattern observed in Lennox–Gastaut syndrome. The epilepsy can be very resistant to treatment; however, novel therapeutic interventions such as the mTOR (mammalian target of rapamycin) inhibitors, a group of immunosuppressant treatments that reduce the hamartomas in this condition, are showing promise in improving seizure control (Curatolo et al., 2016).

6.2.2 Seizure Type

In the past, epidemiological investigations into the association between ID and epilepsy have not focused on detailed descriptions of seizure type or seizure syndromes (Kerr, 1996). What we do know is that generalised tonic–clonic seizures are repeatedly shown to be the most common seizure type in the ID population, irrespective of the sample characteristics (Forsgren et al., 1990; Mariani et al., 1993; Matthews et al., 2008; Shepherd & Hosking, 1989). Moreover, the frequency of generalised tonic–clonic seizures increases with severity of disability. Historically, this may, at least in part be the artefact of less than adequate neurophysiological investigation in individuals with more severe ID. More recent data has demonstrated that multiple seizure types are prevalent throughout the ID population (Matthews et al., 2008). Those individuals who suffer with generalised tonic–clonic seizures are also more likely to experience other seizure types (Airaksinen et al., 2000). An appreciation of seizure type and seizure syndrome will improve clinicians' understanding of treatment options and prognosis for patients.

Epilepsy in the ID population is more severe with lower rates of remission, and higher rates of morbidity and mortality. Poor seizure control is associated with earlier onset of seizures, physical co-morbidities and increased prescription of AEDs (Matthews et al., 2008). Depending upon the sample studied and parameters used, remission rates range between only 19.5% and 32% (Airaksinen et al., 2000; McGrother et al., 2006; Matthews et al., 2008). McGrother et al. (2006) demonstrated that 67.7% of this population continues to have regular seizures on antiepileptic medication. Up to one-quarter of individuals with ID and epilepsy experience daily to weekly seizures (Airaksinen et al., 2000; Forsgren et al., 1990; Matthews et al., 2008).

6.3 Seizure Syndromes (Epileptic Encephalopathies)

6.3.1 Lennox–Gastaut Syndrome

Lennox–Gastaut syndrome is an epileptic encephalopathy with childhood onset. A classic triad has been described (Berg et al., 2010):

(1) seizures – multiple types, treatment resistant;
(2) EEG findings – diffuse slow spike–wave activity (≤2.5 hz), with fast activity during sleep; and
(3) ID and neuropsychiatric problems.

Tonic seizures are thought to be typical of Lennox–Gastaut, but they are often not present at onset and the EEG changes described are not pathognomonic of the disorder (Arzimanoglou et al., 2009). The majority of individuals diagnosed with Lennox–Gastaut syndrome (LGS) will have significant cognitive impairments within five years of diagnosis (Hancock & Cross, 2009). It is unclear whether the cognitive deficits are related to a progressive pathoneurological process or whether it is a result of halted development secondary to continued insults associated with the frequency of seizure activity.

The long-term outcome in terms of both seizure control and social functioning is poor. Almost all will have refractory epilepsy and the premature mortality rate is high (Camfield & Camfield, 2008).

6.3.2 Dravet Syndrome

Originally described by Dravet (1978) as severe myoclonic epilepsy in infancy (SMEI). Dravet is now classified as an epileptic encephalopathy (Engel, 2001). We now understand that Dravet syndrome is a channelopathy, and most affected patients have mutations in the *SCN1A* gene (Claes et al., 2001). There is a subgroup of patients who have little or no myoclonic features, but the course of progression remains similar (Dravet, 2011).

Onset is predominantly within the first year of life, the presence of febrile or afebrile clonic and tonic–clonic generalised and unilateral seizures, which are often prolonged. Later on, individuals develop multiple seizure types, along with a slowing in developmental progression and cognitive skills. Tonic seizures (as in LGS) are uncommon. There is also an association with behavioural disorders (Wolff et al., 2006). Three stages of the disease have been characterised. The febrile stage within the first year, the catastrophic stage between age 1 and 5 years (with frequent seizures and status epilepticus, behavioural deterioration and neurological signs) and the stabilisation period after 5 years (where convulsive seizures decrease and occur mainly in sleep, focal seizures may persist or decrease, mental development and behaviour tend to improve but cognitive impairment persists). This pattern is not always observed (Dravet, 2011). Although the syndrome is frequently treatment resistant, there is some evidence for AEDs (carbamazepine, oxcarbamazepine, eslicarbazepine, phenytoin and lamotrigine, all sodium channel agents that may worsen myoclonic seizures, should be avoided) and the ketogenic diet (see section 6.9). However, a mainstay of treatment is with a view to avoiding temperature fluctuations that may occur with infections and avoiding drugs that may worsen seizures, and treating episodes of status epilepticus.

6.4 Morbidity and Mortality

ID and epilepsy are independently associated with an increased risk of mortality (Heslop et al., 2013; Hitiris et al., 2007). The combination of ID and epilepsy raises standardised mortality ratios significantly. The highest rates of mortality are associated with a high frequency of generalised seizures. The highest rates of epilepsy, seizure frequency and mortality of all causes are associated with profound ID (Forsgren et al., 1996). In those with severe ID and epilepsy, direct seizure-related deaths are also more frequent. Alongside aspiration pneumonia, seizure-related deaths are the most common cause of mortality (Rodway et al., 2014).

There is a specific increased risk of sudden unexplained death in epilepsy (SUDEP) in comparison to the general epilepsy population; reduction of the risk of SUDEP is crucial. Evidence suggests that the greatest risk comes from nocturnal tonic–clonic seizures. All patients should have their SUDEP risk assessed and measures to reduce seizures maximised. It also appears that the ability to identify a night-time convulsive seizure and sit with the individual for an hour may be protective (Devinsky et al., 2016).

Epilepsy alone has a significant impact upon carers, increasing strain and anxiety, without the added complexity of ID (Kerr et al., 2014). Individuals with both ID and epilepsy often have very complex needs and a wide range of co-morbid neuropsychiatric and behavioural difficulties (Cooper et al., 2007,). Unfortunately, they often undergo fewer diagnostic investigations and have less contact with specialist services than the general epilepsy population (Hanna et al., 2002). It has been shown that individuals with ID in particular are more susceptible to bone mineral disorders. This may result from prolonged immobilisation and vitamin D deficiency (Wagemans et al., 1998). There is growing evidence that AEDs themselves may lead to bone mineral disorders in chronic use (Petty et al., 2005). This is of particular importance as people with ID are more likely to have refractory epilepsy, and be prescribed multiple antiepileptic medications for a prolonged period.

6.5 Epilepsy and Mental Health

Epilepsy is strongly associated with an increased risk of mental illness; standards for the neuropsychiatric management exist (Kerr et al., 2011); and there is also guidance when considering behavioural manifestations (Kerr et al., 2016). In people with an ID the active epilepsy population is at greater risk of mental illness (Turky et al., 2011).

In the clinical setting the key is identification and the assessment of the association with the seizure disorder. The clinician needs to identify whether the mental illness is pre ictal, ictal, post ictal or interictal. Pre-ictal disturbance occurs in the days, hours or seconds prior to a seizure and is usually readily identifiable. Ictal psychiatric disturbance in a person with ID is often manifested by the fluctuating levels of consciousness seen in non-convulsive status epilepticus. Post-ictal disturbance may be immediate and is, in essence, a confusional state or may have a later, more severe presentation such as post-ictal psychosis. Finally, inter-ictal disturbances are not temporally associated with the seizures. Pre-ictal, ictal and post-ictal symptoms are initially best managed with AEDs, including benzodiazepines as first-line treatment, whilst interictal symptoms (depression or psychosis) are best managed with the appropriate psychotropic medication.

6.6 Diagnosis

6.6.1 Communication Skills: Management by Proxy

The presence of communication difficulties alters our approach to assessment and diagnosis, and may diminish reliability. The ability to communicate effectively and place an individual at ease is a key skill for any clinician, and there are a number of basic aspects of communication to consider (Table 6.2). Efforts have been made to improve general communication skills through education of medical students and doctors in recent years; however, there is still very limited teaching specific to the communication complexities associated with ID (Kahtan et al., 1994; Trollor et al., 2016). Young people with profound ID are able to discriminate between familiar people and strangers, and are able to form personal relationships. We know that when inexperienced healthcare professionals attempt to communicate with this group they have significantly less interaction and reciprocative communication.

When assessing people with ID we are often reliant, at least in part, on a witness report from a family member or carer. The level of this dependence will be determined by the level of communication, the skills of the interviewer and the reasonable adjustments put in place. When assessing epilepsy, it is important to have a reliable eye-witness account, particularly for first-time seizures. The presence of a family member or carer in clinic should, in principle, inform discussions about the nature, number and frequency of seizures.

Table 6.2 Communication skills for clinicians

1. **Non-verbal** – gaze, appropriate touch, use of gesture
2. **Vocal** – appropriate tone, intelligibility
3. **Verbal** – greeting, using individual's name, balance of communication with carer
4. **Response** – recognising the individual's responses and following leads, respecting information from care giver
5. **Empathy** – showing appropriate respect and empathy

(Kerr et al., 1995)

6.7 Differential Diagnosis: Seizures or Behaviour?

Diagnosis may be confounded by a high prevalence of psychiatric disorders. The point prevalence of mental ill health in the ID population may be up to 54%, with many individuals having more than one diagnosable psychiatric illness (Cooper et al., 2007). Psychiatric disorders are also more prevalent in epilepsy (Tellez-Zenteno et al., 2007). This can impact upon both the assessment and treatment of epilepsy in a number of ways. Firstly, there may be confusion between behaviours that are associated with epilepsy and its treatment, and those that are not. Secondly, we know that antipsychotic and antidepressant medications have epileptogenic potential (Alper et al., 2007).

A seizure disorder is characterised by brief, paroxysmal episodes. In many cases the nature of these episodes is well defined. The semiology of a generalised tonic–clonic seizure does not mimic many other conditions, though cardiac causes and non-epileptic attacks should always be considered. In contrast, the diagnosis of focal seizures is reliant upon a description from the individual and a witness. This may be further complicated by the presence of associated ictal or post-ictal automatisms. Differentiating these more complex seizure presentations from psychiatric disturbance or non-epileptic seizures can be very challenging in the general population. Considering these presentations in the ID population is further complicated by the high prevalence of repetitive stereotyped motor behaviours (Paul, 1997). Between 20% and 25% of patients referred to a specialist epilepsy unit have a misdiagnosis of epilepsy. Observable abnormal movements thought to be of an epileptic nature have frequently been found to be non-seizure-related by neurophysiological testing (Donat & Wright, 1990). Table 6.3 highlights guidelines to this differential diagnosis, although in many cases a detailed functional behavioural analysis will be required.

The ID population should have access to a full range of electrophysiological investigations and neuroimaging. The use of video EEG and telemetry can be particularly useful for this population. However, these investigations are not always easily accessible. We know that there is a high prevalence of abnormalities found with magnetic resonance imaging (MRI) in the ID population (Andrews et al., 1999). Therefore, reasonable adjustments should be put in place for easy access to specialist support for imaging under general anaesthesia (Kerr et al., 2001).

Table 6.3 Differentiating seizure and behaviour disturbance

Seizure	Behaviour disturbance
Identical behaviour during each episode	Variation in behaviour
No precipitant	Precipitant is common – such as demands, or avoidance
Unresponsive to attempts to communicate and calm	Responsive to calming, support and removal from stressor
Investigations:	*Investigations*:
EEG: positive inter-ictal EEG	**EEG:** negative inter-ictal EEG
Video: shows typical seizure features	**Video:** atypical picture seen
Analysis of behaviour: no relationship between environment and behaviour	**Analysis of behaviour:** relationship between environment and behaviour

6.8 Assessment of Risk

Epilepsy is associated with a wide range of risks. The NICE (137) guidelines (2012) state that all individuals and their families should be provided with and have access to information around risk management. Some of the more common risks often discussed include risk of drowning (when bathing or swimming), preparing food using electronic equipment, prolonged seizures, the impact of epilepsy in social settings and more specifically SUDEP.

It is important to remember that the assessment of epilepsy and its associated risk is complex and wide ranging. The impact extends far beyond seizure management. Epilepsy impacts upon every aspect of an individual's day-to-day functioning and affects the interface with many services. We must consider the risk of mortality, and hospitalisation; the emotional, cognitive and behavioural impact; as well as the social and cultural effects of living with a diagnosis of epilepsy.

Therefore, our approach to assessment should be personalised and our management options tailored specifically to manage risk on an individualised basis using evidence-based medicine.

This process can be considered in three stages:

- *identify* the risk

The specific risk should be clearly stated. As for example, when bathing there may be several risks, but they should each be identified, such as 'drowning' or 'scalding'.

- *individualise* the risk

Many characteristics of the individual and their epilepsy may influence the nature of risk. It is crucial that risk is individualised as blanket approaches will miss these nuances. For example, knowing the seizure type and frequency, especially whether there are nocturnal generalised tonic–clonic seizures, can guide the risk of SUDEP.

- *implement* measures to reduce risk

Wherever possible the precise measure to mitigate against the risk should be established. These could include the use of night-time monitors to alert staff or considerations to observe when bathing.

6.9 Treatment

6.9.1 Treatment Choice

When considering treatment options for people with epilepsy and ID it is essential to adopt a person-centred approach. Consideration must be given to seizure type, seizure syndrome and importantly patient and carer choice. Clinicians should be aiming to profile treatment with regard to specific aetiological risk factors, including gender, co-morbidity and epilepsy phenotype.

Patients and carers will have specific concerns over medication that may have cognitive or behavioural side effects. The clinician should clearly describe these potential effects when discussing treatment options. People with ID will often be on multiple therapies and will have tried several AEDs. It is important to place a patient on a treatment pathway that will assess all available treatment options, including those already in place. A simple checklist for a clinician is as follows:

(1) Current therapy – increase current AEDs while monitoring side effects. This is particularly useful if the AED has shown some evidence of efficacy. If on polytherapy, removal of drugs with lack of efficacy.
(2) New AEDs – have all the available AEDs been trialled, including 'new' AEDs?
(3) Surgery – in refractory patients, surgical options should be considered. This should be through referral to an epilepsy surgery service that will assess surgical options and investigations.

6.9.2 Making Your Treatment Work

Many people with ID will have carers who can aid in giving the treatment. The clinician will need to ensure that carers are capable of providing this support. It is also important to identify whether the patient has any swallowing problems that may need consideration when choosing which formulation to prescribe. As a general rule caution in dose escalation is recommended; *start low go slow* is a reasonable policy to adopt. In fact, it is not uncommon to prescribe drugs in the lowest available doses, building up slowly to recommended treatment doses.

Outcome assessment is more complicated due to the refractory nature of epilepsy and concerns over side effects. Treatment outcome frequently focuses on assessing the relative value of any seizure change, alongside judging any potential negative impact of AEDs. The ideal is to establish outcome goals *prior to initiating treatment*, but, unfortunately, we often have to assess outcomes retrospectively. Decisions should be made pre-treatment, aligned to appropriate seizure outcomes. Seizure freedom remains the goal; however, significant seizure reduction, reduction in specific harmful seizures (such as atonic seizures) or changes in cognition may all be goals of treatment.

Seizure recording is important. However, specific help will be needed to count each type of seizure accurately, though it may be very hard to assess alteration in absence seizures. Side effects can also be very difficult to judge, but, for example, a gastrointestinal side effect like nausea may result in a change in behaviour of someone who is non-verbal. However, altered behaviour is likely to be related to behavioural problems already present pre-treatment. Behaviour change can also occur when seizures are reduced (so-called forced normalisation), and this is best approached by managing any change in behaviour through local support services.

To avoid leaving the patient on an increasing number of AEDs it is also good practice to come to a decision on whether the treatment change has been successful. If not then the new treatment should be removed.

6.9.3 Outcome Measures

For individuals with epilepsy and ID it is essential that clinicians consider a wider perspective; epilepsy management is more than monitoring seizures. As clinicians we must take a holistic personalised approach to care. A diagnosis of epilepsy has a broader impact upon quality of life, affecting psychological well-being and impacting upon social functioning. We know that seizure control is not the main determinant of good clinical outcomes (Boylan et al., 2004). This is particularly relevant to those with epilepsy and ID. As we have already described, there are a high number of people in this population with treatment-resistant epilepsy for whom seizure freedom may not be possible.

The Glasgow Epilepsy Outcome Scale (GEOS) is a useful, easy-to-use instrument that may help capture a global range of concerns from individuals and their carers. Items recorded within this instrument were identified directly from carers and health professionals. The GEOS may be used in conjunction with clinical assessment of seizure control and treatment outcome within the process of measuring change. It has been shown to have validity and practical utility for clinicians (Espie et al., 2001).

6.9.4 Special Issues: Assessing the Interaction of Behaviour and Epilepsy

As we have already discussed, the interaction between behaviour and epilepsy is important, not solely for differential diagnosis, but also because side effects of treatment may often have behavioural presentations.

Figure 6.1 sets out guidelines for the clinician to assess the relative likelihood that a behaviour is linked to epilepsy or its treatment. The key element of this assessment is the ability to describe the meaning of the behaviour, the so-called *functional analysis of behaviour*. This may in fact need to be done with such a degree of sophistication that the support of community nurses or psychological services will be necessary. With this a clinician should be able to assess whether a particular behaviour is in fact caused by seizures, caused by medication or independent of both seizures and medication.

The neuropsychiatric side effects of AEDs can often be a concern when prescribing in this population. While there is evidence of adverse cognitive and behavioural effects of some AEDs, there is also evidence that improvement in seizure control may reduce these symptoms (Doran et al., 2016). We will examine the evidence available for the use of AEDs in this population below (Table 6.4).

6.9.5 Pharmacological Interventions

A full review of all AEDs is beyond the scope of this chapter. We will provide detail on evidence that pertains to people with ID.

A Cochrane review into the pharmacological interventions for epilepsy in people with ID highlights the challenge facing those involved in the care of this population. The review demonstrates the paucity of evidence that is available. The evidence we do have demonstrates that in general AEDs demonstrate efficacy in seizure control in this population, even in refractory cases. However, there is a lack of data on many common pharmacological interventions in this population in terms of both efficacy and safety. Making an evidence-based decision between medications is often not possible. The behavioural and cognitive effects, which are often of major concern, require further investigation with robust methodology and appropriate measures of assessment (Beavis et al., 2007).

The majority of data on the pharmacological treatment of epilepsy in the ID population is derived from open, non-randomised trial designs. The results from such trials are open to methodological criticism, and as a result, interpretation can be difficult. There are some exceptions to this. Infantile spasms and Lennox–Gastaut syndrome are two epilepsy syndromes strongly associated with ID. There has been extensive, robust pharmacological research into the efficacy of treatment in these syndromes. The clinical effectiveness data in Lennox–Gastaut syndrome is of particular interest to clinicians dealing with both children and adults with ID.

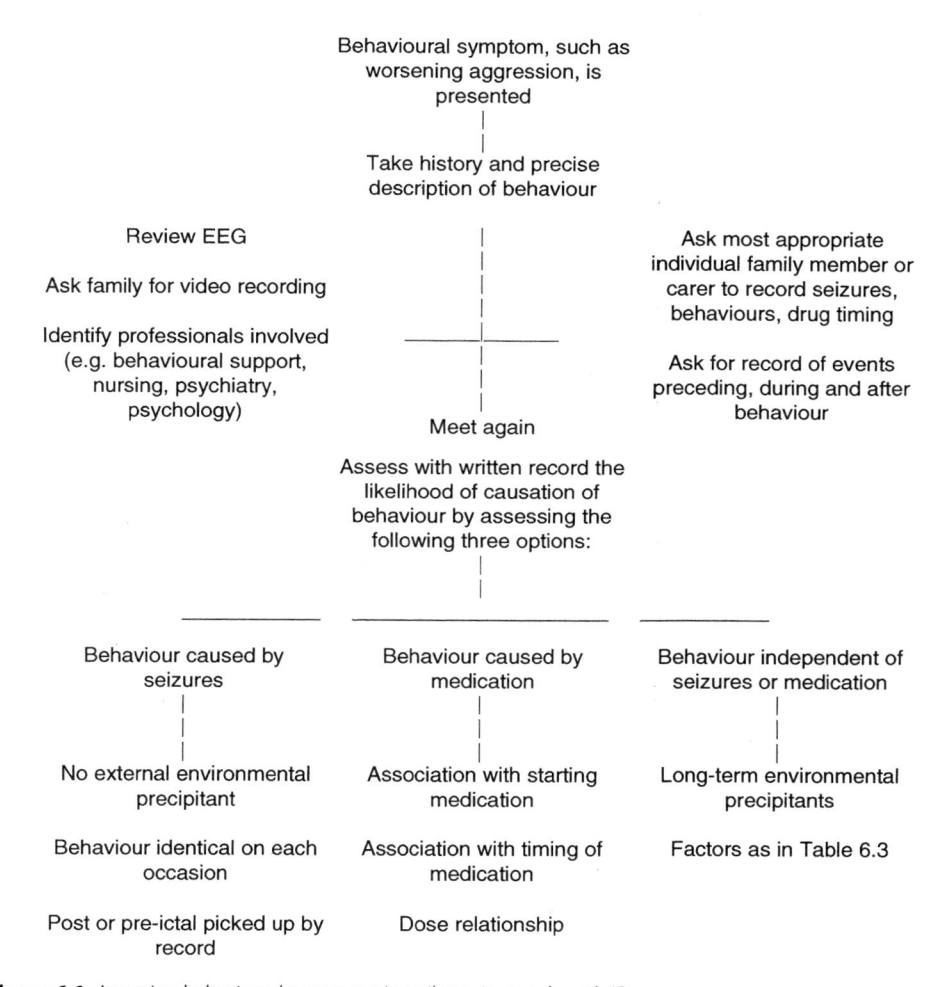

Figure 6.1 Assessing behavioural symptoms in epilepsy in people with ID

```
                    Behavioural symptom, such as
                    worsening aggression, is
                    presented
                              |
                    Take history and precise
                    description of behaviour
                              |
Review EEG                    |                Ask most appropriate
                              |                individual family member or
Ask family for video recording|                carer to record seizures,
                              |                behaviours, drug timing
Identify professionals involved
(e.g. behavioural support,                     Ask for record of events
nursing, psychiatry,                           preceding, during and after
psychology)                                    behaviour
                    Meet again
                    Assess with written record the
                    likelihood of causation of
                    behaviour by assessing the
                    following three options:
```

Behaviour caused by seizures	Behaviour caused by medication	Behaviour independent of seizures or medication
No external environmental precipitant	Association with starting medication	Long-term environmental precipitants
Behaviour identical on each occasion	Association with timing of medication	Factors as in Table 6.3
Post or pre-ictal picked up by record	Dose relationship	

Lamotrigine has been subject to the most rigorous quality-of-life evaluation in the Lennox–Gastaut population. The compound has been investigated through a randomised, placebo-controlled, add-on design with 169 participants. Importantly, this study used a specifically designed quality-of-life scale (ELDQOL) and parental global health evaluation in addition to the usual seizure frequency measures. An improvement in seizure efficacy was observed, with a significant reduction in atonic seizures and total seizures. Parent/carer assessment showed an improvement in global health. Outcome on the ELDQOL showed significant improvement in mood, sociability, with reduced seizure severity but no difference in side-effect profile when compared with placebo group (Trevathan et al., 1996).

The efficacy of topiramate has been investigated through randomised, placebo-controlled, add-on design methodology. This study recruited 98 patients aged 2–42 years. Results showed a statistically significant median reduction in atonic (drop) attacks (placebo increased by 5%, topiramate decreased by 15%; $p = 0.04$) and in parent evaluation of seizure

Table 6.4 Evidence for the use of AEDs for people with an ID and epilepsy: selected example of studies

Antiepileptic drug	Trial design	Outcome	Reference
Gabapentin	Open add-on children mixed intellectual ability (n=32)	Seizure freedom in two cases >50% reduction in seizures in 9 cases No difference between those with ID and those without adverse behavioural events in 15 cases; 3 required dose reduction	Mikati et al. (1998)
Gabapentin and lamotrigine	Randomised open-label adults with ID and resistant epilepsy (n=109)	Gabapentin: 50% had ≥ 50% reduction in seizures Lamotrigine: 48.6% had ≥ 50% reduction in seizures Behavioural improvements	Crawford et al. (2001)
Lamotrigine	Open add-on children (n=32)	74% had ≥50% reduction in seizures 65% enhanced quality of life	Buchanan (1996)
Oxcarbamazepine	Open add-on children (n=40)	48% had ≥50% reduction in seizures 20% dose reduction or discontinuation due to adverse event(s)	Gaily et al. (1998)
Topiramate	Randomised, double-blind, placebo-controlled trial add on adults (n=88)	>30% reduction in seizure frequency from baseline (trend towards statistical significance – 1% in placebo) 12 (7 topiramate) withdrew due to adverse events No effect on behaviour	Kerr et al. (2005)
Zonisamide	Open add-on (6 monotherapy) children mixed intellectual ability (74 with ID) (n=130)	41% had ≥ 50 % reduction in seizure in ID group, with adverse events in 27%; response rate 67% in non-ID	Linumar et al. (1998)

severity (topiramate 52%, placebo 28% improvement). There was no statistically significant decrease in overall median seizure frequency (Sachdeo et al., 1999).

6.9.6 Other Pharmacological Options

There is good evidence to support the use of benzodiazepines as rescue and add-on medication in treatment-resistant epilepsy. Clobazam in particular has evidence to support its use as a rescue treatment for cluster seizures and as an adjunct in all seizure types (Gauthier et al., 2015). Midazolam is used extensively to stop convulsive seizures in the community (McIntyre et al., 2005).

To date levetiracetam has not been trialled in an RCT design within the ID population. In an open study sixty-four patients were given add-on levetiracetam after a three-month baseline. In this study twenty-four patients (38%) became seizure free and there were a further eighteen responders (≥50% reduction in seizures) (Kelly et al., 2004). In general, levetiracetam has been shown to be well tolerated. There is an association with neuropsychiatric disturbance, particularly aggression. However, this may be confined to those biologically vulnerable with a past psychiatric history (Mula et al., 2004). Helmstaedter et al. (2008) have shown that aggressive behaviour associated with levetiracetam may be more frequent in individuals with ID.

There is some emerging evidence from retrospective open studies that newer AEDs such as lacosamide and perampanel may be a useful adjunctive therapy for those with ID and treatment-resistant epilepsy. However, the evidence is very limited to date and caution is required in interpretation (Flores et al., 2012; Grosso et al., 2014; Shah et al., 2016). Rufinamide has been studied in an RCT of patients with Lennox–Gastaut syndrome, in which 138 randomised patients received rufinamide or placebo. Significant improvements were seen in total seizure frequency, atonic (drop) attacks and a 50% responder rate. Common adverse events included somnolence and vomiting (Glauser et al., 2008).

6.10 Non-pharmacological interventions

6.10.1 Diet

There is some evidence to support the use of a ketogenic diet in the management of intractable epilepsy, specifically in Dravet syndrome and glut1 deficiency. Over a three-month follow-up maintenance of a ketogenic diet has been shown to offer seizure freedom in 55% of cases and seizure reduction in 85% (Hee Seo et al., 2007). Essentially a ketogenic diet is high in fat and low in carbohydrate. A recent Cochrane review has examined the current evidence of the diet's efficacy. To date there is a lack of any evidence of the efficacy within the adult population. One of the main drawbacks of the diet is its tolerability. There are more investigations into the efficacy of less restricted diets emerging that show improvement in seizure control.

6.10.2 Epilepsy Surgery

A randomised, controlled trial of surgery for temporal lobe epilepsy has demonstrated a significant improvement in seizure freedom in comparison to medical treatment. The surgical group also reported better quality-of-life measures and a reduction in seizures that impaired awareness. Surgical options should always be considered for people with epilepsy and ID where suitable (Wiebe et al., 2001).

6.10.3 Vagus Nerve Stimulation

A review and meta-analysis conducted into the efficacy and predictors of response of vagus nerve stimulation (VNS) for epilepsy demonstrates that it may be a useful adjunct to treatment in certain patient populations (Englot et al., 2011). It is not a curative intervention and will need long-term monitoring and expect the need for battery replacement. The decision to insert VNS is best made through an epilepsy surgery multidisciplinary team meeting.

6.11 Improving Care Provision and Outcomes

The delivery of epilepsy care to people with ID is complex and services are not always equipped to meet the needs of this population. There is inequality in access to specialist care provision around the UK (Kerr et al., 2014). Collaboration between representative professional bodies would help develop epilepsy care pathways to ensure reasonable adjustments are in place and there is a clear route to access necessary investigations and specialist review. People with epilepsy and ID often have complex needs and numerous co-morbidities. As a result, they require input from a wide range of professionals, it is therefore important that there is one lead team or clinician that is in a position to coordinate person-centred care between primary, emergency and secondary care. Epilepsy specialist nurses are particularly important in the ongoing assessment of seizures and risk. The development of standardised risk assessment tools and protocols, such as the SUDEP and seizure safety checklist (Shankar et al., 2013), should help improve the accuracy of risk assessment and outcomes for patients. Many people with epilepsy and ID are reliant on family members or care staff to support them in their epilepsy management. It is therefore important to improve the education and training provided to these individuals. Standardised seizure-recording forms and clear rescue medication procedures will improve safety and reduce unnecessary hospitalisation (Kerr et al., 2017).

6.12 Conclusion

The broad impact of epilepsy on the lives of people with an ID and their families ensures that many professionals will need an understanding of its impact and management. Psychiatrists, in particular, are often involved in issues of differential diagnosis and assessment of potential adverse treatment effects. It is important that psychiatrists also understand how psychiatric disorders present in people with epilepsy. All providers of care to people with epilepsy and ID will need an understanding of risk and be vigilant to the reduction of risk, in particular that from bathing and SUDEP.

References

Airaksinen, E. M., Matilainen, R., Mononen, T. et al. (2000) A population-based study on epilepsy in mentally retarded children. *Epilepsia*, 41(9), 1214–20.

Alper, K., Schwartz, K. A., Kolts, R. L. & Khan, A. (2007) Seizure incidence in psychopharmacological clinical trials: An analysis of Food and Drug Administration (FDA) summary basis of approval reports. *Biological Psychiatry*, 62(4), 345–54.

Andrews, T. M., Everitt, A. D. & Sander, J. W. A. S. (1999) A descriptive survey of long-term residents with epilepsy and intellectual disability at the Chalfont Centre: Is there a relationship between maladaptive behaviour and magnetic resonance imaging findings? *Journal of Intellectual Disability Research*, 43(6), 475–83.

Arzimanoglou, A., French, J., Blume, W. T. et al. (2009) Lennox–Gastaut syndrome: A consensus approach on diagnosis, assessment, management, and trial methodology. *Lancet Neurology*, 8(1), 82–93.

Bate, L. & Gardiner, M. (1999) Genetics of inherited epilepsies. *Epileptic Disorders*, 1(1), 7–19.

Beavis J, Kerr, M., Marson & A. G., Dojcinov, I. (2007) Pharmacological interventions for epilepsy in people with intellectual disabilities. *Cochrane Database of Systematic Reviews*, issue 3. art. no. CD005399.

Berg, A. T., Berkovic, S. F., Brodie, M. J. et al. (2010) Revised terminology and concepts for organization of seizures and epilepsies: report of the ILAE Commission on Classification and Terminology, 2005–2009. *Epilepsia*, 51(4), 676–85.

Bowley, C. & Kerr, M. (2000) Epilepsy and intellectual disability. *Journal of Intellectual Disability Research*, 44(5), 529–43.

Boylan, L. S., Flint, L. A., Labovitz, D. L. et al. (2004) Depression but not seizure frequency predicts quality of life in treatment-resistant epilepsy. *Neurology*, 62(2), 258–61.

Buchanan, N. (1996) The use of lamotrigine in juvenile myoclonic epilepsy. *Seizure*, 5(2), 149–51.

Camfield, C. & Camfield, P. (2008) Twenty years after childhood-onset symptomatic generalized epilepsy the social outcome is usually dependency or death: A population-based study. *Developmental Medicine & Child Neurology*, 50(11), 859–63.

Chadwick, D. (1994) Epilepsy. *Journal of Neurology, Neurosurgery and Psychiatry* 57, 264–77.

Claes, L., Del-Favero, J., Ceulemans, B. et al. (2001) De novo mutations in the sodium-channel gene SCN1A cause severe myoclonic epilepsy of infancy. *American Journal of Human Genetics*, 68(6), 1327–32.

Cockerell, O. C., Eckle, I., Goodridge, D. M., Sander, J. W. & Shorvon, S. D. (1995) Epilepsy in a population of 6000 re-examined: Secular trends in first attendance rates, prevalence, and prognosis. *Journal of Neurology, Neurosurgery & Psychiatry*, 58(5), 570–6.

Cooper, S. A., Smiley, E., Morrison, J., Williamson, A. & Allan, L. (2007) Mental ill-health in adults with intellectual disabilities:

Prevalence and associated factors. *British Journal of Psychiatry*, 190(1), 27–35

Corbett, J. A., Harris, R., Robinson, R. et al. (1975) Epilepsy. In *Mental Retardation and Developmental Disabilities* (ed. J. Wortis), vol. VII, pp. 79–111. Raven Press.

Crawford, P., Brown, S., Kerr, M. & Parke Davis [clinical trials group] (2001) A randomized open-label study of gabapentin and lamotrigine in adults with learning disability and resistant epilepsy. *Seizure*, 10(2), 107–15.

Curatolo, P., Bjørnvold, M., Dill, P. E. et al. (2016) The role of mTOR inhibitors in the treatment of patients with tuberous sclerosis complex: Evidence-based and expert opinions. *Drugs*, 76(5), 551–65.

Curatolo, P., Verdecchia, M. & Bombardieri, R. (2002) Tuberous sclerosis complex: A review of neurological aspects. *European Journal of Paediatric Neurology*, 6(1), 15–23.

Devinsky, O., Hesdorffer, D. C., Thurman, D. J. Lhatoo, S. & Richerson, G. (2016) Sudden unexpected death in epilepsy: Epidemiology, mechanisms, and prevention. *Lancet Neurology*, 15(10), 1075–88.

Donat, J. F. & Wright, F. S. (1990) Episodic symptoms mistaken for seizures in the neurologically impaired child. *Neurology*, 40(1), 156–156.

Doran, Z., Shankar, R., Keezer, M. R. et al. (2016) Managing anti-epileptic drug treatment in adult patients with intellectual disability: A serious conundrum. *European Journal of Neurology*, 23(7), 1152–7.

Dravet, C. (1978) Les epilepsies graves de l'enfant. *Vie médicale.*, 8, 543–8.

Dravet, C. (2011) The core Dravet syndrome phenotype. *Epilepsia*, 52(s2), 3–9.

Engel, J. (2001) A proposed diagnostic scheme for people with epileptic seizures and with epilepsy: Report of the ILAE Task Force on Classification and Terminology. *Epilepsia*, 42(6), 796–803.

Englot, D. J., Chang, E. F. & Auguste, K. I. (2011) Vagus nerve stimulation for epilepsy: A meta-analysis of efficacy and predictors of response: A review. *Journal of Neurosurgery*, 115(6), 1248–55.

Espie, C. A., Watkins, J., Duncan, R. et al. (2001) Development and validation of the Glasgow

Epilepsy Outcome Scale (GEOS): A new instrument for measuring concerns about epilepsy in people with mental retardation. *Epilepsia*, 42(8), 1043–51

Flores, L., Kemp, S., Colbeck, K. et al. (2012) Clinical experience with oral lacosamide as adjunctive therapy in adult patients with uncontrolled epilepsy: A multicentre study in epilepsy clinics in the United Kingdom (UK). *Seizure*, 21(7), 512–517.

Forsgren, L., Edvinsson, S. O., Hans, K., Heijbel, J. & Sidenvall, R. (1990) Epilepsy in a population of mentally retarded children and adults. *Epilepsy Research*, 6(3), 234–48.

Forsgren, L., Edvinsson, S. O., Nyström, L. & Blomquist, H. K. (1996) Influence of epilepsy on mortality in mental retardation: An epidemiologic study. *Epilepsia*, 37(10), 956–63.

Fryers, T. (1987) Epidemiological issues in mental retardation. *Journal of Intellectual Disability Research*, 31(4), 365–84.

Gaily, E., Granström, M. L. & Liukkonen, E. (1998) Oxcarbazepine in the treatment of epilepsy in children and adolescents with intellectual disability. *Journal of Intellectual Disability Research: JIDR*, 42, 41–5.

Gauthier, A. C. & Mattson, R. H. (2015) Clobazam: A safe, efficacious, and newly rediscovered therapeutic for epilepsy. *CNS Neuroscience & Therapeutics*, 21(7), 543–8.

Glauser, T., Kluger, G., Sachdeo, R., Krauss, G., Perdomo, C. & Arroyo, S. (2008) Rufinamide for generalized seizures associated with Lennox–Gastaut syndrome. *Neurology*, 70(21), 1950–8.

Grosso, S., Parisi, P., Spalice, A., Verrotti, A. & Balestri, P. (2014) Efficacy and safety of lacosamide in infants and young children with refractory focal epilepsy. *European Journal of Paediatric Neurology*, 18(1), 55–9.

Hancock, E. C. & Cross, H. J. (2009) Treatment of Lennox–Gastaut syndrome. *Cochrane Database of Systematic Reviews*, issue 3. art. no. CD003277.

Hanna, N. J., Black, M., Sander, J. W. et al. (2002) report of National Sentinel clinical audit into epilepsy-related death, *Epilepsy – Death in the Shadows*.

Hee Seo, J., Mock Lee, Y., Soo Lee, J., Chul Kang, H. & Dong Kim, H. (2007) Efficacy and tolerability of the ketogenic diet according to lipid: nonlipid ratios – Comparison of 3:1 with 4:1 diet. *Epilepsia*, 48(4), 801–5.

Helmstaedter, C., Fritz, N. E., Kockelmann, E., Kosanetzky, N. & Elger, C. E. (2008) Positive and negative psychotropic effects of levetiracetam. *Epilepsy & Behavior*, 13(3), 535–41.

Heslop, P., Blair, P., Fleming, P., Hoghton, M., Marriott, A. & Russ, L. (2013) Confidential Enquiry into the Premature Deaths of people with Learning Disabilities (CIPOLD). *University of Bristol: Norah Fry Research Centre*, 10(1), 14.

Hitiris, N., Mohanraj, R., Norrie, J. & Brodie, M. J. (2007) Mortality in epilepsy. *Epilepsy & Behavior*, 10(3), 363–76.

Kahtan, S., Inman, C., Haines, A. & Holland, P. (1994) Teaching disability and rehabilitation to medical students. *Medical Education*, 28(5), 386–93.

Kelly, K., Stephen, L. J. & Brodie, M. J. (2004) Levetiracetam for people with mental retardation and refractory epilepsy. *Epilepsy & Behavior*, 5(6), 878–83.

Kerr, M. (1996) Epilepsy in patients with learning disability. *Aspects of Epilepsy*, 3(1), 6.

Kerr, M., Baker, G. A. & Brodie, M. J. (2005) A randomized, double-blind, placebo-controlled trial of topiramate in adults with epilepsy and intellectual disability: Impact on seizures, severity, and quality of life. *Epilepsy & Behavior*, 7(3), 472–80.

Kerr, M., Evans, S., Nolan, M. & Fraser, W. I. (1995) Assessing clinicians' consultation with people with profound learning disability: Producing a rating scale. *Journal of Intellectual Disability Research*, 39(3), 187–90.

Kerr, M., Linehan, C., Brandt, C. et al. (2016) Behavioral disorder in people with an intellectual disability and epilepsy: A report of the Intellectual Disability Task Force of the Neuropsychiatric Commission of ILAE. *Epilepsia Open*, 1(3–4), 102–11.

Kerr, M., Linehan, C., Thompson, R. et al. (2014) A White Paper on the medical and social needs of people with epilepsy and intellectual disability: The Task Force on Intellectual Disabilities and

Epilepsy of the International League Against Epilepsy. *Epilepsia*, 55(12), 1902–6.

Kerr, M. P., Mensah, S., Besag, F. et al. (2011) International consensus clinical practice statements for the treatment of neuropsychiatric conditions associated with epilepsy. *Epilepsia*, 52 (11), 2133–8.

Kerr, M., Scheepers, M., Besag, F. et al. [working group of the International Association of the Scientific Study of Intellectual Disability] (2001) Clinical guidelines for the management of epilepsy in adults with an intellectual disability. *Seizure*, 10(6), 401–9.

Kerr, M. P., Watkins, L. V., Angus-Leppan, H. et al. (2017) The provision of care to adults with an intellectual disability in the UK: A special report from the Intellectual Disability UK Chapter ILAE. ILAE.

Iinuma, K., Minami, T., Cho, K., Kajii, N. & Tachi, N. (1998) Long-term effects of zonisamide in the treatment of epilepsy in children with intellectual disability. *Journal of intellectual disability research: JIDR*, 42, 68–73.

McDermott, S., Moran, R., Platt, T., Wood, H., Isaac, T. & Dasari, S. (2005) Prevalence of epilepsy in adults with mental retardation and related disabilities in primary care. *American Journal on Mental Retardation*, 110(1), 48–56.

McGrother, C. W., Bhaumik, S., Thorp, C. F., Hauck, A., Branford, D. & Watson, J. M. (2006) Epilepsy in adults with intellectual disabilities: Prevalence, associations and service implications. *Seizure*, 15(6), 376–86.

McIntyre, J., Robertson, S., Norris, E. et al. (2005). Safety and efficacy of buccal midazolam versus rectal diazepam for emergency treatment of seizures in children: A randomised controlled trial. *The Lancet*, 366(9481), 205–10.

Mariani, E., Ferini-Strambi, L., Sala, M., Erminio, C. & Smirne, S. (1993) Epilepsy in institutionalized patients with encephalopathy: Clinical aspects and nosological considerations. *American Journal on Mental Retardation*, 98 (suppl.), 27–33.

Martin, K., Jackson, C. F., Levy, R. G. & Cooper, P. N. (2016) Ketogenic diet and other dietary treatments for epilepsy. *Cochrane Database of Systematic Reviews*, issue 2, art. no. CD001903.

Matthews, T., Weston, N., Baxter, H., Felce, D. & Kerr, M. (2008) A general practice-based prevalence study of epilepsy among adults with intellectual disabilities and of its association with psychiatric disorder, behaviour disturbance and carer stress. *Journal of Intellectual Disability Research*, 52(2), 163–73.

Mikati, M. A., Choueri, R., Khurana, D. S., Riviello, J., Helmers, S. & Holmes, G. (1998) Gabapentin in the treatment of refractory partial epilepsy in children with intellectual disability. *Journal of Intellectual Disability Research: JIDR*, 42, 57–62.

Morgan, C. L., Baxter, H. & Kerr, M. P. (2003) Prevalence of epilepsy and associated health service utilization and mortality among patients with intellectual disability. *American Journal on Mental Retardation*, 108 (5), 293–300.

Morgan, V. A., Croft, M. L., Valuri, G. M. et al. (2012). Intellectual disability and other neuropsychiatric outcomes in high-risk children of mothers with schizophrenia, bipolar disorder and unipolar major depression. *British Journal of Psychiatry*, 200(4), 282–9.

Mula, M., Trimble, M. R. & Sander, J. W. (2004) Psychiatric adverse events in patients with epilepsy and learning disabilities taking levetiracetam. *Seizure*, 13(1), 55–7.

NICE (2012) Clinical Guideline 137: The epilepsies: The diagnosis and management of the epilepsies in adults and children in primary and secondary care. NICE.

Owen, M. J. (2014) New approaches to psychiatric diagnostic classification. *Neuron*, 84 (3), 564–71.

Paul, A. (1997) Epilepsy or stereotypy? Diagnostic issues in learning disabilities. *Seizure*, 6(2), 111–20.

Petty, S. J., Paton, L. M., O'Brien, T. J. et al. (2005) Effect of antiepileptic medication on bone mineral measures. *Neurology*, 65(9), 1358–65.

Pueschel, S. M., Louis, S. & McKnight, P. (1991) Seizure disorders in Down syndrome. *Archives of neurology*, 48(3), 318–20.

Richardson, S. A., Koller, H., Katz, M. & McLaren, J. (1981) A functional classification of seizures and its distribution in a mentally retarded population. *American Journal of Mental Deficiency*, 85, 457–66.

Robertson, J., Hatton, C., Emerson, E. & Baines, S. (2015) Prevalence of epilepsy among people with intellectual disabilities: A systematic review. *Seizure*, 29, 46–62.

Rodway, C., Windfuhr, K., Kapur, N., Shaw, J. & Appleby, L. (2014) National Learning Disability Review Development Project Stage 1– Options Development Report. Manchester.

Sachdeo, R. C., Glauser, T. A., Ritter, F. O. et al. and Topiramate YL Study Group (1999) A double-blind, randomized trial of topiramate in Lennox–Gastaut syndrome. *Neurology*, 52(9), 1882–1882.

Sander, J. W. & Shorvon, S. D. (1987) Incidence and prevalence studies in epilepsy and their methodological problems: A review. *Journal of Neurology, Neurosurgery & Psychiatry*, 50(7), 829–39.

Saxena, A. & Sampson, J. R. (2015) Epilepsy in tuberous sclerosis: Phenotypes, mechanisms, and treatments. *Seminars in Neurology*, 35(3), 269–76.

Shah, E., Reuber, M., Goulding, P., Flynn, C., Delanty, N. & Kemp, S. (2016) Clinical experience with adjunctive perampanel in adult patients with uncontrolled epilepsy: A UK and Ireland multicentre study. *Seizure*, 34, 1–5.

Shankar, R., Cox, D., Jalihal, V., Brown, S., Hanna, J. & Mclean, B. (2013) Sudden unexpected death in epilepsy (SUDEP): Development of a safety checklist. *Seizure*, 22 (10), 812–17.

Shepherd, C. & Hosking, G. (1989) Epilepsy in school children with intellectual impairments in Sheffield: The size and nature of the problem and the implications for service provision. *Journal of Intellectual Disability Research*, 33(6), 511–14.

Smith, D., Chadwick, D., Baker, G., Davis, G. & Dewey, M. (1993) Seizure severity and the quality of life. *Epilepsia*, 34(s5), s31–s35.

Stafstrom, C. E. (1993) Epilepsy in Down syndrome: Clinical aspects and possible mechanisms. *American Journal on mental retardation*, 98 (suppl.), 12–26.

Steffenburg, U., Hagberg, G. & Kyllerman, M. (1995). Active epilepsy in mentally retarded children. II. Etiology and reduced pre- and perinatal optimality. *Acta Paediatrica*, 84(10), 1153–9.

Tellez-Zenteno, J. F., Patten, S. B., Jetté, N., Williams, J. & Wiebe, S. (2007) Psychiatric comorbidity in epilepsy: A population-based analysis. *Epilepsia*, 48(12), 2336–44.

Trevathan, E., Motte, J., Arvidsson, J., Manasco, P. & Mullens, L. (1996) Safety and tolerability of adjunctive Lamictal for the treatment of the Lennox–Gastaut syndrome: Results of multinational, double blind, placebo-controlled trial. *Epilepsia*, 37(suppl. 5), s202.

Trollor, J. N., Ruffell, B., Tracy, J. et al. (2016) Intellectual disability health content within medical curriculum: An audit of what our future doctors are taught. *BMC Medical Education*, 16 (1), 1–9.

Turky, A., Felce, D., Jones, G. & Kerr, M. (2011) A prospective case control study of psychiatric disorders in adults with epilepsy and intellectual disability. *Epilepsia*, 52(7), 1223–30.

Wagemans, A. M. A., Fiolet, J. F. B. M., Van Der Linden, E. S. & Menheere, P. P. C. A. (1998) Osteoporosis and intellectual disability: Is there any relation? *Journal of Intellectual Disability Research*, 42(5), 370–4.

Webb, D. W., Fryer, A. E. & Osborne, J. P. (1991) On the incidence of fits and mental retardation in tuberous sclerosis. *Journal of Medical Genetics*, 28(6), 395–7.

Welsh Office (1995) *Welsh Health Survey*. Welsh Office.

Wiebe, S., Blume, W. T., Girvin, J. P. & Eliasziw, M. (2001) A randomized, controlled trial of surgery for temporal-lobe epilepsy. *New England Journal of Medicine*, 345(5), 311–18.

Wilson, S. J., Saling, M. M., Lawrence, J. & Bladin, P. F. (1999) Outcome of temporal lobectomy: Expectations and the prediction of perceived success. *Epilepsy Research*, 36 (1), 1–14.

Wolff, M., Cassé-Perrot, C. & Dravet, C. (2006) Severe myoclonic epilepsy of infants (Dravet syndrome): Natural history and neuropsychological findings. *Epilepsia*, 47(s2), 45–8.

Chapter 7

Complex Physical Health Issues in People with Intellectual Disability

Robyn A. Wallace and Mark Scheepers

7.1 Introduction

It is perhaps uncommon to find a chapter on physical health issues nestled into a psychiatric text. However, increasingly, the confounding impact of hidden physical illness in people presenting with possible mental illness or behaviour change is being recognised. This area of diagnostic overshadowing is particularly important when managing people with intellectual disability (ID).

There is good evidence that adults with ID have higher rates of mental and physical illnesses compared to peers without ID. Given the diversity of such physical and mental illnesses experienced by this population, all health and disability professionals should be well organised, knowledgeable and confident in assisting people with ID achieve their best health possible. Commonly, initial referral to a specialist is triggered by 'challenging behaviour' or 'behavioural change'. It is then the responsibility of the psychiatrist or physician (or both) to work with the person with ID, their carers, their GP and with each other to consider wide differential diagnoses of these behaviours.

Too often, physicians will look no further than the biological (or perhaps feel that behaviours are somehow part of the patient's disability) while psychiatrists may pay much of their attention to the psychosocial (with perhaps a fear that they know insufficient about the biological), and neither will necessarily communicate their formulation well or consider the patient as a whole. Moreover, the patient with ID may also be let down by their carers who may be ill informed and therefore unable to advocate for their charges. This cluster of holes in care results in the patient missing out on appropriate treatment, enduring unnecessary suffering and higher rates of adverse morbidity and mortality.

In this chapter, we aim to shine a light on the relationship between having ID and health status, and the broader interface between health and disability sectors. We will examine the biopsychosocial approach to healthcare for adults with ID, which, when combined with fundamental disability values and good partnerships within health and between health and disability providers, is the most effective means for the person with ID to optimise their overall health and well-being.

7.2 Physical and Mental Health, and ID Interface

There is a significant interplay between ID, mental and physical health. Understanding the relevance of such associations is important for the patient, their carers and for professionals in order to optimise the person's function thereby limiting their disability and preventing handicap. It is also important to acknowledge and address this interface at the systems level of the physical health, mental health, primary care, hospital level care and disability services.

> **Box 7.1** Example of a bidirectional relationship between health and disability
>
> For example, undetected advanced cataracts and the subsequent vision impairment in an adult with Down syndrome can significantly affect their ability to participate and engage in mainstream society, thereby, effectively increasing their disability. Removal of the cataracts can reverse the additional disability of vision impairment, and restore the opportunities available to that person. Going in the other direction, the presence of ID due to Down syndrome may mean that there are delays in recognition of a visual impairment, health services may not be organised to assess vision for people with disability, health professionals may have attitudinal problems or the disability services may not be prepared to support the individual to have a medical procedure. Hence the presence of disability, in this case, works to increase the impact of a (usually treatable) physical health problem, and could additionally lead to more health issues such as falls and fractures, loss of social opportunities and possible depression or other mental health problems.

In the simplest sense, having good physical and mental health can reduce the impact of ID, but the nature of the disability can impact upon health too. Syndromes of ID may be associated with certain physical and mental health conditions. Adding to the trifecta, mental health conditions per se can impact upon physical health outcomes and vice versa. If these mental and physical health conditions are recognised and addressed, then the potential for chronic ill health and suboptimal well-being associated with these conditions is minimised and the opportunities for living a satisfying life are maximised.

Current literature suggests that adults with ID generally endure more negative social determinants of health, including reduced social networks, lower income, less likely to be married or have children, lower education levels leading to loss of any sense of autonomy, chronic sense of frustration, leading to them being attributed, incorrectly, lower social worth (Edwards 1997; Scheepers et al., 2005). They have more medical (physical and mental health) problems (on average five to six each), some of which, but not all, may be syndrome related (Baxter et al., 2006; Beange et al., 1995; Emerson et al., 2016; Hatton et al., 2017; Smiley 2005; Traci et al., 2002; Wallace, 2001).

People with ID:

- are higher users of the hospital system (Balogh et al., 2005, Hsieh, 2005, Janicki et al., 2002);
- have reduced life expectancy by up to twenty years (Bittles et al., 2002, Durvasula et al., 2002, Heslop et al., 2014);
- endure higher rates of preventable in-hospital mortality and morbidity (Heslop et al., 2014);
- are more often allocated palliative care status or a nihilistic approach by health professionals (Mencap, 2002; Mullane, 2002; Tuffrey-Wijne et al., 2014);
- face numerous physical, policy, procedural and attitudinal barriers to access to healthcare (Lagu et al., 2014);
- endure a cluster of negative social determinants of health (Scheepers et al., 2005);
- participate less in healthy living activities (Robertson et al., 2000);
- depending on the level of disability may have lower or higher rates of smoking, excessive and illicit drug use (Robertson et al., 2000; Wallace & Schluter, 2008);

- experience higher rates of physical, sexual, financial and social abuse (Baladerian, 2012); and
- may not be adequately supported by their disability services to undergo health assessments and treatments (Kastner et al., 1993, Tuffrey-Wijne et al., 2014).

Individual participation in the health assessment process for someone with ID may be difficult. They may not be able to independently provide a verbal history, understand the need to undergo examination and tests, and understand the diagnosis and its management. They will often require support to access healthcare, and the healthcare processes within mainstream systems may need to be adapted for their needs. The reliability, credibility and quality of support are not always available, or considered essential, by carers, or fatigued but loving families.

In the education domain, health professionals receive little training as medical students, mainstream clinicians or as training specialists in disability (Duff et al., 2000; Troller et al., 2016). Similarly, the health literacy of carers could also be improved (Australian Commission on Safety and Quality in Healthcare, 2014). Health and disability sectors have traditionally not engaged well, even though it is clear that each party has much to learn from the other, and both presumably have the common goal to optimise the health and well-being of patients or clients with ID. Even within the health sector, in many hospital settings there is little formal collaboration between consultant psychiatrists and physicians, despite the associations between physical and mental health being well described (Royal Australian and New Zealand College of Psychiatrists, 2015).

7.3 Ways to Improve Healthcare Assessment and Delivery for Adults with ID

7.3.1 Biopsychosocial Approach

The biopsychosocial approach, first used by psychotherapists to ensure that the psychosocial aspects of physical health conditions were appropriately evaluated, remains the mainstay of our approach to the health issues in ID. The fundamental algorithm in assessing any person's healthcare is taking a good history, performing a physical examination, doing certain tests, then synthesising the information into diagnoses and management plans. Psychiatrists generally excel in taking a psychosocial history from their patients. Additional consideration of the 'bio' part, however, is really a must in this population in whom physical health problems are so common, and in whom the health assessment is so complex.

The biopsychosocial approach implies that the diagnostic and management issues relating to the assessment of 'challenging behaviour' would include consideration of personality, environment, social, behavioural and functioning aspects of that person along with physical and mental illness considerations.

By the end of a biopsychosocial history, the clinician should have an appreciation of the patient as a person, the impact and nature of their disability and the supports they receive, the life they lead at home, during the day, with family and friends and what their usual personality is like, as well as a comprehensive mental and physical health history.

> **Box 7.2 Values, approach and concepts that should underpin healthcare for people with disability**
>
> **Biopsychosocial:** the biopsychosocial approach to healthcare is one advocated by the World Health Organization in its definition of health. In this approach, consideration of an individual's personality, behaviour, occupation, standing in society, environmental factors and culture forms an essential contribution to the assessment of health and impact of disease for that individual.
>
> **Person-centred approach:** the person-centred approach to healthcare has been defined as 'an innovative approach to the planning, delivery, and evaluation of healthcare that is grounded in mutually beneficial partnerships among health care providers, patients, and families. Patient- and family-centred care applies to patients of all ages, and it may be practiced in any health care setting.'
>
> The dimensions of a patient-centred approach include:
> - respect for patients' preferences and values (not providers);
> - emotional support;
> - physical comfort;
> - information, communication and education;
> - continuity and transition;
> - coordination of care;
> - the involvement of family and friends; and
> - access to care.
>
> **Least-restrictive principle:** refers to the limitation of special intervention in an individual's life to the minimal extent required by the disability.
>
> **Normalisation:** making available to people with ID, patterns and conditions of everyday life; which are as close as possible to the norms and patterns of mainstream society. It is important to use means which are as culturally normative as possible, in order to establish or maintain behaviours and characteristics which are culturally normative as possible.
>
> **Reasonable adjustments:** the way services make their services available to people with disabilities, to make them as accessible and effective as they would be for people without disabilities.
>
> (Australian Commission on Safety and Quality in Healthcare, 2012)

7.3.2 Person-Centred Approach

The person-centred principle is one which makes the patient, the person, the leader of the health management. This practical implementation of this principle means the person (with their family), carers and clinicians all have the opportunity to communicate and work well together.

7.3.3 Least-Restrictive Principle, Normalisation, Reasonable Adjustment, Capacity to Consent and Best Interests

The clinician is obliged to respect the principle of least-restrictive alternative. The principle recognises the right of an individual to live in an environment that is the most supportive and least-restrictive (Turnbull, 1981). In matters of mental and physical healthcare, this principle implies that the least invasive methods of investigations or effective treatments to obtain the required information or health outcome be offered to the person.

The principle of normalisation underscores the point that normal conditions, services and patterns of life should be available for people with ID (Nijrie, 1970; Wolfensberger, 1972). In healthcare terms, this implies that people with ID should be offered the same standard of healthcare and within the same health services as people without disability.

Enshrined in disability legislation is the need for 'reasonable adjustment' which requires that steps are taken to ensure that there is equity of outcome for people with disabilities. In healthcare terms, this may mean longer appointments, accessible investigations, 'trial runs' and a targeted approach (Oulton et al., 2016).

A decision about appropriate investigation and treatment, where someone lacks capacity to make the decision themselves, requires that this is made in the 'best interests' of the person. This would entail discussions and planning with the patient with disability and their family/carers on how usual treatments for that particular health condition in an individual without disability would be offered and adjusted in a person-centred manner. This requires the decision maker to understand the wishes of the individual, those involved in supporting the individual, but, perhaps most importantly, to understand the quality of life that the person enjoys. Too often, the decision maker may think about what they would want personally in this situation, rather than looking at it from the perspective of the individual. This can often lead to a nihilistic approach being taken by the treating clinician.

It is important to highlight the value in taking the time to understand and document the usual cognitive abilities of patients with ID as part of the biopsychosocial approach. This not only helps with application of the above principles but is necessary for clinicians to satisfy government legislative requirements around capacity, and subsequent decisions on physical and mental health treatments.

7.3.4 Engaging with Physical Health Colleagues and the Broader Health Sector

Psychiatrists may feel uncomfortable or insecure in taking a physical health history, because their main contemporary skill is in mental health assessment. We contend that taking a physical health history is a step which must be undertaken in order to provide the complete biopsychosocial review of the person with ID, contributing to the assessment of mental illness (even excluding it) and challenging behaviours. While the history is important, the expectation will not be for the psychiatrist to oversee expert treatment of physical health problems. Treatment should be undertaken via the appropriate channels. However, knowledge of common health problems and how they present in people with ID may trigger earlier referral to colleagues in physical health and open opportunities for efficient multidisciplinary care to provide complete physical and mental healthcare for the individual.

Forming relationships with clinicians in other specialities is tremendously important for the best possible outcomes for people with ID with mental and physical health issues. In secondary care, this may be facilitated by ID specialists attending appointments, for example, ID liaison nurses in a hospital setting, or by ensuring referral letters are detailed yet specific on request. Models of specialised healthcare delivery for adults with ID within mainstream services have also been proposed (Meijer et al., 2004; Wallace & Beange, 2008). Models for such integrated care between psychiatrists and physicians have also been

> **Box 7.3 Key elements of a successful multidisciplinary approach**
>
> - Close-knit peer support for all health professionals and consideration for the complex and sometimes distressing clinical work to be done, i.e. involuntary admissions, violence, suicide, etc.
> - Division of labour to ensure multidisciplinary service delivery, i.e. ensuring that all 'bio-psycho-socio-cultural' components of intervention and care are delivered.
> - Ensuring that all members of the multidisciplinary team are used in a way that is maximally effective (i.e. service users who need a specific input/skill set can have access to that immediately, rather than having multiple assessments); cross-fertilisation of skills between professionals; the team begins to demonstrate the benefits of true multi-skilling without compromising or sacrificing the distinct contribution or professional standards of each discipline
> - Multidisciplinary peer review of all casework at team meetings e.g. formal multidisciplinary debriefing of all service users, peer review at predetermined intervals and each case-manager doing assessments and other work jointly with the psychiatrist or other team professionals as required; this ensures that other team members see and know others' work, can give advice and provide informed cover when people are away.
> - Staff acquire new skills, participate in decision making and take on more responsibility leading to increased job satisfaction.
> - Delivering services that are planned and coordinated.
> - Delivering services that are cost-effective.
> - Enhancing information sharing and streamlining work practices.
>
> Capability includes:
>
> - a *performance* component which identifies 'what people need to possess' and 'what they need to achieve' in the workplace;
> - an *ethical* component that is concerned with integrating a knowledge of culture, values and social awareness into professional practice;
> - a component that emphasises *reflective* practice in action and the capability to *effectively implement* evidence-based interventions in the service configurations of a modern mental health service; and
> - a commitment to working with new models of professional education and responsibility for *lifelong learning*.
>
> (Mental Health Commission, 2006)

developed but are rarely the norm (Royal Australian and New Zealand College of Psychiatrists, 2015).

But even if these services are not in place, a multidisciplinary approach with clear communication, documentation and opportunities for shared learning is essential for clinicians and results in better outcomes for patients.

The development of these relationships is an iterative process and needs to be grown through formal approaches to share learning, case by case, through shared educational events or through clear communication and seeking discussion of clinical dilemmas always advocating for the best outcome for the patient.

As part of the engagement with physical health colleagues, it is also important to outline to colleagues the scope of care provided by psychiatrists and how this is to be undertaken, and equally important to mention what is not going to be covered. The psychiatrist would generally agree to undertake the mental health diagnoses and management plans, but in some circumstances may provide care for some aspects of physical healthcare (e.g. epilepsy); they may make recommendations about refining of disability supports for the particular mental or physical health issue; they may continue to see the patient with ID in the outpatient setting, or refer back to the general practitioner. Communication of organisational matters with colleagues and disability support staff is part and parcel of successful team care.

7.3.5 Engaging with Carers

We know that there is a disparity in access to healthcare for people with ID and that the best outcomes are for those who have an active advocate (Heslop et al., 2014). This can be significantly improved with an increase in health literacy. Unfortunately, the health literacy of people with ID, their families and front-line disability support workers remains low.

The relationships between clinicians, their patients, families and support staff are important in improving outcomes. Each meeting is an opportunity to both listen and to inform. Carers usually know the individual while clinicians know about conditions that affect patients. Disregarding the fact that this is a two-way relationship is done at significant cost to the individual. When making best interest decisions it is important that carers with a good knowledge of the individual with disability and well known by the individual come to the discussion with appropriate information that can be used by clinicians to best understand and explain the condition and the treatment thereof. Inadequate information negates the possibility for a best interest decision and delays treatment while information is collated. Use of the biopsychosocial approach, we contend, is a handy way of opening up to such two-way learning.

In forming such relationships, it is important to distinguish between the roles for disability supports required for the person with ID to access and participate in the mental and physical healthcare plan, and the healthcare plan itself as that provided by the psychiatrist or physician/general practitioner or both. Moreover, when multiple doctors are involved in the care of adult patients with ID, it is important that disability support workers and other carers know the 'line management' for healthcare and where to go for appropriate advice, support and management.

7.4 Using the Biopsychosocial Approach

The art of an appropriate assessment is to take a good history for the individual with ID.

Ensure that you are in a position to be able to complete the assessment in an appropriate setting with appropriate reasonable adjustments. This may require visiting the patient's home, ensuring that the right people are in the room, making longer and more frequent appointments, especially in the beginning, and ensuring that the correct information is available. *Presenting complaint* is noted on the referral but we would recommend starting first with the *developmental* and *psychosocial* history; that is, getting to know the patient as a person, the impact and nature of their ID, and about their daily life, activity levels, strengths and weaknesses.

7.4.1 Take a Developmental History
- At least half of adults with ID will not have a known aetiology, but re-evaluation in an adult is immensely worthwhile.
- New diagnoses in adults are not uncommon; pay attention to the person's phenotype and their behaviours.
- Antenatal, neonatal, family and developmental history may give the diagnosis or rule out some previously held beliefs on aetiology.
- If there are clear markers, consider referral to a geneticist for a molecular karyotype, additional testing and review.
- Useful references: Miller et al. (2010); Wallace (2015).

7.4.2 Obtain a Description of Usual Cognitive and Motor Skills
- Enquire about functional and behavioural ability and, in particular, communication skills, day-to-day self-care, literacy and numeracy and whether these skills are stable, improving or declining.
- Finding out about the person's capacity to understand and participate in their healthcare is vital as this will be used to help formulate what 'person-centred' will entail for this individual.
- Become aware of the local legislative requirements on capacity, restrictive practices, guardianship, financial administration.
- Useful tools: Adaptive Behaviour Scale (Nihira et al.).

7.4.3 Ask about Family Circumstances, Current Home and Support, Recent Major Life Events, Number of Other Residents, History of Institutionalisation, Daytime Employment or Day Service, Social Networks
- These are all important to develop a picture of the person and also to evaluate the stability, satisfaction and networks in their life.
- People with ID endure high numbers of major life events on a regular basis. It could be a death of an elderly parent, seeing a sibling leave home to go to work or a much-loved support worker moving on, a lot of turnover in staff, or co-residents, a sick housemate, a noisy restless household or low satisfaction in daytime activity.
- It is useful to find out how close the person is to their family and other significant relationships.

7.4.4 Find Out about Usual Adult Behaviour, Demeanour and Personality
- What is the patient like as a person? Aim to see through the disability and get to know the person, and about them.
- Determine the baseline for the individual; this is essential, especially if the presenting complaint is about behaviour or if the patient has features of autism.

- Go through the exact circumstances leading to the change, the nature of the change, when it occurs, how often and in what situations it occurs.
- Given that mental illness can be difficult to diagnose, certain validated and reliable scales of mental illness can be used to monitor change, but nothing replaces simple history.
- Knowledge of the aetiology of the ID may help guide the line of questioning and discussion (particularly behavioural phenotypes associated with specific aetiologies). The impact of these behaviours on day-to-day life and what has been tried to treat the behaviour also need to be understood.

A methodical process of physical health assessment comes next in consideration of the presenting complaint. In the grasping of the values, approaches of provision of holistic health and well-being of adults with ID, the essential importance of knowledge should not be underestimated. Psychiatrists need to have the knowledge of the range of physical health problems in their patients with ID, especially those who have common syndromes of ID when undertaking their biopsychosocial review for a challenging behaviour or possible mental illness. It is important to understand what normal looks like for the individual: what is their autonomic function (blood pressure, pulse), what is a raised temperature for this individual, do they become very unwell very quickly, have these changes been seen before?

7.4.5 Ask about Epilepsy
- Epilepsy is so common among adults with ID; in at least 25%, this is the first enquiry.
- Antiepileptic medications – how many, which ones, do levels need to be checked, are there any side effects of these medications or interactions that could explain the behaviour?
- Could some of the behaviours represent an aura or post-ictal event or atypical seizures?
- Useful reference: Kerr et al. (2001).

7.4.6 Ask about Pain
- Pain should be high on the list when evaluating an acute behaviour change such as self-injury or screaming, or dramatic change.
- Particularly relevant at emergency department presentation.
- Consider dental source, including osteonecrosis, ears, limbs or broken bone, headaches, bezoar, gastrointestinal source, painful muscle, hip dislocation, spasm, indigestion, haemorrhoid.
- Where chronic pain is being considered, monitor using validated tools like the Abbey pain scale or the DIS–DAT.
- A very thorough history of the behaviour pattern and a careful and thorough physical history by the psychiatrist will inform later examination, and so it is necessary to consider all of these.
- Useful references: Bosch et al. (1997); Grizenko et al. (1991); Gunsett et al. (1989); de Knegt et al. (2016); McGrath et al. (1998 [Abbey pain scale]); McDermott et al. (1997).

7.4.7 Ask about the Gastrointestinal System
- Frequently a source of pathology in adults with ID.

- Constipation is very common in this population; may be due to lack of exercise, fibre and fluid, an antipsychotic medication side effect, or as a result of years and years of laxative use from institutional days, or related to a syndrome. Working on the bowels is part and parcel of the work for any clinician working with adult patients with ID. There are far too many case reports and series in the literature of acute bowel perforation from volvulus from constipation or appendicitis leading to excruciating deaths or avoidable suffering before a delayed diagnosis.
- H.pylori is likely present in any adult who has ever lived in an institution or still does, in those with more severe levels of behaviour and disability. It can cause discomfort while at the stage of gastritis (present in 100% of those infected), but about 20% of those infected develop peptic ulcer disease, and of those 1 in 100 develop gastric cancer, both complications being potentially painful and making the person feel unwell.
- People with cerebral palsy are particularly prone to oesophagitis, then Barrett's, then oesophageal cancer which could cause pain or obstruction. Increased risk in those taking anticonvulsants, benzodiazepines or antipsychotics.
- Bezoars should be considered where there is a history of pica.
- Adults, who have neurodegenerative conditions of ID, may develop progressive deterioration of the gastrointestinal system and pain and food intolerance.
- Parasitic infections associated with pica, geophagia, coprophagia.
- At least 11% of adults with Down syndrome have celiac disease with, anecdotally speaking, reasonable numbers being diagnosed for the first time as adults, which can, before diagnosis, be associated with many unpleasant gastrointestinal symptoms and secondary nutritional deficiency.
- Useful references: Blankenstein et al. (2004); Bohmer et al. (2000); Khalid & Al-Salamah (2006); Morad et al. (2007); van Erzurumlu et al. (2005); Wallace (2007); Wallace et al. (2002).

7.4.8 Ask about Nutrition, Eating and Choking Symptoms

- The hyperphagia in adults with Prader–Willi syndrome and the associated obesity are not at all inevitable with appropriate treatment.
- Choking has been identified as a relatively common cause of death in people with cerebral palsy and others with disability. Once identified as having this risk in the history, antipsychotic medications which exacerbate dysphagia should be avoided, if possible, and documented as such.
- Overeating and under-nutrition are problems rife in this population. Misinterpretation of disability values permitting people with disability to eat junk food 100% of the time, if that is what they 'choose', is a problem to be addressed in discussion with the patient and their team. All are avoidable, but all contribute to a reduced sense of health and well-being. The multidisciplinary approach may well be called for in these patients and may include allied health professionals such as dieticians and speech therapists.
- Useful reference: New South Wales Ombudsman (2012).

7.4.9 Ask about Respiratory Conditions

- Good dental hygiene is important to reduce the risk of pneumonia, though the risk of infectious disease is common more generally, partly because dental hygiene is harder to manage, and care-givers may not be aware of the importance of processes to optimise dental hygiene.
- Sleep apnoea is common in a number of syndromes, including Prader–Willi and Down syndrome. Irritability, fatigue and apparent disinterest are among the symptoms of untreated sleep apnoea. It must be considered in any mental health review as a possible physical contributor to behavioural issues.
- Frequent chest infections may occur in adults with cerebral palsy; those with mitochondrial and metabolic conditions and chronic infections may contribute to fatigue.
- Useful references: Esbensen (2016); Miller & Wagner (2013); Uppal et al. (2015).

7.4.10 Ask about Cardiac Conditions

- The consequences of treated or untreated congenital heart disease, new onset valvular problems, pulmonary hypertension from sleep apnoea, Eisenmenger's syndrome from longstanding septal defects and the development of coronary artery disease all need to be considered and evaluated in adulthood.
- Changes in exercise tolerance or night-time awakening may be signs of heart failure and should be followed up appropriately. These conditions are largely treatable, if not preventable.
- Assess cardiovascular risk factor profile in older people with ID and be alert to risks and advise.
- Consider the cardiac consequences of antipsychotic medications and avoid if possible.
- Useful references: Troller et al. (2016); Wallace & Schluter (2008).

7.4.11 Ask about the Musculoskeletal System

- Osteoporosis, crush fractures, early onset osteoarthritis, spinal canal stenosis, traumatic fractures, hip dislocations, spasticity management are not the primary responsibility of the psychiatrist, but are within the realm of their biopsychosocial approach.
- Physical fitness, a component of good mental and physical health and well-being, is generally much lower in this population compared to peers without disability.
- Useful references: Center et al. (1998); Schoenecker (2013); Schoufour et al. (2015).

7.4.12 Ask about Endocrine Problems

- Hypogonadism, diabetes, thyroid disorders, infertility, all occur relatively frequently within the population, and certainly can contribute to mental illness and behavioural problems, can occur as a result of antipsychotic medication or contribute to behavioural problems. May be associated with particular syndromes.
- Useful references: Abgulo et al. (2015); Hoyos & Thakur (2017); Jones (2006).

7.4.13 Ask about Hearing and Vision
- Vision and hearing problems are very common in all adults with ID, but can be hard to diagnose and assess. History about day-to-day activity is most helpful.
- Congenital or acquired and when last checked and mechanisms.
- Means of day-to-day adaptation in care and communication. A history from support staff (who know the individual well and whom the individual knows well), or family if the person with disability is unable to describe, helps along with simple tests in the clinic and helps in the diagnosis of congenital sensory impairment.
- The difficulty is with acquired sensory impairment, but knowledge of the aetiology of the syndrome of disability may direct a dedicated search. For example, adults with ID due to congenital rubella may develop retinitis pigmentosa in adulthood.
- Adults with Down syndrome develop cataracts at an earlier age than their peers without disability, and hearing impairment dramatically increases after the age of forty.
An apparent symptom of being less engaged with those around and becoming withdrawn could be due to developed sensory impairment.
- Useful references: Meuwese-Jongejeugd et al. (2006); van Splunder et al. (2006).

7.4.14 Ask about Mental Illness Symptoms
- Relatively common in people with ID compared to their peers without disability but can be difficult to differentiate.
- May present as changes in behaviour. Knowledge of the syndrome of ID can lead to a more focused enquiry.
- If psychotropic medications are already prescribed, the suitability of these should be evaluated. Psychiatrists know how to enquire about symptoms of mental illness; these could be less overt in people with ID.
- Useful references: see chapter 10 on mental illness.

7.4.15 Ask about Medications
- Polypharmacy is very common among people with ID, especially with antiepileptic medications.
- Prevalence of use of antipsychotics among people with ID far exceeds the likely prevalence of true mental illness. Antipsychotics when required for mental illness should be used at the lowest dose possible, and the duration of treatment should be capped, or at least be reviewable.
- Adverse effects are common, could be contributing to the presenting complaint and the efficacy of the drug should be monitored regularly.
- For adults, medications with highest cardiometabolic burden and highest risk for sedation and movement disorder should be avoided. The impact of psychotropic drugs on physical health of adults with ID must be considered given the frequency of their use in this population.
- Useful references: de Kuiper et al. (2013); Troller et al. (2016).

7.4.16 Ask about Age-Related Cognitive Impairment or Slowing Down
- May seem to occur at earlier ages compared to peers without disability.
- Average age of onset of dementia of Down syndrome is mid-fifties, so other causes of skills reduction in younger adults with Down syndrome should be sought.
- Males with permutations of fragile X can present at older ages with an ataxia-dementing condition.
- Adaptive Behaviour Questionnaire of Dementias is a validated and reliable tool to assess for the presence of dementia. It is an easy tool that can be performed in clinic.
- Useful references: Hermans & Evenhuis (2014); Hithersay et al. (2017); Prasher (2004); Schoufour et al. (2015).

7.4.17 Ask about Health Promotion and Healthy Living
- Immunisations, dental review, healthy weight, exercise (as per general population guidelines), vision and hearing assessment may need to occur more frequently.
- Use successful general population strategies with reasonable adjustments: if the patient is smoking ask, advise, assist and include carers; if the patient has too much sun exposure slip, slop, slap.
- Ask if their GP has undertaken an annual health check and action plan, but be aware that overall health assessment requires more than the checklist.
- Useful reference: www.intellectualdisability.info/how-to-guides/articles/annual-health-checks-for-people-with-intellectual-disabilities-in-general-practice [accessed 11 August 2018].

7.4.18 Ask about Physical and Mental Health Issues Related to the Syndrome of Disability
- Double-check any ID syndrome-related physical and mental health issues.
- May require looking up syndrome resources and 'bookmark these'.
- Be aware of physical health conditions in adults with Down syndrome (Wallace & Dalton, 2004).

7.4.19 Ask about Medications, Allergies; Smoking and Alcohol Histories Should Be Sought; Family History of Mental and Physical Health

7.4.20 Ask about How Healthcare Is Managed by the Patient and Their Support Team
- What is the patient's usual role in their own healthcare decisions?
- Who is the person to assist with consent if required?
- Who is the GP, and are other specialists including allied health professionals involved?
- How are health records kept at home, how is the health information shared among the support team and how robust are the processes for supports organisation when the person requires hospitalisation or visits to specialists?

- Who is the patient's main support when it comes to discussions about health issues?
- Does the patient have a health passport, or using an electronic medical record?
- Useful references Western Australia Department of Health (2016); www.england.nhs.uk/wp-content/uploads/2015/01/transform-care-nxt-stps.pdf [accessed 11 August 2018].

7.4.21 What Is the Psychiatrist to Do with This Information Now, Including a Range of Possible Physical Health Co-morbidities?

Having undertaken a complete biopsychosocial review, the psychiatrist is then able to review the presenting complaint in the light of the complete picture of the person with ID, and the impact of their disability and their situation. It is up to the psychiatrist to synthesise and document the various aspects of the presenting complaint to a number of differential diagnoses and potential managements, each involving aspects of the biopsychosocial approach just undertaken. The psychiatrist should be aware of the traps of diagnostic overshadowing and, in turn, iatrogenic illness, especially in the inpatient setting when medications may be incorrectly transcribed, charted or changed, leading to changes in the normal presentation of the individual. Incorporation of disability principles with such a review will facilitate individualised planning of the logistics of supports and reasonable adjustments in the health setting required for the individual to undergo further diagnostic and management assistance required to progress the treatment of the physical health issues raised in the review, and in the most appropriate setting, such as at home, outpatients, an acute medical ward or psychiatric ward. There will be roles to be demarcated by the psychiatrist, for themselves, the GP, other physical health specialists, usually through the GP, the individual patient, their family and carers.

Eventually, at the completion of this initial diagnostic and management plan, the patient and their carers should understand what has gone on, what the possible diagnoses are and, if possible, which ones are excluded, what the treatments are and what the follow-up steps are at outpatients and at home, how urgent they are and if hospitalisation is required.

Clear documentation of all this should be shared with the patient, their carers and all relevant health professionals. At a later appointment, we propose, attention should be given to development of a health action plan. Such a plan would encompass the logistics of healthcare access management from home, especially in crisis admissions to hospitals for mental or physical health conditions, but also helpful processes for outpatient appointments, how to make contact with clinicians outside of appointments, and who is the most appropriate and in what circumstance.

A summary care plan that includes any allergies; what medication they are taking for chronic conditions; what first aid can be performed (recovery position, treatment for low glucose); what an emergency might include (including rescue medication for epilepsy, acute treatment for diabetes or when to call an ambulance); a hospital admission plan (for how to treat a person in hospital when they have physical health problems); and a crisis plan (for mental health-related problems) should be drawn up and shared.

7.5 In the Hospital Setting

Patients with ID who present to the hospital emergency department are likely to have more acute, more urgent and more pressing mental or physical health needs. The necessary components of the biopsychosocial approach are the same as above, though the urgency to involve teamwork with colleagues in physical health is much more urgent. As in outpatient care, there is a need for a high degree of organisation in the process of presentation, admission, inpatient stay and discharge. Data shows that it is in the hospital setting, when the level of health problem is more acute and serious, where people with ID are particularly vulnerable with regard to their health outcomes (Tuffrey-Winje et al., 2013). Delays in diagnoses, poor communication, notes not being available, support staff doing their own thing and not being prepared, poor attitudes towards disability among junior and senior staff all contribute to some very concerning hospital data outcomes (Kastner, 1993). Guides on improving the interface of health and disability staff in this situation are available (Tuffrey-Wijne et al., 2014; Western Australia Department of Health, 2016).

If the psychiatrist is asked to provide a consultation in the emergency department, it should be provided in a timely manner describing what is being considered in terms of mental health conditions or physical health concerns, using biopsychosocial review, clearly documented and clearly requesting physician backup if physical health concerns are considered as being present. Patients with ID and chronic stable mental health conditions presenting with acute medical or surgical problems, we suggest, should be in medical or surgical wards respectively, with the psychiatrist providing as required consultation, also clearly documented. If the patient has an acute mental illness requiring admission but also has chronic physical health conditions, after admission to the mental health unit a routine request for physician consultation is suggested.

Clinicians should understand that the health literacy of their patient with ID may be compromised especially when they are acutely unwell, but to check on this and ensure that as much as possible, the patient and their carers receive the time required for discussion after the emergency treatment, during the inpatient stay for daily updates and on pre-discharge for planning, whenever the psychiatrist has been involved. Disability service providers should be encouraged to understand that for some patients with ID, without their regular support worker present, physical and mental healthcare is much more difficult from the health provider point of view. When required by the individual patient, practical provisions for the carers and family to stay with the individual with ID should be made for 24 hours per day, if required.

On a broader level, psychiatrists, as frequent clinicians of adults with ID, could be considered to have a privileged role and responsibility to promote disability values within the hospital setting and to advocate and help develop reasonable adjustments in hospital systems, policies and protocols, for adults with ID using these services.

7.6 Conclusion

Psychiatrists are well equipped to diagnose and manage mental illness in people with ID. Moreover, many have a good understanding of epilepsy and how this impacts on the individual; some have gone one step further and actively manage epilepsy in their patients.

There is, however, a concern that not enough attention is paid to the general physical well-being of patients with ID, or the role of an acute and chronic medical condition contributing to their referral to the psychiatrist. Physical healthcare is often thought to be the responsibility of GPs or of physicians. However, there is a growing body of evidence that demands that psychiatrists pay more attention to the physical illnesses that may be the cause of some of the behaviours that are seen in their patients and that they are able to understand the symptoms associated with these conditions so as to avoid diagnostic overshadowing where medical conditions are missed and behaviours attributed to the persons ID or, alternatively, diagnosed as a mental illness. There is a need to understand the effects of the medication we prescribe and the long-term consequences of this, particularly where medication is used for purposes other than the intended target for the drug. This is particularly important where antipsychotic drugs are prescribed for behaviours that challenge.

Having a basic framework comprising a biopsychosocial and a multidisciplinary approach (integrating disability principles with which to evaluate a patient and their presentation) allows for a much more holistic approach and allows psychiatrists to advise colleagues in primary and secondary care to pay attention to a particular symptom or to a system that is potentially a cause for concern. This will ensure reasonable adjustments are made and will hopefully lead to equity of outcomes that will mean we can help to close the gap on the premature deaths, and preventable adverse medical events suffered by many people with ID.

References

Abbey, J. De Bellis, A., Piller, N. et al. (1998–2002) Abbey pain scale. JH & JD Gunn Medical Research Foundation.

Angulo, M. A., Butler, M. G. & Cataletto, M. E. (2015) Prader-Willi syndrome: A review of clinical, genetic, and endocrine findings. *Journal of Endocrinological Investigation*, **38**(12), 1249–63. doi: 10.1007/s40618-015-0312-9

Australian Commission on Safety and Quality in Healthcare (2012) www.safetyandquality.gov.au/wp-content/uploads/2012/01/PCCC-DiscussPaper.pdf [accessed 11 August 2018]

(2014) Health literacy statement.

Baladerian, N., Coleman, T. & Stream, J. (2012) Report on the 2012 national survey on abuse of people with disabilities. Spectrum Institute Disability and Abuse Project. Available at: www.disabilityandabuse.org [accessed 11 August 2018]

Balogh, R., Hunter, D. & Ouellette-Kuntz, H. (2005) Hospital utilization among persons with an intellectual disability, Ontario, Canada, 1995–2001. *Journal of Applied Research in Intellectual Disability*, **18**, 181–90.

Baxter, H., Lowe, K., Houston, H. et al. (2006) Previously unidentified morbidity in patients with intellectual disability. *British Journal of General Practice*, **56**, 93–8.

Beange, H., McElduff, A. & Baker, W. (1995) Medical disorders of adults with mental retardation: A population study. *American Journal of Mental Retardation*, **99**, 595–604.

Bittles, A. H., Petterson, B. A., Sullivan, S. G. et al. (2002) The influence of intellectual disability on life expectancy. *Journals of Gerontology. Series A, Biological Sciences and Medical Sciences*, **57**(7), M470–2.

Böhmer, C. J., Klinkenberg-Knol, E. C., Niezen-de Boer, M. C. et al. (2000) Gastroesophageal reflux disease in intellectually disabled individuals: How often, how serious, how manageable? *American Journal of Gastroenterology*, **95**(8), 1868–72.

Bosch J., Van, Dyke, C., Smith, S. M. et al. (1997) Role of medical conditions in the exacerbation of self-injurious behavior: An exploratory study. *Mental Retardation*, **35**(2), 124–30.

Center, J., Beange, H. & McElduff, A. (1998) People with mental retardation have an increased prevalence of osteoporosis: A population study. *American Journal of Mental Retardation*, **103**, 19–28.

de Knegt, N. C., Lobbezoo, F., Schuengel, C. et al. (2016) Self-Reporting Tool on Pain in People with Intellectual Disabilities (STOP-ID!): A Usability study. *Augmentative and Alternative Communication*, **32**(1), 1–11.

de Kuijper, G., Mulder, H., Evenhuis, H. et al. (2013) Determinants of physical health parameters in individuals with intellectual disability who use long-term antipsychotics. *Research in Developmental Disabilities*, **34**(9), 2799–809. doi: 10.1016/j.ridd.2013.05.016

Duff, M., Hoghton, M. & Scheepers M. (2000) More training is needed in health care of people with learning disabilities. *BMJ Clinical Research*, **321**(7257), 385–6.

Durvasula, S., Beange, H. & Baker, W. (2002) Mortality of people with intellectual disabilities in northern Sydney. *Journal of Intellectual and Developmental Disability*, **27**, 255–64.

Edwards, S. D. (1997) The moral status of intellectually disabled individuals. *Journal of Medical Philosophy*, **22**, 29–42.

Emerson, E., Hatton, C., Baines, S. et al. (2016) The physical health of British adults with intellectual disability: Cross sectional study. *International Journal of Equity Health*, **15**, 11.

Engel, G. L. (1978) The biopsychosocial model and the education of health professionals. *Annals of the New York Academy of Sciences*, **310**, 169–81.

Erzurumlu, K., Malazgirt, Z., Bektas, A. et al. (2005) Gastrointestinal bezoars: A retrospective analysis of 34 cases. *World Journal of Gastroenterology*, **11**(12), 1813–7.

Esbensen, A. J. (2016) Sleep problems and associated comorbidities among adults with Down syndrome. *Journal of Intellectual Disability Research*, **60**(1), 68–79. doi: 10.1111/jir.12236

Giacometti, A., Cirioni, O., Balducci, M. et al. (1997) Epidemiologic features of intestinal parasitic infections in Italian mental institutions. *European Journal of Epidemiology*, **13**, 815–30.

Grizenko, N., Cvejic, H., Vida, S. et al. (1991) behaviour problems of the mentally retarded. *Canadian Journal of Psychiatry*, **36**, 712–17.

Gunsett, R. P., Mulick, J. A., Fernald, W. B. et al. (1989) Indications for medical screening prior to behavioural programming for severely and profoundly mentally retarded clients. *Journal of Autism and Developmental Disorders*, **19**, 167–72.

Hatton, C., Emerson, E., Robertson, J. et al. (2017) The mental health of British adults with intellectual impairments. *Journal of Applied Research in Intellectual Disability*, **30**(1), 188–97.

Hermans, H. & Evenhuis, H. M. (2014) Multimorbidity in older adults with intellectual disabilities. *Research in Development Disabilities*, **35**(4), 776–83. doi: 10.1016/j.ridd.2014.01.022

Heslop, P., Blair, P., Fleming, P. et al. (2014) Rates of in hospital mortality and morbidity: The confidential inquiry into premature deaths of people with intellectual disabilities in the UK: A population-based study. *The Lancet*, **383**, 889–95.

Hithersay, R. Hamburg, S. Knight, B. et al. (2017) Cognitive decline and dementia in Down syndrome. *Current Opinion in Psychiatry*, **30**, 102–7.

Hoyos, L. R. & Thakur, M. (2017) Fragile X premutation in women: recognizing the health challenges beyond primary ovarian insufficiency. *Journal of Assisted Reproduction and Genetics*, **34**(3), 315–23. Available at: www.ncbi.nlm.nih.gov/pmc/articles/PMC5360682 [accessed 11 August 2018]

Hsieh, K. (2005) Analysis of hospital utilisation among adults with intellectual disability in one American state. *Journal of Policy and Practice in Intellectual Disabilities*, **2**, 199.

Janicki, M., Davidson P., Henderson, C. et al. (2002) Health characteristics and health services utilisation in older adults with intellectual disability living in community residences. *Journal of Intellectual Disability Research*, **46**, 287–98.

Jones, K. L. (2006) *Smith's Recognizable Patterns of Human Malformation* (6th edn). Elsevier.

Kastner, T., Nathanson, R. & Friedman, D. L. (1993) Mortality among individuals with mental retardation living in the community. *American Journal of Mental Retardation*, **98**, 285–92.

Kerr, M., Scheepers, M., Besag, F. et al. [working group of the International Association of the Scientific Study of Intellectual Disability] (2001) Clinical guidelines for the management of epilepsy in adults with an intellectual disability. *Seizure*, **10**(6), 401–9.

Khalid, K. & Al-Salamah, S. M. (2006) Surgery for acute abdominal conditions in intellectually-disabled adults. *ANZ Journal of Surgery*, **76**(3), 145–8.

Lagu, M. P. H., Iezzoni, L. I. & Lindenauer, P. K. (2014) The axes of access – Improving care for patients with disabilities, *New England Journal of Medicine*, **370**(19), 1847–51.

McDermott, S., Breen, R., Platt, T. et al. (1997) Do behaviour changes herald physical illness in adults with mental retardation? *Community Mental Health Journal*, 33, 85–97.

McGrath, P. J., Rosmus, C., Canfield, C. et al. (1998) Behaviours caregivers use to determine pain in non-verbal, cognitively impaired individuals. *Developmental Medicine Child Neurology*, 40, 340–3.

Meijer, M., Carpenter, S. & Scholte, F. A. (2004) European manifesto on basic standards of health care for people with intellectual disabilities. *Journal of Policy and Practice in Intellectual Disabilities*, 1, 10–15.

Mencap (2002) *Death by Indifference*.

Mental Health Commission (2006) *Multidisciplinary Team Working: From Theory to Practice*. Available at: www.mhcirl.ie/file/discusspapmultiteam.pdf [accessed 11 August 2018]

Meuwese-Jongejeugd, A., Vink, M., van Zanten, B. et al. (2006) Prevalence of hearing loss in 1598 adults with an intellectual disability: cross-sectional population based study. *International Journal of Audiology*, 45(11), 660–9.

Miller, D. T., Adam, M. P., Aradhya, S. et al. (2010) Consensus statement: Chromosomal microarray is a first-tier clinical diagnosis test for individuals with developmental disabilities or congenital anomalies. *American Journal of Human Genetics*, 86, 749–64.

Miller, J. & Wagner, M. (2013) Prader–Willi syndrome and sleep-disordered breathing. *Pediatric Annals*, 42(10), 200–4.

Morad, M., Nelson, N. P., Merrick, J. et al. (2007) Prevalence and risk factors of constipation in adults with intellectual disability in residential care centers in Israel. *Research in Development Disabilities*, 28(6), 580–6.

Mullane, C. (2002) *Young Deaths – Children with Disabilities in Care*. Community Services Commission New South Wales.

New South Wales Ombudsman (2015) *Report of Reviewable Deaths in 2012 and 2013* (vol. II, Deaths of People with Disability in Residential Care).

Nihira K, Leland, H, & Lambert, N. (1993a) *Adaptive Behaviour Scale*. American Association on Mental Retardation, Washington, DC.

Nihira K, Leland, H, & Lambert, N. (1993b) *Adaptive Behaviour Scale-Residential and Community Examiner's Manual*. ProEd, Austin, Texas.

Nijrie, B. (1970) The normalization principle: Implications and comments. *Journal of Mental Subnormality*, 16, 62–70.

Oulton, K., Wray, J., Carr, L. et al. (2016) Pay more attention: A national mixed methods study to identify the barriers and facilitators to ensuring equal access to high-quality hospital care and services for children and young people with and without learning disabilities and their families. *BMJ Open*, 6(12), e012333. doi: 10.1136/bmjopen-2016-012333

Prasher, V. (2004) Adaptive Behaviour Dementia Questionnaire (ABDQ). *Research in Development Disabilities*, 25(4), 385–97.

Robertson, J., Emerson, E., Gregory, N. et al. (2000) Lifestyle related risk factors for poor health in residential settings for people with intellectual disabilities. *Research in Developmental Disabilities*, 21, 469–86.

Royal Australian and New Zealand College of Psychiatrists (2015) *Keeping Body and Mind Together: Improving the Physical Health and Life Expectancy of People with Serious Mental Illness*. RANZCP.

Scheepers, M., Kerr, M., O'Hara, D. et al. (2005) Reducing health disparity in people with intellectual disabilities: A report from health issues special interest group of the international association for the scientific study of intellectual disabilities. *Journal of Policy and Practice in Intellectual Disabilities*, 2, 249–255.

Schoenecker, J. G. (2013) Pathologic hip morphology in cerebral palsy and Down syndrome. *Journal of Pediatric Orthopedics*, 33 (suppl. 1), S29–32.

Schoufour, J. D., Echteld, M. A., Bastiaanse, L. P. et al. (2015) The use of a frailty index to predict adverse health outcomes (falls, fractures, hospitalization, medication use, comorbid conditions) in people with intellectual disabilities. *Research in Development Disabilities*, 38, 39–47. doi: 10.1016/j.ridd.2014.12.001

Smiley, E. (2005) Epidemiology of mental health problems in adults with learning disability. *Advances in Psychiatric Treatment*, 11, 214–22.

Troller, J., Eagleson, C., Turner, B. et al. (2016) Intellectual disability health content within nursing curriculum: An audit of what our future nurses are taught. *Nurse Education Today*, 45, 72–9.

Trollor, J., Salomon, C., Curtis, J. et al. (2016) Positive cardiometabolic health for adults with intellectual disability: An early intervention framework. *Austin Journal of Primary Health*, 22. doi: 10.1071/PY15130

Trollor, J. N., Salomon, C. & Franklin, C. (2016) Prescribing psychotropic drugs to adults with an intellectual disability. *Australian Prescriber*, 39(4), 126–30.

Tuffrey-Wijne, I., Giatras, N., Goulding, L., et al. (2013) Identifying the factors affecting the implementation of strategies to promote a safer environment for patients with learning disabilities in NHS hospitals: A mixed-methods study. *Health Services and Delivery Research*, 1.13.

Tuffrey-Wijne, I., Goulding, L., Gordon, V. et al. (2014) The challenges in monitoring and preventing patient safety incidents for people with intellectual disabilities in NHS acute hospitals: Evidence from a mixed-methods study. *BMC Health Services Research*, 14, 432.

Turnbull, H. (1981) *The Least Restrictive Alternative: Principles and Practices*. American Association of Mental Retardation.

Uppal, H., Chandran, S., & Potluri, R. (2015) Risk factors for mortality in Down syndrome. *Journal of Intellectual Disability Research*, 59(9), 873–81.

van Blankenstein, M., Böhmer, C. J. & Hop, W. C. (2004) The incidence of adenocarcinoma in Barrett's esophagus in an institutionalized population. *European Journal of Gastroenterology & Hepatology*, 16(9), 903–9.

van Splunder, J., Stilma, J. S., Bernsen, R. M. & Evenhuis, H. M. (2006) Prevalence of visual impairment in adults with intellectual disabilities in the Netherlands: cross-sectional study. *Eye (London)*, 20(9), 1004–10.

Wallace, R. A. (2001) Biopsychosocial profile of adults with intellectual disability. *Medical Journal of Australia*, 174, 200–1.

Wallace, R. A. (2007) Clinical audit of gastrointestinal conditions occurring among adults with Down syndrome attending a specialist clinic. *Journal of Intellectual and Developmental Disability*, 32(1), 45–50.

Wallace, R. A. (2015) Genetic testing of aetiology of intellectual disability in a dedicated physical healthcare outpatient clinic for adults with intellectual disability. *Internal Medicine Journal*. doi.org/10.1111/imj.12946

Wallace, R. A. & Beange, H. (2000) On the need for a specialist service within the generic hospital setting for the adult patient with intellectual disability and physical health problems. *Journal of Intellectual and Developmental Disability*, 33, 354–61.

Wallace, R. A. & Dalton, A. (2006) Clinician's guide to physical health problems of older adults with down syndrome (supplement 1). *Journal on Developmental Disabilities*, 12(1), 1–92.

Wallace, R. A. & Schluter, P. (2008) Audit of cardiovascular disease risk factors among supported adults with intellectual disability attending an ageing clinic. *Journal of Intellectual and Developmental Disability*, 33 (1), 48–58.

Wallace, R. A., Schluter, P. J. & Webb, P. M. (2004) Effects of helicobacter pylori eradication among adults with intellectual disability. *Journal of Intellectual Disability Research*, 48 (7), 646–54.

Wallace, R. A., Webb, P. M., & Schluter, P. J. (2002) Environmental, medical, behavioural and disability factors associated with Helicobacter pylori infection in adults with intellectual disability. *Journal of Intellectual Disability Research*, 46(1), 51–60.

Western Australia Department of Health (2016) *Hospital Stay Guideline for Hospitals and Disability Service Organisations*. Perth Health Networks Directorate.

Wolfensberger, W. (1972) The principle of normalisation in human services. Toronto: National Institute of Mental Retardation.

Chapter 8
Mortality in People with Intellectual Disability

Pauline Heslop and Matthew Hoghton

8.1 Introduction

This chapter outlines the emergence of understanding mortality as a key issue in the care of people with intellectual disability (ID). Analysis of mortality data to improve the health of the population has a long history, but not so in the case of people with ID. In the UK, William Farr used mortality data in the 1850s to stimulate debate about why some cities were less healthy than others (Szreter, 1991), and at about the same time in the US, the Massachusetts Sanitary Commission highlighted differences in age at death between farmers and mechanics, urging doctors to make more inquiries into the causes of death which prematurely shortened lives (Shattuck, 1850). Reliable and timely information on cause-specific mortality has now become a fundamental component of evidence-based health policy development, implementation and evaluation (Heslop et al., 2015). However, it was not until the 1990s that the mortality of people with ID came into question, and this chapter highlights some of the seminal pieces of work in England in this respect.

The chapter then moves on to describe patterns of mortality in people with ID with a particular focus on age and cause of death. Age and cause-of-death data is essential for pinpointing the diseases and injuries that may be associated with premature mortality, and for planning preventive services to avoid these causes of death. But the data is also useful for highlighting health (and mortality) disparities between subgroups in the population, something that in England has not been possible until recently for people with ID. This chapter provides up-to-date information in this respect, reporting on data from general practitioner (GP) records that have been linked with national mortality data.

The chapter ends with a consideration of avoidable deaths of people with ID. The concept of avoidable mortality was first introduced by Rutstein and others in the 1970s, who argued that in order to develop effective indicators of healthcare, lists of diseases which should not (or only infrequently) give rise to death or disability should be drawn up (Rutstein, 1976). The UK Office for National Statistics subdivides avoidable deaths into those that are preventable by public health interventions in the broadest sense and those that are amenable to good-quality care. It is the category of amenable deaths that is of concern in relation to people with ID, and which this chapter focuses on. By addressing issues underpinning deaths amenable to good-quality care, we can start to make reductions in the unacceptably high level of premature deaths of people with ID.

8.2 The Emergence of Mortality as a Key Issue in the Care of People with ID

In England since the 1990s there have been a number of key research reports and case studies that have consistently expressed concern that people with ID die younger than people in the general population, that they may die from different causes of death from people in the general population and that a large proportion of the deaths of people with ID are preventable by improved health and social care.

The first significant report was by Professor Hollins and her colleagues (Hollins et al., 1998), who followed 2,000 people with ID in two London districts for eight years. During the period 1982 to 1990, 270 (13.3%) died. These people with ID died at a much younger age than the general population; more than half had died before the age of 65 compared with just 17% of the general population. People with cerebral palsy, incontinence, mobility problems or those living in hospital all died at younger ages. The researchers reported that cause-of-death certificates were not a reliable source of information about the factors contributing to a person's cause of death and recommended an extension to the format of cause-of-death certificates that would include recording chronic disabling conditions.

In 2004 the National Patient Safety Agency (NPSA) investigated patient safety issues for people with ID and highlighted the problem of choking during feeding (National Patient Safety Agency, 2007). Subsequently, over a three-year period, 2004–7, the NPSA received 605 reports of choking-related incidents involving adults with ID. In 2005, the NPSA commissioned a scoping report for a confidential inquiry into excess mortality in people with ID. The report, led by the University of Birmingham, concluded that a confidential inquiry was desirable because of apparent excess mortality, evidence of poor access to some healthcare and the increased likelihood of detecting errors of care (Stoddart et al., 2005).

A significant catalyst for the inquiry came from the bereaved families who had reported to Mencap concerns about the healthcare of their relatives with ID. The Mencap report *Death by Indifference*, published in 2007, described the circumstances of the deaths of six people with ID while they were in the care of the NHS, exposing 'institutional discrimination' (Mencap, 2007: 1). It remains a distressing account of the deaths of Emma (26 years), Mark (30 years), Martin (43 years), Ted (61 years), Tom (20 years) and Warren (30 years). The families wanted to fully understand why their relatives died and improve the access to healthcare for others.

The Parliamentary and Health Service Ombudsman and Local Government Ombudsman reviewed the deaths of the six adults reported in *Death by Indifference* and published the results of their investigation (2009). The report *Six Lives: The Provision of Public Services to People with Learning Disabilities* concluded that one of the deaths was avoidable, and one was likely to have been avoidable. It confirmed maladministration and service failure for disability-related reasons in relation to a number of the NHS bodies and local councils involved, and that there had been unnecessary distress and suffering for the aggrieved families. It stated:

> Our findings contrast markedly with the first principle of the recently published NHS Constitution for England and Wales, which says that 'The NHS provides a comprehensive service, available to all irrespective of gender, race, disability, age, sexual orientation, religion or belief. It has a duty to each and every individual it serves and must respect their human rights.'
> (Parliamentary and Health Service Ombudsman, 2009: 3)

Running concurrently with the Ombudsman investigation into the six deaths was an independent inquiry into the wider issue of access to health services for people with ID, chaired by Sir Jonathan Michael. The report (Michael, 2008) found that:
- People with ID found it harder to access assessment and treatment for general health problems that were unrelated to their disability than people without ID.
- There was insufficient attention given to making reasonable adjustments to support the delivery of equal treatment, as required by the Disability Discrimination Act.
- Parents and carers of people with ID often had their opinions and assessments ignored by healthcare professionals, even though they often had the best information about, and understanding of, the people they support.
- Health service staff, particularly those working in general healthcare, had very limited knowledge about ID and the legislative framework within which they should work. Staff were not familiar with what help they should provide or from whom to get expert advice.

The report recommended the establishment of the learning (intellectual) disabilities Public Health Observatory, and a time-limited confidential inquiry into premature deaths of people with learning (intellectual) disabilities.

The Confidential Inquiry into Premature Deaths of People with Learning Disabilities in England (CIPOLD) ran from 2010 to 2013, and reviewed the deaths of all people with ID in five (former) Primary Care Trust areas in south-west England over a two-year period, 2010–12. It focused on the care that people received in the period leading up to their deaths to identify errors or omissions that may have contributed to the deaths, to illustrate good practice and to provide improved evidence on avoiding premature deaths of people with ID. Significantly, it included the views of all those involved in supporting each person who died, including the bereaved families and friends. CIPOLD confirmed the early deaths of people with ID and evidence of potentially avoidable deaths (Heslop et al., 2014). It also highlighted the absence of national mortality data relating to people with ID, and that without this information, it is difficult to assess the extent of health inequalities faced by this population nationally, to monitor a reduction in premature deaths or to understand where targeted resources could be most effective. It concluded:

> The quality and effectiveness of health and social care given to people with learning disabilities has been shown to be deficient in a number of ways. Despite numerous previous investigations and reports, many professionals are either not aware of, or do not include in their usual practice, approaches that adapt services to meet the needs of people with learning disabilities. (Heslop et al., 2013: 5)

The Mencap report *Death by Indifference: 74 Deaths and Counting* (2012) concluded that the NHS continued to be unsafe for people with ID with particular lack of focus on the identification of people with ID within the health service and a lack of tracking of their care pathways. Mencap called on the NHS to act to stop more people with ID dying unnecessarily.

Connor Sparrowhawk, an 18-year-old man with ID, drowned after an epileptic seizure under the care of Southern Health NHS Foundation Trust, in 2013. Following his death there was considerable campaigning by his family after they were dissatisfied with the Trust's care and by the internal investigation into Connor's death. NHS England commissioned Mazars to review all the deaths of people with ID or mental health needs in receipt of services from Southern Health NHS Foundation Trust between April 2011 and March 2015, and the Trust's own internal investigation process. Mazars (2015) reported a lack of leadership, focus and time spent on carefully reporting and investigating unexpected deaths of mental health and ID service users, and that the Trust could not demonstrate a comprehensive, systematic approach to learning from deaths as evidenced by action plans, board review and follow-up, high-quality thematic reviews and resultant service change.

The Mazars report was published soon after the national Learning Disabilities Mortality Review Programme (LeDeR) was established in England. LeDeR aims to improve the quality of health and social care delivery for people with ID through a retrospective review of their deaths. The case reviews support health and social care professionals, and others, to identify and take action on the avoidable contributory factors leading to premature deaths in this population. The programme, which has been commissioned by NHS England and is being led by the University of Bristol, has now been fully rolled out across England. The headline findings of these reports are summarised in Table 8.1.

8.3 Mortality Surveillance

Mortality surveillance is an essential component for planning and allocating health resources and identifying targets for health and service improvement strategies (NHS Clinical Commissioning Group, 2013). Further, examination of mortality over time can demonstrate patterns in causes of deaths and can help assess the impact of initiatives to improve the health and well-being of the population. Individual-level case reviews can provide a complementary perspective to population trends and can help elucidate explanatory qualitative factors (Barbieri et al., 2013). Reviewing the circumstances and contributing factors of individual deaths facilitates the identification of potentially modifiable factors associated with deaths that may not be apparent in population-level surveillance (Lauer et al., 2015). They can provide a rich source of information about legal, policy and institutional-level barriers to quality care, and can illustrate positive examples of best practice.

Information about the age and cause of death of the general population is routinely reported at national and cross-national levels, but it is not usually possible to extract data about people with ID from this information (Heslop et al., 2015). There are a number of reasons why this is the case:

- A lack of recording that a person had ID on their cause-of-death certificate. World Health Organization rules for completing the cause-of-death certificate requires a record of the sequential train of events leading to death, plus a record of any other diseases, injuries, conditions or events that contributed to the death but were not part of the direct sequence of events leading to death (World Health Organization, 1992). In many cases, a person's ID may not cause or contribute to the person's death, so would not therefore be recorded. In England, the proportion of deaths of people known to have ID whose cause-of-death certificate mentioned this ranged from was 41% (Tyrer & McGrother, 2009) to 23% (Heslop et al., 2013).
- Coding errors on cause-of-death certificates have been noted in a number of research studies and are an additional factor precluding the identification of people with ID. Landes and Peek (2013) reported that 20% of the 2,278 cases where ID was recorded on a cause-of-death certificate were coded erroneously by stating 'mental retardation' as the underlying cause of death. They concluded that diagnostic overshadowing may be obscuring the true cause of death of some people with ID.

Table 8.1 Key research reports about mortality of people with ID

Report	Headline findings
Hollins et al. (1998) Mortality in people with learning disability: Risks, causes and death certification findings in London. *Developmental Medicine & Child Neurology*, 40 (1), 50–6	More than half of people with learning disabilities died before the age of 65 compared with just 17% of the general population
Mencap (2007) *Death by Indifference*	Described the circumstances of the deaths of six people with ID while they were in the care of the NHS, exposing 'institutional discrimination'. There was considerable family and carer involvement in the preparation of this report.
Parliamentary and Health Service Ombudsman (2009) *Six Lives: The Provision of Public Services to People with Learning Disabilities* (Stationery Office). This report was the Parliamentary and Health Service Ombudsman response to *Death by Indifference*.	Significant and distressing failures were identified across both health and social care, in which people with learning disabilities experienced prolonged suffering and inappropriate care. There was evidence of maladministration, service failure and unremedied injustice in relation to a number of the NHS bodies and local councils. Several failed to live up to human rights principles, especially those of dignity and equality.
Michael, J. (2008) *Healthcare for All: Report of the Independent Inquiry into Access to Healthcare for People with Learning Disabilities* (Department of Health)	People with ID found it harder to access assessment and treatment for general health problems that were unrelated to their disability than people without ID
Mencap (2012) *Death by Indifference: 74 Deaths and Counting. A Progress Report 5 Years on*	Concluded that the NHS continued to be unsafe for people with ID
Heslop et al. (2014) The confidential inquiry into premature deaths of people with ID in the UK: A population-based study. *Lancet*, 383, 889–95	Confirmed the early deaths of people with ID and evidence of potentially avoidable deaths. Reported that the quality and effectiveness of health and social care given to people with ID has been shown to be deficient in a number of ways
Mazars (2015) Independent review of deaths of people with a learning disability or mental health problem in contact with Southern Health NHS Foundation Trust April 2011 to March 2015, London	Reported a lack of leadership, focus and time spent on carefully reporting and investigating unexpected deaths of people using mental health and ID services

Additional complexity is caused by a lack of consistency in the identification of people with ID, with some agencies using administrative criteria (eligibility for particular services) and others using psychological testing such as IQ tests. This can lead to incomplete and incompatible registers of people with ID, and considerable disjoint between different registers. Finally, multiple coding options for the existence of ID are problematic: Glover and Ayub (2010), for example, identified 48 ICD10 codes for medical conditions usually associated with ID.

8.4 The Age of Death of People with ID

8.4.1 Age at Death and Life Expectancy

Multiple studies have reported an earlier age at death of people with ID than the general public. CIPOLD (Heslop et al., 2013, 2014) reported that in England men with ID died thirteen years sooner than men in the general population and women with ID died twenty years sooner than women in the general population. These findings are supported by analysis of Clinical Practice Research Database data from April 2010 to March 2014 (CPRD GOLD, September 2015) comprising roughly 5% of the population of England in the period studied, linked with national death certification data (Glover et al., 2017). Death rates were higher in those with ID than those without at all ages and for both sexes, significantly so except for men aged 18 to 24, and 85 and older. The life expectancy at birth for people with ID was 19.7 years lower than for people without ID. Most recently in England, data from almost half of all GP practices in England collected from 2014 to 2015 suggests that females with ID had an eighteen-year lower life expectancy than the general population, while males with ID had a fourteen-year lower life expectancy than the general population (NHS Digital, 2016).

International studies have also reported disparities in the age at death of people with ID when compared with the general population. Data from three US states suggested an average age at death of people with intellectual and developmental disabilities to be between 59 and 62 years, compared with the average age at death of US residents at birth (78.5 years) and US residents after 20 years (84.2 years) (Lauer & Bonardi, 2013). In Ireland over the period 2003–12, there was a 19 years disparity in life expectancy: the average age at death of people with ID was 55 years, compared with 74 years in the general population, with the gap between age at death for females with and without ID being larger than for males (McCarron et al., 2015).

8.4.2 Standardised Mortality Rates

The standardised mortality rate reports how many people, per thousand of the population, will die in a given year. Glover et al. (2017) usefully compared the all-cause directly standardised mortality rates across different countries for adults with ID. Data from nationally representative linked data in England suggest a standardised mortality rate of 26.6 deaths per 1,000 population for people with ID. This is higher than data provided by Ouellette-Kuntz et al. (2015) in Manitoba, Canada (22.5), and SE Ontario, Canada (19.0); and Arvivo et al. (2016) in Finland (19.5). It is lower than data provided by Lauer (2016) in Massachusetts, USA (33.6); and McCarron et al. (2015) in the Republic of Ireland (42.2).

8.4.3 Standardised Mortality Ratio

The standardised mortality ratio (SMR) is perhaps a more informative measure as it estimates the ratio of age-specific observed deaths in a particular group in relation to expected deaths in the general population. This is important given the difference in age profiles of people with ID compared with the general population. However, comparisons of SMR also show excess mortality in people with ID compared to the general population.

Data from 1993 to 2006 suggested that the SMR for adults with moderate-to-profound ID to be almost three times as high (SMR 2.77, 95% CI: 2.53–3.03) as the general population (Tyrer & McGrother, 2009). Glover et al. (2017) in their analysis of nationally representative linked data from England reported an SMR for people with ID as being 3.18 (95%CI 2.94–3.43), and that it was higher for women (3.40–3.02 to 3.81) than for men (3.03–2.73 to 3.35).

Internationally too, the SMR for people with ID has been found to be consistently greater than in the general population. Most recently in Finland, Arvivo et al. (2016) used administrative data-based national insurance benefits paid to people with a diagnosis of ID and reported SMR for females with a mild ID (IQ 50–69) to be 2.8 and for males 2.0. For females with a severe ID (IQ <50) the SMR was 5.2 and for males 2.6.

8.5 Cause of Death

Understanding the cause of death can help us to better understand the health of a population and how it can be improved. It can help us to identify who is at risk of particular diseases, what disparities exist between subgroups in the population and where we should best target public health interventions and improvements in the delivery of care.

Cause-of-death certificates are divided into two parts. In part 1 causes of death are entered sequentially, starting with immediate cause and ending with the underlying cause. The underlying cause of death is defined by the World Health Organization (1992) as the disease or injury that initiated the train of events leading directly to death, or the circumstances of the accident or violence which produced the fatal injury. As a general rule, mortality statistics report the *underlying* cause of death, not the immediate cause of death. Part 2 of the cause-of-death certificate documents all diseases or conditions contributing to the death that were not reported in the chain of events in part 1, and that did not result in the underlying cause of death.

There are a number of challenges to the accuracy of cause-of-death reporting in people with ID (Glover & Ayub, 2010; Tyrer & McGrother, 2009). Landes and Peek (2013) in their review of cause-of-death certificates for people with ID in the US described 'death by mental retardation', with 'mental retardation' being inappropriately coded as the underlying cause of death particularly when the death certificate provided little information about other disease processes; when the person died in an outpatient or emergency setting; or when the person had either abnormal symptomatology or died as a result of injury, accident or other external cause.

Despite such challenges, cause-of-death certificates remain one of the best sources of information about why people with ID die.

8.5.1 Cause-Specific Mortality

As with the general population, the most common causes of death in people with ID are heart disease, cancer and respiratory diseases. However, these three causes account for a lower proportion of deaths of people with ID than for the general population. This results in a more varied profile of underlying causes of death in people with ID, including some conditions much less commonly seen in the general population, such as seizures and aspiration of solids or liquids.

The most recent comprehensive data about cause of death of people with ID in England have come from linking data held by GPs with mortality data. Both Glover et al. (2017) and Hosking et al. (2016) used data from the Clinical Practice Research Database, a large, validated primary care database that has been shown to be representative of the UK population (Herrett et al., 2015). Linkage to Office for National Statistics death certification data provided mortality data for people with and without ID, overall and by cause.

Diseases of the circulatory system were responsible for the largest number of deaths of people with ID in England, accounting for 21.6% of all underlying causes of death (Hosking et al., 2016). Glover et al. (2017) reported that within this category, when compared with the general population, people with ID had more deaths than would be expected from ischaemic heart disease, cerebrovascular disease, phlebitis and thrombophlebitis, cardiomyopathy and pulmonary embolism.

Diseases of the respiratory system were responsible for the second largest number of deaths of people with ID in England, accounting for 18.8% of all underlying causes of death (Hosking et al., 2016). Glover et al. (2017) reported that within this category, the most common cause was pneumonia, followed by pneumonitis due to solids and liquids. The death rates among adults with ID for these two causes were more than ten times higher than were rates among matched controls (Hosking et al., 2016).

Neoplasms were responsible for the third largest number of deaths of people with ID in England, accounting for 14.9% of underlying causes of death (Hosking et al., 2016). What is of interest here is the different distribution of types of cancer in people with ID compared with the general population. Glover et al. (2017) reported that within this category, when compared with the general population, people with ID had more deaths than would be expected from malignant neoplasms of the digestive organs, particularly cancers of the colon and rectum, and cancers of the uterine body.

In addition to exploring the ICD chapters accounting for the largest numbers of deaths of people with ID, Glover et al. (2017) also looked for any other causes that were responsible for 2% or more of deaths of people with ID. The three other causes identified were dementia (of unspecified type), epilepsy and infantile cerebral palsy.

8.5.2 Potentially Avoidable Deaths, and Those Amenable to Good-Quality Care

The concept of avoidable deaths is based on the assumption that 'premature deaths from certain conditions should be rare, and ideally should not occur in the presence of timely and effective health care' (Office for National Statistics, 2016: S16). Identifying some deaths as avoidable was originally designed to highlight areas of potential weaknesses in healthcare that could benefit from further in-depth investigation. The Office for National Statistics categorises deaths as avoidable if they are preventable, amenable (treatable) or both.

Preventable deaths are those that could largely be avoided by public health interventions in the broadest sense. Amenable deaths are those where, in the light of medical knowledge and technology at the time of death, all or most deaths from that cause (subject to age limits if appropriate) could be avoided through good-quality healthcare. Table 8.2 summarises the Office for National Statistics definitions.

Heslop et al. (2013), using data from CIPOLD, first reported an excess of deaths of people with ID that were potentially avoidable by reason of being amenable to good-quality care, as categorised by the Office for National Statistics. CIPOLD data indicated that 36.5%

Table 8.2 Office for National Statistics categories of avoidable deaths

Preventable deaths	Amenable deaths
A death is preventable if, in the light of understanding of the determinants of health at the time of death, all or most deaths from that cause (subject to age limits if appropriate) could be avoided by public health interventions in the broadest sense	A death is amenable (treatable) if, in the light of medical knowledge and technology available at the time of death, all or most deaths from that cause (subject to age limits if appropriate) could be avoided through good-quality healthcare
Avoidable deaths	
All those defined as preventable, amenable (treatable) or both, where each death is counted only once; where a cause of death is both preventable and amenable, all deaths from that cause are counted in both categories when they are presented separately	

of deaths of people with ID could have been avoided through good-quality healthcare, compared with just 13% in the general population.

Hosking et al. (2016) undertook a similar analysis based on national linked data, also reporting a higher percentage of deaths amenable to good-quality care among people with ID (37%), than among matched controls (22.5%). The most prominent causes of amenable deaths in people with ID reported by Glover et al. (2017) were deaths from congenital malformations, deformations and chromosomal anomalies, and deaths from pneumonia, ischaemic heart disease, epilepsy and cerebrovascular disease; however, Hosking et al. (2016) cautioned that the current categories of amenable deaths do not include some important treatable causes of deaths in people with ID, such as urinary tract infections or aspiration, and thus 'are likely to underestimate the true burden of amenable mortality' in this population (Hosking et al., 2016: 1488).

The issue of potentially amenable deaths is one of national importance, and particularly so for those supporting the health of people with ID. A number of reasons have been proposed as to why there is such a disparity between people with ID and the general population in this respect. Arguably the best insights into this come from in-depth case reviews of the circumstances leading to deaths. The deaths reviewed as part of CIPOLD indicated three important factors that were related to deaths amenable to good-quality care: a lack of reasonable adjustments to help people to access health services; a lack of coordination of care across and between different disease pathways and service providers; and a lack of effective advocacy.

8.6 Reducing Premature Deaths in People with ID

The CIPOLD team proposed that there were four key factors that professionals should consider for helping reduce premature mortality.

8.6.1 Identify People with ID, Anticipate Their Likely Needs and Make Reasonable Adjustments

A significant issue identified in the reviews of deaths conducted by CIPOLD was the lack of identification that a person had ID in any referral letters or records, and a resulting lack of the provision of 'reasonable adjustments' to their care as is required for all disabled people under the Equality Act 2010. 'Flagging' that a person has ID in their health and care records should lead to an individual assessment of their needs and the identification of what reasonable adjustments are required for the person to be able to access any health or care services. Adjustments such as longer appointment times, familiarisation visits to hospital departments or the attendance of a specialist liaison nurse at appointments to ensure that the person understands their condition and treatment can be vital for people with ID.

8.6.2 Diagnose and Treat Illness Quickly

CIPOLD reported significant concerns about delays in the care pathways of people who had died. The majority of people with ID had been identified as unwell prior to their death and sought medical attention in a timely way. Where problems then arose was in the diagnosis and treatment of their illness. Particular recommendations from the CIPOLD study included treating people with ID as a high-risk group for deaths from respiratory problems, being cautious if 'watching and waiting' to see how an illness develops and proactively referring the person to specialist ID services for advice and support if there are any problems in diagnosing or treating the person's illness.

8.6.3 Coordinate Care and Share Information Appropriately

A striking finding of the CIPOLD reviews of deaths was the multiplicity and complexity of clinical conditions that people with ID had. This resulted in people's needs being served by a range of different specialists, sometimes in different hospitals, with no designated or responsible coordinator for their care, thus limiting the opportunity for a holistic focus on their health and effective coordination of the different specialists involved. Ensuring good coordination of care across and between different disease pathways and service providers is essential when supporting people with ID who may be unable to do so for themselves. For those with complex or multiple needs, multi-morbidity or long-term health conditions and living with little support in the community, a named healthcare coordinator is advisable. It is also vital for practitioners to look at the whole picture and overall pattern of a person's illnesses, not just single discrete episodes of illness, so that, for example, recurrent chest infections suggesting problems aspirating food or fluids can be identified early.

8.6.4 Listen to People with ID and Their Family and Carers

An important aspect of responding appropriately and effectively to the health needs of people with ID is to have a good understanding of them as a person, as well as their medical histories. Listening to the views of the person and their family is crucial to this. However, CIPOLD reported that family members (and paid carers) often struggled to get their voice heard when they tried to advocate for their family member, feeling ignored, dismissed or lacking credibility. Recognising people with ID, family and paid carers as partners in care alongside healthcare professionals is vital; they have expert knowledge of the person, and this knowledge should be utilised respectfully and carefully. Table 8.3 summarises these recommendations.

8.7 Summary

Mortality surveillance exposes significant health inequalities in access to healthcare for children and adults with ID. It is important to monitor their healthcare, particularly because

Table 8.3 Key factors that professionals should consider for helping reduce premature mortality in people with ID

(1) Identify people with ID, anticipate their likely needs and make reasonable adjustments
(2) Diagnose and treat illness quickly
(3) Coordinate care and share information appropriately
(4) Listen to people with ID and their family and carers

deinstitutionalisation in both developed and developing countries allows the potential for people with ID to become hidden and their support poorly resourced in the community while more populist healthcare concerns are addressed by national governments. In England the Learning Disabilities Mortality Review (LeDeR) Programme aims to make improvements to the lives of people with ID. It clarifies any potentially modifiable factors associated with a person's death and works to ensure that these are not repeated elsewhere. For further information, see www.bristol.ac.uk/sps/leder.

References

Arvio, M., Salokivi, T., Tiitinen, A. & Haataja, L. (2016) Mortality in individuals with intellectual disabilities in Finland. *Brain and Behavior*, 6, e00431. Available at: http://onlinelibrary.wiley.com/doi/10.1002/brb3.431/epdf [accessed 24 November 2016]

Barbieri, J. S., Fuchs, B. D., Fishman, N. et al. (2013) The mortality review committee: A novel and scalable approach to reducing inpatient mortality. *Joint Commission Journal on Quality and Patient Safety*, 39, 9, 387–95.

Glover, G. & Ayub, M. (2010). *How People with Learning Disabilities Die*. Improving Health & Lives: Learning Disabilities Observatory. Available at: www.improvinghealthandlives.org.uk/publications/928/How_people_with_learning_disabilities_die [accessed 24 November 2016]

Glover, G., Williams, R., Heslop, P., Oyinlola, J. & Grey, J. (2017) Mortality in people with intellectual disabilities in England. *Journal of Intellectual Disability Research*, 61(1), 62–74.

Herrett, E., Gallagher, A. M., Bhaskaran, K. et al. (2015) Data resource profile: Clinical Practice Research Datalink (CPRD). *International Journal of Epidemiology*, 4(3), 827–36.

Heslop, P., Blair, P. S., Fleming, P., Hoghton, M., Marriott, A. & Russ, L. (2013). *Confidential Inquiry into Premature Deaths of People with Learning Disabilities (CIPOLD): Final Report.* Norah Fry Research Centre, University of Bristol.

Heslop, P., Blair, P. S., Fleming, P., Hoghton, M., Marriott, A. & Russ, L. (2014) The Confidential Inquiry into premature deaths of people with intellectual disabilities in the UK: A population-based study. *The Lancet*, 383(9920), 889–95.

Heslop, P., Lauer, E. & Hoghton, M. (2015) Mortality in people with intellectual disabilities. *Journal of Applied Research into Intellectual Disabilities*, 28, 367–72.

Hollins, S., Attard, M., van Fraunhofer, N., McGuigan, S. M. & Sedgwick, P. (1998). Mortality in people with learning disability: Risks causes, and death certification findings in London. *Developmental Medicine and Child Neurology*, 40(1), 50–6.

Hosking, F. J., Carey, I. M., Shah, S. M. et al. (2016) Mortality among adults with intellectual disability in England: Comparisons with the general population. *American Journal of Public Health*, 106 (8), 1483–90. doi: 10.2105/AJPH.2016.303240

Landes, S. D & Peek, C. W. (2013) Death by mental retardation? The influence of ambiguity on death certificate coding error for adults with intellectual disability. *Journal of Intellectual Disability Research*, 57(12), 1183–90.

Lauer, E. (2016) (2012–13) *Mortality Report.* Available at: http://shriver.umassmed.edu/sites/shriver.umassmed.edu/files/2012-13%20DDS%20Mortality%20Report%20Final_v2.pdf [accessed 24 November 2016]

Lauer E. & Bonardi, A. (2013). Utility of mortality surveillance in adults with intellectual and developmental disabilities. Presented at American Public Health Association 141st Annual Meeting & Expo, Boston, MA.

Lauer, E., Heslop, P. & Hoghton, M. (2015) Identifying and addressing disparities in mortality: US and UK perspectives. In *International Review of Research in Developmental Disabilities: Health Disparities and Intellectual Disabilities* (eds. Chris Hatton & Eric Emerson), pp. 195–245. Elsevier.

McCarron, M., Carroll, R., Kelly, C. & McCallion, P. (2015) Mortality rates in the general Irish population compared to those with an intellectual disability from 2003 to 2012. *Journal of Applied Research in Intellectual Disabilities*, **28**, 406–13.

Mazars (2015) *Independent Review of Deaths of People with a Learning Disability or Mental Health Problem in Contact with Southern Health NHS Foundation Trust April 2011 to March 2015.* Available at: www.england.nhs.uk/south/wp-content/uploads/sites/6/2015/12/mazars-rep.pdf [accessed 24 November 2016]

Mencap (2007) *Death by Indifference.* Available at: www.mencap.org.uk/sites/default/files/documents/2008-03/DBIreport.pdf [accessed 24 November 2016]

Mencap (2012) *Death by Indifference: 74 deaths and counting. A Progress Report 5 Years on.* Available at: www.mencap.org.uk/sites/default/files/documents/Death%20by%20Indifference%20-%2074%20Deaths%20and%20counting.pdf [accessed 24 November 2016]

Michael, J. (2008) *Healthcare for All: Report of the Independent Inquiry into Access to Healthcare for People with Learning Disabilities.* Department of Health. Available at: http://webarchive.nationalarchives.gov.uk/20130107105354/http:/www.dh.gov.uk/prod_consum_dh/groups/dh_digitalassets/@dh/@en/documents/digitalasset/dh_106126.pdf [accessed 24 November 2016]

National Patient Safety Agency (2004) *Understanding the Patient Safety Issues for People with Learning Disabilities.* Available at: www.nrls.npsa.nhs.uk/resources/clinical-specialty/learning-disabilities/?entryid45=59823&p=2 [accessed 24 November 2016]

National Patient Safety Agency (2007) *Problems Swallowing? Ensuring Safer Practice for Adults with Learning Disabilities Who Have Dysphagia.*

Available at: www.nrls.npsa.nhs.uk/resources/?entryid45=59823 [accessed 24 November 2016]

NHS Clinical Commissioning Group (2013) CCG outcomes indicator set. Available at: http://content.digital.nhs.uk/catalogue/PUB11718/ccg-ind-toi-sep-13-toi.pdf [accessed 24 November 2016]

NHS Digital (2016) Health and care of people with learning disabilities experimental statistics, 2014–15. Available at: www.content.digital.nhs.uk/catalogue/PUB22607/Health-care-learning-disabilities-2014-15-summary.pdf [accessed 24 November 2016]

Office for National Statistics (2016) Avoidable mortality in England and Wales: 2014. Available at: www.ons.gov.uk/peoplepopulationandcommunity/healthandsocialcare/causesofdeath/bulletins/avoidablemortalityinenglandandwales/2014 [accessed 24 November 2016]

Ouellette-Kuntz, H., Shooshtari, S., Balogh, R. & Martens, P. (2015) Understanding information about mortality among people with intellectual and developmental disabilities in Canada. *Journal of Applied Research in Intellectual Disabilities*, **28**, 423–35.

Parliamentary and Health Service Ombudsman (2009) *Six Lives: The Provision of Public Services to People with Learning Disabilities.* Stationery Office. Available at: www.ombudsman.org.uk/_data/assets/pdf_file/0013/1408/six-lives-part1-overview.pdf [accessed 24 November 2016]

Rutstein, D. D., Berenberg, W., Chalmers, T. C., Child, C. G., Fishman, A. P. & Perrin, E. B. (1976) Measuring the quality of healthcare: A clinical method. *New England Journal of Medicine*, **294**, 582–8.

Shattuck, L. (1850) *Report of the Sanitary Commission of Massachusetts.* Available at: www.deltaomega.org/documents/shattuck.pdf [accessed 24 November 2016].

Stoddart, S., Griffiths, E. & Lilford, R. (2005) *A Confidential Inquiry into Excess Mortality in Learning Disability. Scoping Report to the National Patient Safety Agency.* University of Birmingham.

Szreter, S. (1991) The General Register Office and the Public Health Movement in Britain, 1837–1914. *Social History of Medicine*, **4**, 465–94.

Tyrer, F. & McGrother, C. (2009) Cause-specific mortality and death certificate reporting in adults with moderate to profound intellectual disability. *Journal of Intellectual Disability Research*, **53**, 898–904.

World Health Organization (1992) *International Statistical Classification of Diseases and Related Health Problems: 10th Revision* (vol. II). Available at: www.who.int/classifications/icd/en [accessed 24 November 2016]

Section 3 Psychiatric and Behavioural Disorders

Chapter 9

Children with Intellectual Disabilities and Psychiatric Problems

Pru Allington-Smith

9.1 Introduction

We know that 40% of people who have an intellectual disability (ID) develop significant behavioural problems (Emerson & Hatton, 2007) during their lifetime. These problems often start early in life and if not addressed during the developmental period can become entrenched and extremely difficult to treat by the time the individual reaches adulthood.

Within the United Kingdom services for children with an ID now lie within CAMHS (Child and Adolescent Mental Health Services); in the past it was more usual to have lifespan ID services. The move is largely welcome as it emphasises that all children should be able to access mental health services and not be discriminated against by virtue of their disability. The change has, however, not been without its problems. Hard-pressed CAMHS services have been asked to accept this group of patients with very little extra funding and with a shortage of skilled professionals to do the work. Although most CAMHS professionals are comfortable working with young people with a mild ID, many lack the skills to work with non-verbal children, who may present with very difficult behaviours and they often struggle to recognise how mental illness presents in these children.

The situation continues to improve but there are still areas where services remain poor and all too often parents are turned away when they try to seek help. When services fail, the result all too often, is a child moving away from home into vastly expensive care settings with little prospect of moving back home. If some of the funds spent on paying for these placements were invested into skilled local services, many more children would be able to remain within their homes and communities.

Working with children and their families is highly rewarding. Children have the greatest capacity to change, and parents are usually motivated to engage with the therapist. Relatively little is done directly with the child, as more often it is by working with their families, their teachers and all those who help care for the child that change can be effected. Individual work can be invaluable in some circumstances, but for the most part, more is accomplished by influencing the management strategies of those around the young person.

Education is a key part of this, working with the parents and wider family to understand the reason why the child behaves as it does, and by giving them the management strategies to change behaviours for the better. Helping parents understand autism, where present, is particularly important. Parents may also overestimate or underestimate what their child is capable of, and communicate with them at a level that the child cannot fully comprehend. Parents often need help to utilise objects, photographs or symbols alongside speech to aid understanding. These communication strategies will help the young person to be able to start indicating their needs in a more appropriate manner.

Support to families has to start early in order to detect those children who are at high risk of developing serious behavioural issues. These include children who self-injure, those with syndromes we know are associated with high rates of difficult behaviours such as Smith–Magenis, Cornelia de Lange and Prader–Willi syndromes, to name but a few. Another high-risk group are children with severe autism who have no functional communication. Parents may need help to learn how to interact with their children and encourage them to play. Behaviours become harder to change as the child grows older and bigger and are especially difficult once a child can physically overpower their parents.

Aggression is one of the most common presenting complaints in a clinic situation. Thinking about why this is helps with management. Getting our needs and wants met is a basic drive in all of us. As we get older we learn to communicate these needs, to find our own ways to satisfy them and to gain a degree of autonomy. A child with an ID may have little or no speech to ask for what they need. They cannot always successfully problem-solve well and may rely on adults to help them. If they also have an autism spectrum disorder (ASD), then they may be especially poor at verbal and non-verbal communication.

Without useful communication, crying, screaming or hitting gets attention from the adult who then has to try and work out what the child is after. If they guess successfully, the child may repeat the behaviour when they want something else. Aggression can become the child's main form of communication especially if their desires continue to be fulfilled by the parent in response. Normally developing youngsters can also be aggressive but slowly learn to model their behaviour on their peers and learn alternative strategies to get what they want. They also realise that their behaviour causes distress to others.

A child with an ID, especially if they also have ASD, will usually not model their behaviour on others. Those with ASD may lack theory of mind/empathy and will not know that they are causing distress. Aggression is one of the few skills that such a child can perform as well as their normally developing peers and they will keep on employing strategies that work successfully for them to get their needs met. Under these circumstances they will not give up violence as a strategy unless they are taught other more adaptive and socially acceptable ways to get what they are after. The problem, predictably, gets a lot worse when the child is big enough to overpower the adults, especially if the parent's main management technique, up until this point, has been to simply employ physical means of control without offering an alternative communication solution.

Self-injury is seen as self-directed aggression and may develop very early in some youngsters. Children with additional sensory impairments or specific syndromes are at particularly high risk. The behaviour may fulfil a sensory need for stimulation, be in response to physical pain or it may become a form of communication, in a particular situation, that the child wants something. Most parents will respond immediately to a child who is hurting themselves and then try to second-guess why the child is distressed. As time goes on, the behaviours may generalise and be shown whenever the child wants anything at all from the parent. The longer the behaviours go on, the harder it is to intervene successfully. Early behavioural intervention in self-injury is vital but, sadly, all too often is unavailable.

9.2 Family Issues

The birth of a disabled child is a devastating event for any parent and usually results in them going through a grieving process for the child they were expecting. Nearly all will come to terms with what has happened quickly, but a few may take a long time. This grief may resurface at significant milestones which emphasise societal expectation with reality.

A failure to negotiate grief may show itself in an unwillingness to accept the child's level of functioning, with resultant unrealistic expectations placed upon the young person. A few parents will seek tirelessly for a cure, spending all their time and energy scouring the internet for the latest breakthrough or raising money to send the child for the latest radical treatment, but sometimes avoiding spending time with their offspring. Time spent helping the parent to understand their child's needs and encouraging them to play with the child can make a big difference.

Having a child with an ID may make it much harder for parents to work and many do struggle financially and have housing difficulties. Practitioners need to keep these potential issues firmly in mind when dealing with families. A parent facing imminent eviction is not going to be able to concentrate on behavioural strategies. Signposting to social services, housing and voluntary services may be a more important action.

Some parents will themselves have an ID and/or mental illness and will need a lot of support to overcome behavioural difficulties in their children. Working closely with social services with such families is essential. Social care may be able to provide sessional or residential respite care for parents through personal budgets and ensure that they are receiving the correct benefits to which they are entitled.

Where there are child protection concerns balancing the needs of the parent with the needs of the child, it is the latter which must take precedence. Physical and sexual abuse and neglect are more common in children with ID reflecting their vulnerability and often their inability to protect themselves or speak up about what is happening to them. Particularly difficult situations can arise with a child who is significantly more able than their parent where it is often the parent who is at risk.

Parenting groups are an important cornerstone of treatment strategies. Structured courses such as Triple P (Positive Parenting Programme) and the Cygnet (education on autism for children diagnosed after school age; see Stuttard et al. (2016)) are generally very well received. Generally, joining with parents of normal ability children, whose needs are often very different, is not successful.

Work with parents may be clinic based but community nurses often favour working in the home particularly when modelling appropriate behaviour with the child for the parent. Flexibility to work with the child in all its environments is a hallmark of a successful service. The psychiatrist is more likely to be clinic based because of time constraints but school clinics are a good option and allow the child to be observed in a more natural environment. The input of teachers and school nurses there is invaluable.

The needs of siblings can sometimes be overlooked. Many become carers themselves, at an early age, supporting their parents. It is often hard for them to be able to socialise with peers because their parents are unable to take them out. Parents can have enormous expectations of the 'normal' child which are unrealistic. Some siblings feel deeply resentful that their needs are often overlooked by their parent who has to spend all their time with their disabled brother or sister. Young carers groups can be an invaluable source of support and enjoyment for them.

No matter how good a service, there will always be circumstances where either the child's behaviour or the family circumstances make it impossible for the child to continue to be cared for in the family home. Fostering may be possible for some children, but finding skilled foster carers, able to manage challenging children is extremely difficult. Specialist children's homes exist and are more likely to operate in areas where they are offered support by the local children's community learning disability team. Residential schools are often clustered in rural areas where large houses are affordable for conversion and therefore often far from the child's home, making it harder for families to stay in close contact with their child. Once a child is in residential provision, then most will remain out of their families for the remainder of their childhood. The emphasis should be on preventing this from happening by supporting the parents to care for their child.

9.3 School

For most children with an ID, school is a positive experience where they can learn new skills in a supportive environment. Some thrive in a 'special' educational environment and others in mainstream school with support. Around the UK the proportion of children in special schools and those in mainstream schools with additional support varies hugely according to local policies.

Not every child will thrive in a special school, and those that do not may be referred to services with severe anxiety, depression and/or or challenging behaviours. Some children become very fearful of very loud and overbearing classmates to the point that they may be physically sick with fear each morning before school. Others may mimic the behaviours they see in other children.

In a mainstream school setting there may be a place where, on a daily basis, it is clear to the child that they are not like their normally developing peers. Even with dedicated adult support they may not be able to follow the class lesson and become disruptive in order to be able to leave and to go somewhere more enjoyable. The other children in a mainstream environment, at best, protect and support their classmates with ID, particularly when they are young. As the child and his classmates grow, this support usually diminishes and sometimes turns to overt hostility and bullying, especially as the gap in ability between the child and their companions widens. It is not unusual for children to then start refusing to go to school, sometimes resorting to increasingly dramatic behaviours in order to ensure that their parents cannot get them there.

It is more common for children to be excluded from mainstream schools, or even worse be placed on substantially reduced educational hours. Some children are only allowed into school for as little as an hour a day and may then be taught in complete isolation from their peers.

School needs to be a place where every child can learn at the pace that suits them and where they can succeed according to their abilities. It should be a place where the child can make true friendships, not just be looked after. It is also vital that life skills are incorporated into the curriculum as these ultimately will be of more use to a child who does not have the potential to become functionally literate. The school also needs to be a place where teachers have good behavioural techniques and training in teaching children with ASD who especially need structure and predictability. Teachers in most special schools operate in a 'total communication' environment, supported by speech and language therapists, for those children who have little or no verbal ability.

For parents choosing the right sort of school for their child is extremely stressful. Most will quickly recognise when their child is not thriving, but a few will insist on a mainstream environment, even when it is clear that their child is very unhappy. For parents who want their child to change schools the process that they have to go through is a daunting one. The recent introduction of the EHCP (education, health and care plan) in England has been a move to improve the integration of education, social care and health needs for young people up to the age of 25 who have significant special educational needs. Although still in its early stages, it does seem to be improving the coordination of these three statutory services vitally important when dealing with children and young adults. Other jurisdictions have their own laws for educational support, for example, Scotland uses a Co-ordinated Support Plan (CSP) for children with additional support needs (ASN), bringing together social care, education and health; and there is a new Special Educational Needs and Disability Act in Northern Ireland (2016), which will also use an Education Health and Care Plan approach due for implementation in 2019.

9.4 Transition

Most young people in the UK with a substantial ID are entitled to education until the school year in which they become 19 years old. Increasingly many now go on to college courses designed for their needs for up to three years.

Leaving school is often a traumatic time for young adults. For most disabled children, school has been the place where their friends are, where they are treated with respect and where they have had fun. They are often extremely fearful about a new environment and the increasing demands that will be made of them. College placements are seldom full-time, and the young people and their families have to cope with the extra unoccupied time.

Around the same time that they are in their final year at school there may be other major changes. A new doctor to see, a new social worker and for some young adults a move away from home to some form of supported accommodation. It is not surprising therefore that these years are a peak time for the emergence of psychiatric illness.

In an ideal world, transition planning should start at 14 years of age with initial discussion with parents and the young person as to what they would like for their future. Person-centred planning is an excellent way to do this. All too often though the process is started much later and may not even be concluded until after the young person has left school.

There is a risk that young people will be lost to services at transfer. Joint appointments with the adult services before transfer will reduce that risk. Transition clinics held in special schools where child and adult ID professionals and community paediatricians meet together with parents and children, work well.

9.5 The Community Children's ID Team

Guidance for providing a psychiatric service for children with an ID can be had in the Royal College of Psychiatrists (2016) CR 200 report.

The mainstay of most multidisciplinary teams is usually community nurses, clinical psychologists and the psychiatrist. A dedicated speech and language therapist and sensory trained occupational therapist are also highly recommended. The team may be embedded in a wider CAMHS team or operate semi-independently.

Many of the children seen by the team will have chronic issues and may need interventions at various times in their childhood, particularly around times of transition. The move between primary and secondary school is often when children present to services for the first time. Going from a small school where they spend the majority of their time with one teacher and their classmates to a huge school where they are expected to move around the school independently and be taught by a large number of teachers is a significant change which many youngsters with ID find too difficult, resulting in them becoming anxious and school avoidant.

Liaison with education, social services and other health professionals especially paediatricians is a major part of the work. Children are seen in a variety of settings including their home, respite services and in school. In practice most schools have little input from educational psychologists who have to use their limited hours doing assessments rather than being able to support schools around serious behavioural difficulties.

The functions of a service include diagnosis and assessment, counselling for the young person and family work. Specific therapies will include a variety of behavioural and psychodynamic approaches including positive behavioural support, functional analysis and modified cognitive behavioural therapy (CBT).

The speech and language therapist will assess the level of the child's communication and provide appropriate resources for the family to use and guidance on simplifying language and instructions where needed.

The psychiatrist has a particular role in assessment, looking for additional co-morbid conditions such as anxiety, depression, ASD and attention deficit hyperactivity disorder (ADHD) and investigating physical illness as a reason for behavioural difficulties. Where medication is indicated, then they need to supervise this closely.

9.6 Commonly Encountered Problems

Sleep disorders are common in young children with an ID especially if they also have autism. Sleep-onset problems are the most common with the child being unable to wind down enough to sleep. Parents often report having to stay with the child for a couple of hours before they can settle.

Simple sleep hygiene measures such as having regular bed-time routines and a wind-down time free of the TV or computer games can help. If behavioural measures on their own are unsuccessful, then melatonin may be indicated. Once a routine has been established, then it may be possible to withdraw the medication, but many children stay on it for much longer periods. Sleep usually improves around puberty and by then medication is needed much less often.

Medication for sleep is generally ineffective where a child goes to sleep well but then wakes repeatedly. Behavioural measures are generally successful if implemented consistently, but environmental issues and possible physical disorders, causing discomfort, need to be considered.

9.6.1 ASD

The majority of children who have an ID referred to a child psychiatrist with serious behavioural issues are likely also to have ASD (author's own audit). Screening for this condition is therefore vital. Not all young people with ASD will avoid eye contact; some will be very friendly and chatty. Others will have no obvious signs of ASD-like behaviour, but elements of the history will suggest that screening is necessary. The method of diagnosis will depend on what is agreed locally, or on the practitioner's training. Many children with ASD will have significant problems with anxiety and this may underlie behavioural problems. Poor communication and sensory problems can also be key to understanding the behavioural presentation.

9.6.2 ADHD

ADHD is relatively common and should be thought about with any child struggling with behaviour and attention in school. Unfortunately, there is no ADHD screening tool specific to ID. The existing tools based on a normal population sample will show if the behaviours are pervasive across home and school and can be useful when taken in conjugation with a good clinical history and bearing in mind the ability level of the young person. Appropriate treatment of ADHD can have a huge impact on the child's ability to learn and on their behaviour. It is sometimes impossible to tell whether a child, with a severe ID and autism and who cannot settle, has treatable ADHD. Under such circumstances a closely observed trial of a stimulant medication such as methylphenidate may be indicated.

Non-stimulant treatment of ADHD can be very helpful in those children where the home behaviour is more problematic than in school. It is also indicated in those children with an ID, autism and ADHD in whom behaviour is especially difficult as stimulant medication is wearing off.

9.6.3 Epilepsy

Epilepsy is much more common in children with an ID and may present with inattention or behavioural problems. Anti-epileptic medications may also be associated with problematic behaviours as a result of side effects. While the psychiatrist may not be managing the epilepsy, they should be aware of the diagnosis and the treatment in order to take these into account when assessing the child.

9.6.4 Tics and Tourette's Syndrome

Tics and Tourette's syndrome are not uncommon as in the mainstream population. There is an overlap with all of the neurodevelopmental conditions, including ADHD and ASD. Where things differ is that the tics are often more distressing for the parent to witness than the child to experience. Where the child is distressed, behavioural measures such as utilising competing responses can be tried, or medication can be considered, however, this is rarely needed.

9.6.5 Depression

Depression, it is rare for less able children to be able to voice depressive thoughts; fortunately, suicidal ideas or behaviours are rare. Most children present with withdrawn behaviour, persistent lack of enjoyment and sometimes an increase in stereotypical behaviour. However, depression may manifest itself as restlessness and irritability. Anhedonia (lack of enjoyment in a previously favoured activity) is a fairly constant symptom. Biological features of depression such as early morning wakening may be present. A good question to ask is when the child last smiled. More able children may benefit from modified CBT, but others will usually require antidepressants.

9.6.6 Anxiety

Simple phobias are common in children, but some may cause significant problems. It is not uncommon to come across children who have been knocked down by a car running away, in terror, from a dog. Treatment is usually by graded exposure, although it can take considerably longer than with normally developing children. Anxiety management techniques can be taught to many children but need to be repeatedly rehearsed as children may struggle to apply the techniques when they are needed.

Anxiety levels in children with autism are usually very high. Heightened anxiety may show itself with a worsening of repetitive questioning and a reluctance to go out. The child may 'play up' and refuse to leave the house or even strip off their clothes so that being made to go out is impossible. Some children may be so anxious that they will vomit. Preparing the child for where they are going using pictures or symbols can help as can ending the trip with a known pleasurable activity as an incentive. The child may need a timetable to help them understand their day. Social stories which personalise what is going to happen and what the child will be expected to do when out can also be very useful. These may use words, symbols or pictures depending on the child's level of understanding, but require that it is communicated in the same way by all. In some children sensory strategies can be effective in reducing anxiety. These may include weighted rucksacks, hug vests or by including strenuous activities into the timetable before the child is expected to settle to work in the classroom. Assessment by a suitably qualified sensory practitioner is advised.

Only when communication, behavioural, environmental and, where indicated, sensory measures have been unsuccessful in managing the child's anxiety should medication be considered. This is especially true when the anxiety is significantly impacting on their life or where there is risky aggression or self-injury.

9.6.7 Medication

Medication that reduces anxiety is the mainstay of drug treatment. In the history it is important to look for the links between behaviour and stress-inducing situations. If these are not present and the young person's behaviour is more about trying to control their environment and family or to get at things they want, then medication may be less effective. It should go without saying that medication should only be used in anxiolytic doses and never to sedate the child.

In autism, as anxiety is usually a chronic condition, medication often ends up being given long term. This has serious implications in terms of inevitable dose escalation over time and the risk of significant side effects. There is serious concern about the number of people with an ID who end up on medication for behavioural reasons with no evidence for its efficacy in the long term. In the short term though, it has its place in serious situations where the young person is a significant risk to themselves or to others or where behaviour risks them having to move out of the home. Before embarking on medication, practitioners need to have a long conversation with parents about the risks and alternative options. If medication is to be used, it must be closely monitored and only continued if there is clearly a positive response. There is no role for the use of benzodiazepines in chronic anxiety as dependence and loss of efficacy will occur in a short time.

Neuroleptic medications such as risperidone and aripiprazole can be useful in very small doses, but these also have a significant risk of side effects such as weight gain, sedation and extra pyramidal side effects such as muscle stiffness and spasm. Aripiprazole is often used as it is slightly less likely to result in major weight gain. However, it can cause akathisia, a sense of inner restlessness which is particularly hard to detect in children who have a severe ID. The lowest dose possible of the neuroleptic should be started and not escalated quickly. Screening bloods and an electrocardiogram prior to treatment are good practice if the child is able to cooperate.

It is often better to start with alternatives such as beta blockers or the selective serotonin reuptake inhibitors (SSRI) antidepressants. Beta blockers can be very helpful in less able children who have obvious physical symptoms of anxiety. By blocking many of the somatic symptoms of anxiety beta blockers can sometimes prevent anxiety escalating into externalized behaviours such as aggression.

SSRI antidepressants have good properties against anxiety and seem to be particularly helpful in more able young people with autism and symptoms of social anxiety. When given as a liquid it is possible to start at a low dose and titrate up to an effective dose.

9.6.8 Self-talk

Self-talk – failure to internalise our thoughts – is a developmental phenomenon. In early childhood we stop saying everything we are thinking and choose when to speak our thoughts. Some children with an ID never attain this developmental stage or revert to it when under stress. These children are occasionally referred to psychiatric services querying auditory hallucinations. Self-talk is particularly common in people who have Down syndrome. The most common scenario is a young person who returns from school and goes straight to their bedroom. Their parent then hears their child having an animated conversation with himself/herself. This conversation is usually a re-enactment of an encounter the child had earlier that day that didn't go well. This time round the child either changes the ending to suit them better or tells the other person off in the heated tones they didn't use the first time round.

9.6.9 Psychosis

Early onset psychosis is fortunately rare in young people and usually presents with hallucinations which can be in any modality (auditory, visual or tactile) paranoia and a significant change in personality and functioning. Children with autism and those who have had suffered significant life events are particularly at risk. Many go on to develop schizoaffective-type picture and end up needing antipsychotic medication and a mood stabiliser. Epilepsy should be thought about in the differential diagnoses.

9.6.10 Atypical Mood Disorders

Some children being presented to services turn out, on questioning, to go through phases of agitated and overactive behaviour associated with a decreased need for sleep and/or periods when they become withdrawn and sleep more than usual. In between, they may be settled for a few weeks or months. The information about times when behaviour is fine is often not volunteered by parents who are understandably keen for the therapist to understand the seriousness of the difficult phases. Where such a history is present, it is useful for the parent to keep a mood and sleep diary. Treatment with a mood stabiliser such as carbamazepine, sodium valproate or lamotrigine may help such young people. Lithium is rarely used because of the need for frequent blood tests in the early stages of therapy.

9.7 Conclusion

Working with young people who have an ID and their families is very rewarding. Seeing young people improve and gain in confidence is a wonderful thing. We get to know some families very well and develop a good working relationship with schools, social care and our paediatric colleagues.

Contrary to most people's expectations there is a lot that can be done to improve the lives of our patients and their families. But we need to continue to struggle to get the resources we require to carry out our work within hard-pressed CAMHS services and to maintain our strong bonds with adult ID services.

References

Emerson, E. & Hatton, C. (2007) Mental health of children and adolescents with intellectual disabilities in Britain. *British Journal of Psychiatry*, **191**, 493–9.

Stuttard, L. et al. (2016) An evaluation of the Cygnet parenting support programme for parents of children with autism spectrum conditions. *Research in Autism Spectrum Disorders*, 23 March, pp. 166–78.

Royal College of Psychiatrics (2016) CR200. Psychiatric services for young people with intellectual disabilities. Available at: www.rcpsych.ac.uk/usefulresources/publications/collegereports/cr/cr200.aspx [accessed 11 August 2018]

Triple P [Positive Parenting Programme] available at: www.triplep-parenting.uk.net/uk-en/blog-and-videos/blogs-and-news/post/triple-p-programme-shown-to-help-families-of-kids-with-disabilities [accessed 11 August 2018]

Further Reading

Bernard, S. & Turk, J. (eds.) (2009) *Developing Mental Health Services for Children and Adolescents with Learning Disabilities: A Toolkit for Clinicians*. Royal College of Psychiatrists. Available at: www.rcpsych.ac.uk/PDF/DevMHservCALDbk.pdf [accessed 11 August 2018]

Department for Education, Department of Health (2015) *Special Educational Needs and Disability Code of Practice: 0–25 Years*. Stationery Office. Available at: www.gov.uk/government/publications/send-code-of-practice-0-to-25 [accessed 11 August 2018]

National Autism Society www.autism.org.uk/about/strategies/social-stories-comic-strips.aspx [accessed 11 August 2018]

National Institute for Health and Care Excellence (2015) *Challenging Behaviour and Learning Disabilities: Prevention and Interventions for People with Learning Disabilities Whose Behaviour Challenges* (NG11). Available at: www.nice.org.uk/guidance/ng11 [accessed 11 August 2018]

— (2015) *Learning Disabilities: Challenging Behaviour* (QS101). Available at: www.nice.org.uk/guidance/qs101 [accessed 11 August 2018]

Chapter 10
Adults with Intellectual Disabilities and Psychiatric Disorders

Sally-Ann Cooper

10.1 Introduction

Psychiatric disorders are commonly experienced by adults with intellectual disabilities (ID), and can impact on the quality of life of the person with ID, and that of their family and paid carers. This chapter focuses on the main classes of psychiatric disorders in adults with ID, excepting dementia, autism, forensic psychiatry and specific behavioural phenotypes which feature in other chapters of this book.

Adults with ID can experience all of the types of psychiatric disorders that the rest of the population experience. They require specific consideration because there are distinctions to the rest of the population:

- they are often overlooked, or misattributed to the person's ID or other conditions;
- they typically co-occur with other health conditions and disabilities, making assessment and diagnosis more complex, and with implications for treatment due to drug–drug, drug–disease and disease–disease interactions;
- assessments typically need to include family and paid carers as well as the person with ID, and may require information gathering from several carers or teams of carers;
- the presentation often differs from that found in the general population;
- psychiatric classification systems have been refined specifically for people with ID;
- treatments need to be tailored to their requirements; and
- problem behaviours are common, out of keeping with findings in the general population.

10.2 Epidemiology

Psychiatric disorders are common in adults with ID (Buckles et al., 2013). A wide range of prevalence rates have been reported, and need to be interpreted within the context of each individual study (Smiley, 2005). For example, studies conducted within psychiatric services are likely to overrepresent people with psychiatric conditions; studies conducted within administratively defined populations of people with ID (e.g. people receiving support from local authorities) are more likely to be representative of the wider population of people with ID; while population-based studies are fully representative. However, identifying a full population is not straightforward, as it would require everyone to be assessed for whether or not they had ID. Therefore, there is a compromise between broad-brush assessments of whole populations, or more detailed assessments of people identified to have ID through means likely to identify most of the population.

An example of the latter is a study in Scotland, in which the local population with ID was identified via multiple sources, including GP records; GPs were financially incentivised to identify their population with ID and all in the locality did so (Cooper et al., 2007c). In this study, 1,023 adults with ID were included, and each person had detailed psychiatric assessments, physical health assessments and assessment for ID. It reported that 40.9% of adults had current psychiatric disorders, or 28.3% excluding problem behaviours, or 22.4% excluding both problem behaviours and autism (Cooper et al., 2007c), but does not have a comparison general population rate. In the same study, 22.5% were reported to have problem behaviours (Smiley et al., 2007), and of those, 10% had aggressive behaviour (Cooper et al., 2009b), and 5% had self-injurious behaviour (Cooper et al., 2009a). This is similar to results from previous smaller studies within England (Cooper & Bailey, 2001; Corbett, 1979; Bailey, 2007).

An example of a broad-brush large-scale whole population study is Scotland's Census, 2011. The whole population of Scotland completed a national census on 27 March 2011 (Scotland's Census, 2011); 94% of the population are believed to have a record in the Census. The Census asked the question 'Do you have any of the following conditions which have lasted, or are expected to last, at least 12 months? Tick all that apply.' There was a choice of ten conditions, which included 'intellectual disability (for example, Down's syndrome)', and also explicitly distinguished this from specific learning difficulties such as dyslexia, and autism spectrum disorder, and also included 'mental health conditions'. While this approach is reliant on self- (or proxy) report information, it has the advantage of large-scale coverage, and allows direct comparisons to be drawn between the population with ID and the rest of the population. It found that 5,038/21,115 (23.9%) of adults with ID reported having an additional psychiatric disorder, compared with 224,584/4,357,930 (5.2%) of adults without ID (Scottish Learning Disabilities Observatory, 2016). So a higher rate was found when detailed individual assessments were conducted (Cooper et al., 2007c), although the two studies reported rates that were not that dissimilar, and a direct comparison with the general population could be made using the Census (Scottish Learning Disabilities Observatory, 2016).

Other approaches to reporting prevalence of psychiatric disorders have included using existing cohorts (e.g. birth cohorts). These have the attraction of allowing comparisons with the general population, but in view of their size, tend to include few people with ID, particularly more severe ID; unfortunately, they are prone to differential loss to follow-up of people with ID (Maughan et al., 1999; Richards et al., 2001; Wadsworth et al., 1992).

Other considerations when comparing results from prevalence studies are the disorders included within the studies, particularly whether or not problem behaviours and autism are included, as this can account for substantial differences in reported rates. These disorders also vary with level of ID, as both problem behaviours and autism increase in prevalence with increasing degree of ID.

Other factors that can influence reported prevalence rates include the age of the population (some studies do not separate out children and young people from adults - rates are higher in adults), and the types of assessments and diagnostic criteria used. The classification used influences rates if they are strictly operationalised, particularly for problem behaviours which are not appropriately included in the two standard classificatory manuals, *The ICD-10 Classification of Mental and Behavioural Disorders* (ICD-10; World Health Organization, 1993), and *Diagnostic and Statistical Manual of Mental Disorders* (DSM5; American Psychiatric Association, 2013).

Some particular types of psychiatric disorders are more common in adults with ID than other adults, including problem behaviours (Smiley et al., 2007), dementia (Cooper, 1997; Strydom et al., 2007), autism (Brugha et al., 2017), schizophrenia (Cooper et al., 2007a; Turner, 1989), bipolar affective disorder (Cooper et al., 2007b) and attention deficit hyperactivity disorder (ADHD) (Emerson & Hatton, 2007).

For adults with ID, the most common types of psychiatric disorders experienced are problem behaviours (Cooper et al., 2007c) autism (Baird et al., 2006; Emerson & Hatton, 2007), depression (Cooper et al., 2007b), anxiety disorders (Reid et al., 2011) and schizophrenia (Cooper et al., 2007a), though this does vary with the underlying cause of their ID. For example, affective psychosis is particularly common in adults with Prader–Willi syndrome (Beardsmore et al., 1998; Soni et al., 2007) and dementia in middle-aged adults with Down syndrome (Oliver & Holland 1986; Prasher, 1995). Behavioural phenotypes are detailed in Chapter 3.

10.3 Awareness of Psychiatric Disorders and Diagnostic Overshadowing

Accurate identification of psychiatric disorders is important so the adult with ID:
- can receive appropriate treatment and support;
- does not receive inappropriate treatment needlessly or with potentially harmful consequences; and
- does not have initiation of treatment delayed, which may result in poorer outcomes in the long term, and may cause needless stress in the short term for the person and their carers, in severe cases possibly putting their home and support package at risk.

It is well recognised that psychiatric disorders are under-detected in adults with ID (Hassiotis & Turk, 2012). In view of their communication needs, they may not be able to report distressing symptoms, instead being reliant on their carers to observe that they may have a problem. For paid carers this may be particularly difficult as they may share caring with several adults all with different types of needs, and may not know the individual well, depending upon how long they have worked with the person. A person's baseline behaviours may not be the same as for the average person (e.g. long-standing poor sleep, compulsions or problem behaviours), and hence recognising changes are important, but can be challenging depending upon how well the carers know the person. Piecing together aspects of the person's health and symptoms will be influenced by how well information is shared between carers and care teams (e.g. carers at the person's home, and carers at a day centre), and between staff at night (e.g. sleep problems) and during the day (e.g. appetite problems). Problem behaviours can be a feature of other psychiatric disorders. As problem behaviours can be challenging for carers and can be the focus of considerable carer attention, other symptoms or changes in a person may be overlooked, and not reported to the health professionals, leading to an inaccurate diagnosis and care plan if the professional is not vigilant.

Diagnostic overshadowing – attributing symptoms and signs to the person's ID rather than to the additional health need – is a common phenomenon. This occurs with some paid carers, primary and secondary healthcare professionals; it is an issue throughout the whole system for people with ID, leading to under-recognition and under-treatment of psychiatric disorders.

If an adult with ID changes in their behaviour, loses skills or needs more prompting with tasks, this is likely to indicate onset of a psychiatric disorder (or physical disorder), and they should have a thorough health assessment.

In view of the high levels of untreated health problems in adults with ID, and typically multi-morbidity, England and Wales are currently paying GPs to conduct annual health checks with their registered adults with ID. The National Institute for Health and Care Excellence (NICE) recently published two clinical guidelines for people with ID: one on problem behaviours (NG11; NICE, 2015), and one on psychiatric disorders (NG54; NICE, 2016). One of its recommendations in both guidelines is for annual health checks to be conducted in primary care for adults and young people with ID; the psychiatric disorder guideline (NG54; NICE 2016) specifically states that these should include assessment for psychiatric disorders.

10.4 Assessment

Assessment follows the same principles as for the general population, including history and collateral history, mental state examination, physical examination, investigations, risk assessment, to determine the diagnosis, differential diagnosis, aetiology and to draw up the care plan. However, it is more complex and time-consuming in view of:

- communication needs and understanding;
- the need to always include carers, and for people living with paid carer support to include both paid carers, and family carers (as the family can provide the background information that current paid carers may not know, and may be the key decision makers for adults with ID who do not have capacity to make the decisions around the assessment and treatment options);
- the need to negotiate the care plan with paid carers who are likely to have a role in delivering it, as well as with the adult with ID and their family;
- the cause of ID must always be assessed as it may guide the differential diagnosis and prognosis, and level of ID should be assessed as it affects the presentation of symptoms (e.g. preoccupation with death or guilt is unlikely in a person with a developmental level equivalent to fewer than seven years, i.e. severe or profound ID), and the suitability of treatments and supports (e.g. talking therapies) needs to be considered;
- pre-existing disabilities (e.g. visual and/or hearing impairments which are common) and physical disabilities, which may require specific accommodations during the assessment, and need to influence treatment decisions;
- concomitant neurodevelopmental disorders (e.g. autism and/or ADHD), which can affect the presentation of other psychiatric disorders, and delineation of symptoms (e.g. what is a new symptom, or what is a long-standing symptom or trait);
- pre-existing physical disorders, which are common. For example, epilepsy is common in people with ID; complex partial seizures can be confused with anxiety, anti-epileptic drug side effects can mimic depressive symptoms, many psychotropic drugs lower seizure threshold and so the interplay between these conditions and their treatments need to be understood and monitored. Treatment options also need to consider other disorders, e.g. treatments for osteoporosis may not be tolerated by adults with gastro-oesophageal disorders, both of which are common in people with ID; postural disabilities may affect gastrointestinal disorders and contribute to anxiety; and

- polypharmacy, and, in particular, anticholinergic burden, which can impair cognition, and may result in drug–drug interactions, in addition to adding to the diagnostic complexity.

Co-occurring conditions and polypharmacy are so common that they are the norm for people with ID (Carey et al., 2016; Cooper et al., 2015), and a key reason for the complexity of assessments with people with ID. Indeed, some symptoms are so closely associated that the term ESSENCE has been coined (early symptomatic syndromes eliciting neurodevelopmental clinical examinations; Gillberg, 2010), and genetic information appears to substantiate this (Moreno-De-Luca et al., 2013).

Symptoms are influenced by the level of ID, but the same broad classes of psychiatric disorders can be seen. A study that used exploratory and confirmatory factor analyses on two large datasets of psychopathology in adults with mild-profound ID (n=457; n=274) extracted a model of psychopathology with five factors: depressive, anxiety, cognitive decline, psychosis and affect dysregulation–problem behaviour (Melville et al., 2016a, 2016b). This latter factor was distinct from the depressive and other factors, with good discriminate validity and predictive validity (over a five-year follow-up period). It includes the symptoms of:

- increased physical aggression;
- increased verbal aggression;
- increased mood lability;
- irritable mood;
- diurnal variation – worse in the morning;
- self-harm; and
- specific phobia.

Further details on assessment are provided by Simpson et al. (2016).

10.5 Psychiatric Symptoms and Classification

Psychiatric symptoms can be affected by developmental level. Change in behaviour, and/or loss of skills/requiring more prompting, can be key symptoms of psychiatric disorders. Symptoms requiring complex intellectual functioning or linguistics do not usually feature, such as delusional perception, distorted body image, guilt or preoccupation with death. Psychotic symptoms are usually appropriate to developmental level, so should not be dismissed if they have a childlike quality, the abnormal form is more important diagnostically than the content. Sometimes no background information is available, if there are no family members still in contact with the adult with ID, which presents difficulties in establishing what normal behaviour is for the person, and for meeting age-of-onset restrictions in some categories of standard diagnostic criteria (e.g. autism and ADHD). For these reasons, the *Diagnostic Criteria for Psychiatric Disorders for Use with Adults with Learning Disabilities/Mental Retardation* (DC-LD; Royal College of Psychiatrists, 2001) and *The Diagnostic Manual – Intellectual Disability 2* (DM-ID2; Fletcher et al., 2016) were developed.

DC-LD (Royal College of Psychiatrists, 2001) is a classificatory manual designed to be complementary to the ICD10, is specifically for adults with ID, and particularly those with more severe levels of ID (as the presentation of psychiatric symptoms in adults with mild ID is closer to that seen in the general population). The classification has three axes: severity of

ID, cause of ID and psychiatric diagnosis; with five levels within the psychiatric diagnosis axis: developmental disorders, psychiatric illness, personality disorders, problem behaviours and other disorders. It also provides information on behavioural phenotypes and on associated medical conditions. It provides guidance for the clinician, with diagnosis proceeding through a hierarchy.

DM-ID2 (Fletcher et al., 2016) is a classificatory manual designed to be complementary to DSM-5. It interprets the operationalised criteria within the DSM-5 categories for clinicians working with adults with ID. There are two versions, one also being a textbook, providing updated information on each of the psychiatric disorder categories. The previous edition of DM-ID2 was field-tested and found to have good clinical utility (Fletcher et al., 2016).

10.6 Aetiology

When considering aetiology of psychiatric disorders, a similar framework as for the general population can be followed, with the addition of developmental history (i.e. biological, psychological, social and developmental aetiologies). Often multiple, interacting aetiologies exist, and some of these are transactional; linear cause and effect directions cannot usually be inferred. ACORNS (accessible cause–outcome representation and notation system; Moore & George, 2011) provides a detailed model to conceptualise these factors across dimensions and across the life course. This can be helpful in finding ways to prevent or reduce psychiatric disorders, or to aid recovery.

Behavioural phenotypes are one of the most striking forms of biological/developmental aetiologies for psychiatric disorders; these are considered in more detail in Chapter 3 of this book. While they are genetically determined, treatments can often be helpful.

Other biological factors may be implicated in psychiatric disorders in adults with ID. Some disorders have familial genetic inheritance and so the person may have acquired the condition even if they did not have ID (e.g. schizophrenia). Epilepsy is common in people with ID, and may increase the risk of psychiatric disorders, although research findings are rather mixed on this point. Other physical health problems and pain may increase risk of psychiatric disorders, but, once again, research is limited, and what research there is, is largely with older people with ID. Polypharmacy can also be implicated in psychiatric disorders. There is preliminary evidence that people with ID have higher levels of inflammatory cytokines and increased level of oxidative stress (Carmelli et al., 2012), so these biological mechanisms may be involved in psychiatric disorders in adults with ID. Some personal characteristics also appear to relevant, e.g. with autism and ADHD commencing in childhood and more so in boys than girls, and schizophrenia typically having onset in adulthood.

Psychological factors affect personality development, and experiences in formative years can have lasting affects lifelong. Abuse, neglect or exploitation have been shown to predict incident episodes of psychiatric disorders in adults with ID (Smiley et al., 2007), and low self-esteem is associated with depression in adults with ID (MacMahon & Jahoda, 2008). These factors are all thought to be more common in people with ID than in the general population.

Child–environment transactions are key in developing secure attachments, and forming relationships, and secure and sensitive early relationships are predictors of later psychiatric disorders (Murray et al., 1996). Attentional control is likely to be relevant in children with ID in these transactions.

Social and environmental factors may influence the onset and development of psychiatric disorders. Lone-parent family, poor family functioning, lack of parental educational qualifications, income poverty and households with no paid employment have been shown to be associated with mental health problems in children and young people with ID (Emerson & Hatton, 2007). Additionally, the children and young people were more likely to experience all of these types of social disadvantage. Transactional models are likely to occur – the behaviour of the child with ID affecting the parents' behaviour which in turn affects the child's behaviour.

Life events are associated with, and predictive of, psychiatric disorders in general (Cooper et al., 2007c; Emerson & Hatton, 2007; Hulbert-Williams et al., 2008), depression (Esbensen & Benson, 2006; Hastings et al., 2004) and anxiety (Reid et al., 2011) in particular. Life events are more common for people with ID, and when they do occur they tend to be multiple, for example the death of a parent-carer leading to multiple changes in the person's life and care, move of home and dislocation from former environment, family friends and occupation.

Most adults with ID lack paid employment and some have poverty of environment and recreational opportunities. Adults with ID can be socially excluded, and experience bullying, harassment, stigma and hate crimes, which may impact upon psychiatric disorders (Ali et al., 2012; 2015; Cooney et al., 2006 Jahoda & Markova, 2004).

'A problem shared is a problem halved': adults with ID and communication needs are disadvantaged in this regard. Communication is important in most functions of life, and poses particular difficulties for adults with ID, which can be compounded if the people they are interacting with do not work on reciprocity to maximise understanding and expression. Being dependent upon others in daily tasks can be restrictive upon what an individual can achieve and aspire to, which may impact upon their health.

10.7 Interventions

NG11 (NICE, 2015) outlines the evidence-based treatments for problem behaviours, which are also considered in Chapter 15 of this book. For other types of psychiatric disorders, drug treatments should typically follow those used in the general population (except where there are genetically determined physiological differences), but being mindful that people with ID may not be able to report side effects, and that carers may not observe them until they are more severe. A general guidance would therefore be to monitor carefully, perhaps starting on a lower dose and increasing in smaller increments, with more frequent reviews than for the general population, but being careful to ensure an effective (not sub-therapeutic) dose is ultimately used.

The evidence base for psychological interventions is limited (NG54; NICE, 2016) through lack of research rather than negative trial findings. A sensible approach would be that interventions should be tailored to an individual's need, taking account of their level of ability, communication needs, and other disabilities, and amount of support they have. There is some evidence to suggest that cognitive behaviour therapy-based approaches may be helpful in depression and anxiety, and a recently completed randomised controlled trial suggests that both behavioural activation and guided self-help are useful treatments for depression in adults with ID (Jahoda et al., 2017). Developmental approaches using skills training can be useful adjuncts to the care plans, to help build trusting relationships and build confidence, as well as developing skills.

10.8 Prognosis

Research on the prognosis of psychiatric disorders in people with ID is limited. Longitudinal research with general population cohorts has suggested that anxiety and depressive symptom tend to be more enduring in people with ID (Collishaw et al., 2004; Maughan et al., 1999; Richards et al., 2001); these findings relate to predominantly people with mild ID, given that few with more severe ID are included in these cohorts.

The incidence of psychiatric disorders in adults with ID, excluding problem behaviours, has been reported to be 12.6% over a two-year period; 8.3% for affective disorders, 1.7% for anxiety disorders and 1.4% for psychotic disorders (Cooper et al., 2007a; Smiley et al., 2007). Two-year incidence of aggression was reported as 1.8% and of self-injury 0.6% (Cooper et al., 2009a, 2009b). Full remission of psychosis after two years was only 14.3% (Cooper et al., 2007a), and for aggression it was 27.7% and self-injury 38.2% (Cooper et al., 2009a, 2009b). These findings suggest that while incidences are higher than those found in the general population, much of the current high prevalence of psychiatric disorders is due to enduring disorders, rather than new episodes. The extent to which this is intrinsic to the disadvantages of having ID, or reflects that interventions are not optimised needs to be better understood; either way, improved interventions need to be developed to address this inequity and improve the quality of life of people with ID who have psychiatric disorders.

References

Ali, A., Hassiotis, A., Strydom, A. & King M. (2012) Self stigma in people with intellectual disabilities and courtesy stigma in family carers: A systematic review. *Research in Developmental Disabilities*, **33**, 2122–40.

Ali, A., King, M., Strydom, A. & Hassiotis, A. (2015) Self-reported stigma and symptoms of anxiety and depression in people with intellectual disabilities: Findings from a cross sectional study in England. *Journal of Affective Disorders*, **187**, 224–31.

American Psychiatric Association (2013) *The Diagnostic and Statistical Manual of Mental Disorders* (5th edn). American Psychiatric Publishing.

Bailey, N. (2007) Prevalence of psychiatric disorders in adults with moderate to profound learning disabilities, *Advances in Mental Health and Learning Disabilities*, **1**, 36–44.

Baird, G., Simonoff, E., Pickles, A. et al. (2006) Prevalence of disorders of the autism spectrum in a population cohort of children in South Thames: The Special Needs and Autism Project (SNAP). *The Lancet*, **368**(9531), 210–15.

Beardsmore, A., Dorman, T., Cooper, S.-A. & Webb, T. (1998) Affective psychosis and Prader–Willi syndrome. *Journal of Intellectual Disabilities Research*, **42**, 463–71.

Brugha, T. S., Spiers, N., Bankart, J. et al. (2016) Epidemiology of autism in adults across age groups and ability levels. *British Journal of Psychiatry*, **209**, 498–503.

Buckles, J., Luckasson, R. & Keefe, E. (2013) A systematic review of the prevalence of psychiatric disorders in adults with intellectual disability, 2003–2010. *Journal of Mental Health Research in Intellectual Disabilities*, **6**, 181–207.

Carey, I. M., Shah, S. M., Hosking, F. J. et al. (2016) Health characteristics and consultation patterns of people with intellectual disability: A cross-sectional database study in English general practice. *British Journal of General Practice*, **66**(645), 264–70.

Carmelli, E., Imass, B., Bacher, A. & Merrick, J. (2012) Inflammation and oxidative stress as biomarkers of premature aging in persons with intellectual disability. *Research in Developmental Disabilities*, **33**, 369–75.

Collishaw, G., Maughan, B. & Pickles, A. (2004) Affective problems in adults with mild learning disability: The roles of social disadvantage and ill health. *British Journal of Psychiatry*, **185**, 350–1.

Cooney, G., Jahoda, A., Gumley, A. & Knott, F. (2006) Young people with learning disabilities attending mainstream and segregated schooling:

perceived stigma, social comparisons and future aspirations. *Journal of Intellectual Disability Research*, 50, 432–45.

Cooper, S.-A. (1997) High prevalence of dementia amongst people with learning disabilities not attributed to Down's syndrome. *Psychological Medicine*, 27, 609–16.

Cooper, S.-A. & Bailey, N. M. (2001) Psychiatric disorders amongst adults with learning disabilities – Prevalence and relationship to ability level. *Irish Journal of Psychological Medicine*, 18, 45–53.

Cooper, S.-A., McLean, G., Guthrie, B. et al. (2015) Multiple physical and mental health comorbidity in adults with intellectual disabilities: Population-based cross-sectional analysis. *BMC Family Practice*, doi:10.1186/s12875-015-0329-3

Cooper, S.-A., Smiley, E., Allan, L. et al. (2009a) Adults with intellectual disabilities: Prevalence, incidence and remission of self-injurious behaviour, and related factors. *Journal of Intellectual Disability Research*, 53, 200–16.

Cooper, S-A., Smiley, E., Jackson, A. et al. (2009b) Adults with intellectual disabilities: Prevalence, incidence, and remission of aggressive behaviour, and related factors. *Journal of Intellectual Disability Research*, 53, 217–32.

Cooper, S-A., Smiley, E., Morrison, J. et al. (2007a) Psychosis and adults with intellectual disabilities: Prevalence, incidence, and related factors. *Social Psychiatry and Psychiatric Epidemiology*, 42, 530–6.

Cooper, S-A., Smiley, E., Morrison, J. et al. (2007b) An epidemiological investigation of affective disorders with a population-based cohort of 1,023 adults with intellectual disabilities. *Psychological Medicine*, 37, 873–82.

Cooper, S-A., Smiley, E., Morrison, J. et al. (2007c) Prevalence of and associations with mental ill-health in adults with intellectual disabilities. *British Journal of Psychiatry*, 190, 27–35.

Corbett, J. A. (1979) Psychiatric morbidity and mental retardation. In *Psychiatric Illness and Mental Handicap* (eds F. E. James & R. P. Snaith), pp. 11–25. Gaskell.

Emerson, E. & Hatton C. (2007) Mental health of children and adolescents with intellectual disabilities in Britain. *British Journal of Psychiatry*, 191, 493–9.

Esbensen, A. J. & Benson, B.A. (2006) A prospective analysis of life events, problem behaviours, and depression in adults with intellectual disability. *Journal of Intellectual Disability Research*, 50, 248–58.

Fletcher, R., Barnhill, J. & Cooper, S.-A. (2016) *The Diagnostic Manuel – Intellectual Disability 2* (eds. R. Fletcher, J. Barnhill & S.-A. Cooper). NADD Press.

Fletcher, R., Havercamp, S., Ruedrich, S. et al. (2009) Clinical usefulness of the diagnostic manual-intellectual disability for mental disorders in persons with intellectual disability. *Journal of Clinical Psychiatry*, 70, 967–74.

Gillberg C. (2010) The ESSENCE in child psychiatry: Early symptomatic syndromes eliciting neurodevelopmental clinical examinations. *Research in Developmental Disabilities*, 31, 1543–51.

Hassiotis, A. & Turk, J. (2012) Mental health needs in adolescents with intellectual disabilities: Cross-sectional survey of a service sample. *Journal of Applied Research in Intellectual Disabilities*, 25, 252–61.

Hastings, R. P., Hatton, C., Taylor, J. & Maddison, C. (2004) Life events and psychiatric symptoms in adults with intellectual disabilities. *Journal of Intellectual Disability Research*, 52, 95–106.

Hulbert-Williams, L., Hastings, R. P., Crowe, R. & Pemberton, J. (2011) Self reported life events, social support and psychological problems in adults with intellectual disabilities. *Journal of Applied Research in Intellectual Disabilities*, 24, 427–36.

Jahoda, A., Hastings, R., Hatton, C. et al. (2017) A randomised controlled trial comparing a behavioural activation treatment for depression in adults with intellectual disabilities with guided self-help. *The Lancet Psychiatry*, 4, 909–19.

Jahoda, A. & Markova, I. (2004) Coping with social stigma: People with intellectual disabilities moving from institutions and family home. *Journal of Intellectual Disability Research*, 48, 719–29.

MacMahon, P. & Jahoda, A. (2008) Social comparison in depressed and non-depressed people with mild and moderate intellectual disability. *American Journal on Mental Retardation*, **113**, 307–18.

Maughan, B., Collishaw, S. & Pickles, A. (1999) Mild mental retardation: Psychosocial functioning in adulthood. *Psychological Medicine*, **29**, 351–66.

Melville, C. A., Smiley, E., Simpson, N. et al. (2016b) Statistical modelling studies examining the dimensional structure of psychopathology experienced by adults with intellectual disabilities. Systematic review. *Research in Developmental Disabilities*, **53–4**, 1–10.

Melville, C., McConnachie, A., Johnson, P. et al. (2016a) Problem behaviours and symptom dimensions of psychiatric disorders in adults with intellectual disabilities: An exploratory and confirmatory factor analysis. *Research in Developmental Disabilities*, **55**, 1–13.

Moore, D. G. & George, R. (2011) ACORNS: A tool for the visualisation and modelling of atypical development. *Journal of Intellectual Disability Research*, **55**, 956–72.

Moreno-De-Luca, A., Myers, S. M., Challman, T. D. et al. (2013) Developmental brain dysfunction: Revival and expansion of old concepts based on new genetic evidence. *Lancet Neurology*, **12**, 406–14.

Murray, L., Fiori-Cowley, A., Hooper, R. & Cooper, P. (1996) The impact of postnatal depression and associated adversity on early mother–infant interactions and later infant outcome. *Child Development*, **67**, 2512–26.

NICE (2015) Challenging behaviour and learning disabilities: Prevention and interventions for people with learning disabilities whose behaviour challenges (NG11). Available at: www.nice.org.uk/guidance/ng11 [accessed 9 August 2018]

NICE (2016) Mental health problems in people with learning disabilities: Prevention, assessment and management (NG54). Available at: www.nice.org.uk/guidance/ng54 [accessed 9 August 2018]

Oliver, C. & Holland, A. J. (1986) Down's syndrome and Alzheimer's disease: A review. *Psychological Medicine*, **16**, 307–22.

Prasher, V. P. (1995) Age-specific prevalence, thyroid dysfunction and depressive symptomatology in adults with down syndrome and dementia. *International Journal of Geriatric Psychiatry*, **10**, 25–31.

Reid, K., Smiley, E. & Cooper, S.-A. (2011) Prevalence and associations with anxiety disorders in adults with intellectual disabilities. *Journal of Intellectual Disability Research*, **55**, 172–81.

Richards, M., Maughan, B., Hardy, R. et al. (2001) Long-term affective disorder in people with learning disability. *British Journal of Psychiatry*, **170**, 523–7.

Royal College of Psychiatrists (2001) *DC-LD [Diagnostic Criteria for Psychiatric Disorders for Use with Adults with Learning Disabilities/ Mental Retardation]*. Gaskell Press.

Scotland's Census (2011) www.scotlandscensus.gov.uk/supporting-information [accessed 9 August 2018]

Scottish Learning Disabilities Observatory (2016) www.sldo.ac.uk/census-2011-information/learning-disabilities/topics/health [accessed 9 August 2018]

Simpson, N., Mizen, L., Cooper, S.-A. (2016) Intellectual disabilities. *Medicine*, **44**, 679–82.

Smiley, E. (2005) Epidemiology of mental health problems in adults with learning disability: An update. *Advances in Psychiatric Treatment*, **11**, 214–22.

Smiley, E., Cooper, S-A., Finlayson, J. et al. (2007) The incidence, and predictors of mental ill-health in adults with intellectual disabilities. Prospective study. *British Journal of Psychiatry*, **191**, 313–19.

Soni, S., Whittington, J., Holland, A. J. et al. (2007) The course and outcome of psychiatric illness in people with Prader–Willi syndrome: Implications for management and treatment. *Journal of Intellectual Disability Research*, **51**, 32–42.

Strydom, A., Livingston, G., King, M. & Hassiotis, A. (2007) Prevalence of dementia in intellectual disability using different diagnostic criteria. *British Journal of Psychiatry*, **191**, 150–7.

Turner, T. H. (1989) Schizophrenia and mental handicap: An historical review, with implications for further research. *Psychological Medicine*, **19**, 301–14.

Wadsworth, M. E., Mann, S. L., Rodgers, B. et al. (1992) Loss and representativeness in a 43 year follow up of a national birth cohort. *Journal of Epidemiology and Community Health*, **46**, 300–4.

World Health Organization (1993) *The ICD-10 Classification of Mental and Behavioural Disorders: Diagnostic Criteria for Research.*

Chapter 11
Management of Dementia in Intellectual Disability

Vee P. Prasher and Hassan Mahmood

11.1 Introduction

Dementia in older persons with intellectual disability (ID) is becoming a major public health concern. Dementia in Alzheimer's disease (DAD), along with other forms of dementia, are emerging as a significant concern for local authorities and health services who provide care for the ID population. A number of western countries have now published specific guidance to increase public and professional awareness (Bishop et al., 2015; British Psychological Society, 2015; Moran et al., 2013). The management of dementia in the ID population remains an ongoing challenge to carers, health service managers and clinicians (Evans et al., 2013; Nieuwenhuis-Mark, 2009; Prasher et al., 2015). Particular issues include the high prevalence of co-morbidities in older adults with dementia, the lack of internationally recognised diagnostic criteria, limited number of clinical experts and the lack of advocacy for patients.

Dementia is the progressive loss of cognitive ability and defined as a chronic disorder of the brain which adversely affects higher cortical functions, including memory, language and orientation (American Psychiatric Association, 2013; World Health Organization, 1992). For the ID population, most research and clinical information has focussed on dementia in the Down syndrome (DS) population (Janicki & Dalton, 1999; Prasher, 2005). There is less known about the epidemiology of dementia in non-DS ID individuals (Cooper, 1997; Strydom et al., 2013) and of the occurrence in the ID population of the differing types of dementia; vascular dementia, dementia with Lewy bodies, dementia in Pick's disease, frontotemporal dementia and mixed dementia.

This chapter highlights the incidence, prevalence, diagnosis and treatment of dementia in people with ID as a whole and not just in older persons with DS.

11.2 Epidemiological Issues

Among people with ID, older persons with DS are the most at risk of developing dementia, with a mean age of onset of 50–55 years (Evans et al., 2013; Oliver & Holland; 1986; Prasher, 1995). Persons with DS have an earlier onset of DAD than the general population. Prevalence rates for dementia increase with age; 2–5% in those aged 30–39 years, 8–15% aged 40–49 years, 20–40% for those aged 50–59 years and 35–50% of DS adults over the age of 60 years (Prasher, 2005). Holland et al. (2000) reported on age-specific incidence rates of dementia over an 18-month period; 26% for persons aged 30–39 years, 26% for 40–49 years and 22% for 50–59 years. Over a five-year follow-up period in a population of females with DS, Cosgrave et al. (2000) found the incidence rate rose from 8.7% at the start of the study to 44% at the end of the study. McCarron et al. (2014), in a fourteen-year follow-up study, found that females with DS had a 20% risk of dementia at 50 years, 45% at age 55 years and 80% at 65 years.

There is limited information available on the epidemiology of dementia in the non-DS ID population. Research suggests similar or increased prevalence rates (18–22% over 65 years) as compared to the non-ID population (Cooper, 1997; Strydom et al., 2009; Zigman et al., 2004). Incidence of dementia in the non-DS ID population was reported to be up to five times higher than in the non-ID population (Strydom et al., 2013).

The majority of literature in the field of dementia and ID has focused on 'dementia' as a general disorder and few on DAD as a discrete disorder. Some caution is required when reviewing the literature on dementia in the DS population as to exactly what is being discussed. As mentioned previously, very few studies have investigated other forms of dementia in the ID population such as vascular dementia, frontotemporal dementia (FTD) and dementia with Lewy bodies.

The association between DS and AD is due in part to the genetic link between the amyloid precursor protein gene (*APP*) found on chromosome 21 and the risk of DAD. Resultant over-expression of the *APP* gene leads to the increase in neuropathology of AD in persons with DS. Other genetic factors such as apolipoprotein E, S100 calcium binding protein beta and superoxide dismutase I may play a significant role, leading to a common pathway of development of AD in the DS and general populations (Hartley et al., 2015). Non-genetic factors such as brain reserve, brain trauma, emotional trauma, diet, season of birth, exercise and co-morbid medical conditions have, to date, not been fully investigated in the ID/DS populations (Evans et al., 2013).

11.3 Diagnosis and Evaluation of Dementia

Dementia is characterised by a decline in cognitive and non-cognitive brain functions associated with loss of adaptive skills from a pre-morbid level. Diagnosis of dementia is relatively straightforward for the non-ID population, but for persons with ID, a number of diagnostic challenges exist (British Psychological Society, 2015; Moran et al., 2013; Nagdee, 2011). There is currently no internationally agreed approach to the diagnosis and/or screening of dementia in the ID population (Zeilinger et al., 2013). In the USA, the National Task Group on Intellectual Disabilities and Dementia Practices was convened to address this topic (Moran et al., 2013).

The Task Group recommended a number of procedural steps to improve the evaluation, diagnosis, treatment and follow-up of DAD in persons with ID. A nine-step approach in the evaluating process was recommended:

(1) gathering a pertinent psychiatric and medical history;
(2) obtaining a historical description of the patient's baseline functioning;
(3) obtaining a current description of the patient's functioning, and comparing it with baseline;
(4) performing a focused systems review;
(5) thoroughly reviewing the patient's medication list;
(6) obtaining a pertinent family history;
(7) assessing for other psychosocial issues or changes – including identification of coexisting mood disorders such as untreated anxiety or depressed mood that could strongly influence a person's cognition and functioning;

(8) reviewing the social history, living environment and the level of support; and
(9) synthesising the information.

The Task Group highlighted the need for cognitive and physical examinations to be conducted in addition to the above evaluating process. At least one cognitive or behavioural assessment should be undertaken and used to track a decline in scores over time. A number of instruments were mentioned but no one test was recommended. It was more important for clinicians to choose an instrument that they felt could recognise change and detect decline in relation to a premorbid baseline.

Nagdee (2011) further reviewed the challenges in diagnosing dementia in patients with ID. These included (i) lack of recognised diagnostic criteria such as DSM-IV and ICD-10, (ii) assessment techniques and tools not being appropriate for some patients with ID, (iii) signs of dementia seen in the non-ID population such as dyspraxia or agnosia may not be recognised in persons with ID, especially early in the illness, (iv) subtle symptoms of dementia potentially being concealed by pre-existing cognitive impairment and (v) greater importance may need to be given to disturbances in personality, changes in emotions and decline in adaptive behaviour.

The British Psychological Society in collaboration with the Royal College of Psychiatrists published in 2015 some guidance on the assessment and management of dementia in people with ID (British Psychological Society, 2015). The document highlighted key factors to be considered in the assessment process:

(1) History and information gathering – establishing the pre-morbid level and signs of 'change'.
(2) Mental state examination – excluding depression and psychosis, and assessing cognition.
(3) Physical examination – including screen for hormonal disorders.
(4) Physical investigations – standard laboratory tests (full blood count, urea and electrolytes, blood sugar, thyroid function tests, liver function tests, B12 and folate level, lipid profile), sensory screening (vision and hearing) and optional tests (EEG, ECG and neuroimaging).
(5) Environmental assessment – life events and safety issues.

Given the difficulties in conducting a complete physical examination and undergoing brain scans in a number of ID patients with dementia, the guidance gave a helpful guide to essential assessments that should be done.

The guidance emphasises the importance of following the Mental Capacity Act (2005) and its code of practice guidelines where investigation is considered, and the person is unable to consent and cooperate. If a person lacks the capacity to consent to investigations, it is important to consider using the Mental Capacity Act to carry out the investigations in the person's best interest.

It is important to weigh up the risks of benefits in carrying out investigations (e.g. asking for neuroimaging against causing undue distress to an individual). Magnetic resonance imaging has an important but limited role to play in the management of Alzheimer's disease in the population with Down syndrome (Prasher et al., 2003).

The British Psychological Society (2015) highlighted a number of assessments/tests which can provide additional information to support the diagnostic process, which are set out in the following sections.

11.3.1 Direct Tests with the Person with ID

CAMCOG-DS

Neuropsychological Assessment of Dementia in Adults with Intellectual Disabilities (NAID)

Severe Impairment Battery (SIB)

Test for Severe Impairment

Dalton Brief Praxis Test

11.3.2 Informant Questionnaires

CAMDEX-DS informant interview

Dementia Questionnaire for people with Learning Disabilities (DLD)

Dementia Scale for Down's syndrome (DSDS)

Dementia Screening Questionnaire for Individuals with ID (DSQIID)

Adaptive Behaviour Dementia Questionnaire (ABDQ)

A number of other assessments include those for the assessment of mental health, the assessment of depression, carer burden, life events and adaptive behaviour.

Zeilinger et al. (2013) undertook a systematic review on assessment instruments for dementia in persons with ID. Existing instruments were collected and described. The review determined which concepts the instruments assessed, whether they were especially developed or adapted for persons with ID, and whether they were designed to assess dementia. The review identified 114 instruments with 79 to be completed by the person with ID and 35 were informant-based. Four test batteries were found. The authors highlighted that some of the instruments were neither designed for the assessment of dementia nor for persons with ID. The authors concluded that there was a wide variety of different tools used for the assessment of dementia in ID. No agreed-upon approach or instrument was in use.

A number of researchers have now emphasised the importance of ascertaining a change from premorbid functioning in order to determine cognitive decline and to consider non-cognitive features such as personality, behaviour and executive dysfunction changes as early indicators of the onset of dementia. Lack of information on 'normal' ageing for the ID population remains an important issue for professionals caring for persons with ID. Further research is required on age-related cognitive decline and how this can be distinguished from dementia. The role of the severity of ID on the detection and subsequent treatment of dementia is unclear.

11.4 Treatment

Once the diagnosis of dementia and in particular DAD is made, a professional discussion should take place about the ongoing management plan. Best practice would suggest the need for a multidisciplinary team (MDT) approach throughout the process of a dementia care pathway. Antidementia medication may play a role but not necessarily in all persons with dementia and ID. Underlying cardiac abnormalities, severity of dementia, placement and family views are important factors to consider. Overall, the treatment of dementia in patients with ID is not too different to patients within the general population (Prasher et al., 2016) with both pharmacological and non-pharmacological approaches. However, the underlying ID can make the management of DAD more challenging in older adults with ID.

11.4.1 Pharmacological Treatment

11.4.1.1 Antidementia Drugs

A number of reviews by the Cochrane collaboration (Mohan et al., 2009a, 2009b, 2009c, 2000d) have reported on how there have been only a few drug trials assessing the possible benefits of acetylcholinesterase inhibitors in patients with DS and dementia. There is no published research on the pharmacological treatment of non-DS ID patients with dementia. To date, four antidementia drugs have been given a licence for treatment. Donepezil, rivastigmine and galantamine increase the availability of acetylcholine. Memantine blocks the role of the neurotransmitter glutamate. All are administered orally as a tablet, capsule, oral solution or orodispersible tablet, except rivastigmine, which can also be administered as a transdermal patch. Donepezil, rivastigmine and galantamine are indicated for those with mild-to-moderate DAD, whereas memantine is indicated for those with moderate-to-severe DAD.

A non-statistically significant reduction in deterioration in the assessment of DAD or modest improvement in dementia scores with the use of donepezil and transdermal rivastigmine as compared to non-treated individuals has been reported (Johnson et al., 2003; Kishnani et al., 2009; Lott et al., 2002; Prasher, 2013). Hanney et al. (2012) reported findings from a large prospective randomised double-blind trial of memantine in older persons with DS. No statistically significant benefit was identified using the antidementia drug.

As there were a number of methodological flaws with antidementia studies in the ID population, the Cochrane Collaboration reviews (Mohan et al., 2009a, 2009b, 2009c, 2000d) of donepezil, galantamine, rivastigmine and memantine could not recommend the use of antidementia drugs. NICE guidance (2012) has recommended the use of acetylcholinesterase inhibitors for mild-to-moderate dementia and the use of memantine for severe dementia or in moderate dementia where acetylcholinesterase inhibitors have not been beneficial.

As with the use of other drugs for persons with ID, antidementia medications should be used with vigilance in older persons with dementia and ID. Donepezil, rivastigmine and galantamine should be used with caution in those with sick sinus syndrome, supraventricular conduction abnormalities, history of peptic ulcers, asthma and chronic obstructive airways disease. Memantine should be used with caution in those with renal impairment, epilepsy and cardiovascular disorders.

11.4.1.2 Antipsychotic Medication

Behavioural problems can be a common feature of dementia in persons with ID. Aggression, anxiety, agitation, mood changes and irritability can occur. Initially such problems should be managed with environmental and/or psychosocial approaches (Kalsy-Lillico et al., 2012). Use of psychotropic medications to control behaviour problems in dementia may be necessary. NICE guidelines on dementia approves the use of an antipsychotic drug but only if a number of conditions have been met:

(1) Full discussion with the person with dementia and/or carers about possible benefits and risks of treatment.

(2) Changes in cognition should be assessed and recorded at regular intervals. Alternative medication should be considered if necessary.
(3) Target symptoms should be identified, quantified and documented.
(4) Changes in target symptoms should be assessed and recorded regularly.
(5) The effect of co-morbid conditions, such as physical illness, pain and depression should be considered.
(6) The choice of antipsychotic should be made after an individual risk–benefit analysis.
(7) The dose should be low initially and then titrated upwards.
(8) Treatment should be time-limited and regularly reviewed (every three months or according to clinical need).

Eady et al. (2015), in a large survey of antipsychotic prescribing to adults with ID in the UK, found that the most common indications for medication prescribing were psychotic illness (42%), anxiety (42%) and behavioural problems (38%). In this survey, risperidone was the most commonly prescribed antipsychotic. Others included olanzapine and quetiapine. The study was undertaken prior to the wide availability of aripiprazole. Eady et al. (2015) highlighted the need to use antipsychotics with caution in older adults with ID. Olanzapine and quetiapine have potential antimuscarinic activity, metabolic syndrome is a well-known complication of newer antipsychotics and clozapine, quetiapine, olanzapine and risperidone may cause hypotension. An increased risk of cerebrovascular events secondary to the prescribing of antipsychotic medication in older ID persons with dementia is of concern.

11.4.1.3 Treatments of Co-morbidities

11.4.1.3.1 Depression and Use of Antidepressants

It is not uncommon in the ID population for depression to present as dementia or for it to occur as part of a dementing illness (Tsiouris et al., 2014; Wark et al., 2014). Subsequent treatment of the depressive illness can significantly improve the quality of life and also increase longevity. To date there is evidence to recommend any specific antidepressant drug and all may be efficacious. Selective serotonin reuptake inhibitors (SSRIs; e.g. fluoxetine, fluvoxamine, paroxetine, sertraline) are often the drugs of choice. As with other medication, starting the medication at a low dose with a gradual increase in dosage and close monitoring for side effects is important. Rarely have mood stabilisers such as lithium, sodium valproate and carbamazepine been used for rapid swings in mood.

11.4.1.3.2 Insomnia and Hypnotics

Difficulties in trying to fall asleep, waking up in the early hours, being fully awake all night and sleeping excessively during the day but being awake at night are not uncommon complaints made by families or carers looking after a person with dementia and ID. If good sleep hygiene (e.g. limiting evening caffeine, black-out curtains, avoidance of daytime sleeping) has not proved to be beneficial, night sedative medication may be prescribed for a short period. Drugs used to aid sleep include melatonin, lorazepam, zopiclone, zaleplon and zolpidem. Oversedation can worsen cognitive function and lead to unsteadiness, falls, confusion and apathy, as a result, this medication should be carefully considered.

11.4.1.3.3 Seizures and Antiepileptic Drugs

An association between seizures and dementia in adults with ID is well established (Lott et al., 2012; McCarron et al., 2005; Prasher 2014; Pueshel et al., 1991). Late-onset seizures have been reported to be a strong indicator of an underlying dementing process and a poor prognostic factor (Prasher & Corbett, 1993); the mean life expectancy after the onset of seizures in persons with DS and DAD is 1.5 years. The drug treatment of seizures is not too dissimilar to the treatment of seizures in younger adults with ID and it should follow standard epilepsy treatment pathways.

11.4.2 Non-Pharmacological

Non-pharmacological interventions used to manage dementia in the non-ID population can be adapted for use in people with dementia and ID. The British Psychological Society (2015) summarised interventions and categories in several domains:

- person-centred approaches to support
- mobility
- eating/drinking
- continence
- communication
- environment
- self-help skills
- occupation/activity
- orientation/confusion
- work with families and carers

It is important to remember that epilepsy has an impact on the quality of life and therefore psychosocial well-being in adults with an ID (Kerr et al., 2009).

An increasing number of non-pharmacological interventions are available for people with dementia. They can be divided into standard therapies, alternative therapies and brief psychotherapies. Standard therapies include behavioural therapy, reality orientation, validation therapy and reminiscence therapy. Alternative therapies include art therapy, music therapy, activity therapy, complementary therapy, aromatherapy, bright-light therapy and multisensory approaches. Brief psychotherapies include cognitive behavioural therapy and interpersonal therapy (Douglas et al., 2004).

11.4.2.1 Psychological Approaches

Psychological interventions can be classified as behaviour-orientated, emotion-orientated, cognition-orientated and stimulation-orientated (Kalsy-Lillico et al., 2012). Stimulation-orientated treatments include recreational activities and art therapies that are designed to provide stimulation and enrichment. Various practical principles of care practices that aim to facilitate more enabling care experiences include embracing positive philosophies of care, taking a life-story perspective and consideration of carer characteristics. Kalsy-Lillico et al. (2012) focused on key areas in terms of general guidance in relation to this area. These areas included use of the individual's preferred communication form, identifying potential benefits of knowing (and not knowing) the diagnosis, tailoring the approach according to the individual and using a multidisciplinary approach to answer any questions and make recommendations. A more open discussion on the diagnosis of dementia, its prognosis and changing needs as the disease progresses can reduce carer burden.

Positive behavioural support (PBS) is a favoured intervention in patients who present with challenging behaviour. According to Lavigna et al. (2012), PBS was effective with both severe and high-rate behaviour problems. It was also cost-effective and the methodology used could easily be trained and widely disseminated in institutional settings.

11.4.2.2 Environmental Factors

The environmental design for patients with dementia should not hinder an individual. They should have beneficial effects for the individual and staff. Compensating for the disability, maximising independence and reinforcing personal identity are examples of how an environment should have beneficial effects. The environments require to be calm, familiar, suitably stimulated and safe and risk assessed. An environmental assessment should include looking at the quality of the person's physical environment, staffing levels and staff characteristics and competence (British Psychological Society, 2015; Marshall et al., 1998).

11.4.2.3 Carers

While looking after an individual with dementia, family members and paid carers experience considerable stress. There are numerous carer interventions available, which include education, financial consideration, home environment changes and easy access to services. Professional carers' experiences of caring for individuals with dementia and ID have previously highlighted a number of themes such as staff knowledge of dementia, staff training in dementia, caregiving, challenging behaviour, pain management, mealtime support and coping strategies. Education includes providing the carer with a wide breadth of information. Emotional support includes joining local support groups, community nursing support or individual psychological counselling. Access to day care and/or respite care can enable carers to have time for themselves and for other members of the family (Cleary et al., 2016; Prasher, 2005). Cleary et al. (2016) found that the relationship between a carer and the person with dementia is fundamental to person-centred care and it enables staff to tailor care to the person with dementia. To be effective, a collaborative approach is central from diagnosis to end-of-life care.

It remains essential that carers have a good understanding of the key issues affecting a person with dementia and ID. This is more than knowledge of the symptoms and signs of dementia, but also includes an awareness of the roles of different professionals, how to access specialist services and how to receive appropriate training. The National Task Group on Intellectual Disabilities and Dementia Practices (Bishop et al., 2015) published guidelines to enable caregivers (whether they are family members or paid carers) to prepare for and advocate during health visits. The challenges for healthcare advocacy and access included information and awareness of symptoms (caregivers and practitioners), the referral and assessment process, follow-up and clinical assistance communication with healthcare personnel and training.

11.5 Conclusion

Dementia in older persons with ID is becoming, as per the non-ID population, an increasing concern to health and social care providers. Older persons with DS are most at risk of developing DAD. They have an earlier onset of DAD than the general population and prevalence rates dramatically increase with age. Virtually all persons with DS over the age of 40 years will have the neuropathology of Alzheimer's disease but not all will inevitably develop the clinical features of DAD.

The accurate diagnosis of dementia in ID by clinical and neuropsychological means has been the focus of research over the last thirty years. However, a number of diagnostic challenges still remain, no more so than expert recommendations not yet being widely implemented into routine clinical practice. There remains high variability both nationally and more so internationally in the quality of the assessment process for dementia in persons with ID. The diagnostic process should include a detailed clinical assessment, physical investigations and at least one cognitive or behavioural assessment which should be undertaken to track a decline in scores over time.

The management of dementia should involve the MDT and a holistic approach is important. Pharmacological treatment includes antidementia drugs, antipsychotic use and treatment of co-morbidities such as depression, insomnia and seizures. Antidementia medications consist of donepezil, rivastigmine, galantamine and memantine, but their efficacy remains unclear. Antipsychotic medications can be prescribed to manage behavioural problems. Antidepressants should be used to treat depressive illness, with SSRI medications often being the treatments of choice. All medication in older adults with dementia and ID should be commenced at a low dose and gradually increased in dosage with close monitoring for side effects. Late-onset seizures strongly indicate an underlying dementing process and a poor prognostic factor in those with DS, but should not preclude the individual from treatment of their dementia symptoms. The drug treatment of seizures should follow standard epilepsy treatment pathways.

Non-pharmacological interventions play a significant role in the management of dementia in people with ID. Psychological interventions can be classified as behaviour-orientated, emotion-orientated, cognition-orientated and stimulation-orientated. PBS is a favoured intervention in people with challenging behaviour. The environment for people with dementia and ID is important to provide optimum care. It should benefit both the individual with dementia and their carers.

The management of dementia in older persons with ID remains the responsibility of many interested parties; families, paid carers, health and social care professionals may have a 'hands-on' role but health and social care commissioning agencies, along with the private sector will also determine the quality of future care. As per the non-ID population, closer working and a more integrated approach to care is very much the way forward.

References

American Psychiatric Association (2013) The Diagnostic and Statistical Manual of Mental Disorders (5th edn). American Psychiatric Publishing.

Bishop, K. M., Hogan, M., Janicki, M. et al. (2015) Guidelines for dementia-related health advocacy for adults with intellectual disability and dementia: National Task Group on Intellectual Disabilities and Dementia Practices. *Intellectual and Developmental Disabilities*, 53, 2–29.

British Psychological Society (2015) *Dementia and People with Intellectual Disabilities: Guidance on the Assessment, Diagnosis, Interventions and Support of People with Intellectual Disabilities Who Develop Dementia*. British Psychological Society.

Cleary, J. & Doody, O. (2016) Professional carers' experiences of caring for individuals with intellectual disability and dementia: A review of the literature. *Journal of Intellectual Disability.* Epub, 14 March.

Cooper, S-A. (1997) High prevalence of dementia among people with learning disabilities not attributable to Down's syndrome. *Psychological Medicine,* 27, 609–16.

Cosgrave, M. P., Tyrrell, J., McCarron, M. et al. (2000) A five year follow-up study of dementia in persons with Down's syndrome: Early symptoms and patterns of deterioration. *Irish Journal of Psychological Medicine,* 17, 5–11.

Douglas, S., James, I. & Ballard, C (2004) Non-pharmacological interventions in dementia. *Advances in Psychiatric Treatment,* 10, 171–7.

Eady, N, Courtenay, K. & Strydom, A. (2015) Pharmacological management of behavioral and psychiatric symptoms in older adults with intellectual disability. *Drugs Aging,* 32, 95–102.

Evans, E., Bhardwaj, A., Brodaty, H. et al. (2013) Dementia in people with intellectual disability: Insights and challenges in epidemiological research with an at-risk population. *International Review of Psychiatry,* 25, 755–63.

Hanney, M., Prasher, V., Williams, N. et al. (2012) Memantine for dementia in adults older than 40 years with Down's syndrome (MEADOWS): A randomised, double-blind, placebo-controlled trial. *The Lancet,* 379, 528–36.

Hartley, D., Blumenthal, T., Carrillo, M. et al. (2015) Down syndrome and Alzheimer's disease: Common pathways, common goals. *Alzheimer's & Dementia,* 11, 700–9. Epub, 12 December.

Holland, A. J., Hon, J., Huppert, F. A. et al. (2000) Incidence and course of dementia in people with Down's syndrome: Findings from a population based-study. *Journal of Intellectual Disability Research,* 44, 138–46.

Janicki, M. P. & Dalton, A. J. (eds) (1999) *Aging, Dementia and Intellectual Disabilities: A Handbook.* Taylor & Francis.

Johnson, N., Fahey, C., Chicoine, B. et al. (2003) Effects of donepezil on cognitive functioning in Down syndrome. *American Journal of Mental Retardation,* 108, 367–72.

Kalsy-Lillico, S., Adams, D. & Oliver, C. (2012) Older adults with intellectual disabilities: issues in ageing and dementia. In *Clinical Psychology and People with Intellectual Disabilities* (2nd edn) (eds. E. Emerson, C. Hatton, K. Dickson, R. Gone, A. Caine & J. Bromley). Wiley.

Kerr, M. P., Turky, A. & Huber, B. (2009) The psychosocial impact of epilepsy in adults in adults with an intellectual disability. *Epilepsy and Behaviour,* 15 (suppl. 1), S26–3.

Kishnani, P. S., Sommer, B. R., Handen, B. L. et al. (2009) The efficacy, safety, and tolerability of donepezil for the treatment of young adults with Down syndrome. *American Journal of Medical Genetics Part A,* 149A, 1641–54.

Lavigna, G. W. & Willis, T. J. (2012) The efficacy of positive behavioural support with the most challenging behaviour: The evidence and its implications. *Journal of Intellectual and Developmental Disability,* 37, 185–95.

Lott, I. T., Doran, E., Nguyen, V. Q. et al. (2012) Down syndrome and dementia: Seizures and cognitive decline. *Journal of Alzheimer's Disease,* 29, 177–85.

Lott, I. T., Osann, K., Doran, E. et al. (2002) Down syndrome and Alzheimer disease: Response to donepezil. *Archives of Neurology,* 59, 1133–6.

McCarron, M., Gill, M., McCallion, P. et al. (2005) Health co-morbidities in ageing persons with Down syndrome and Alzheimer's dementia. *Journal of Intellectual Disability Research,* 49, 560–6.

McCarron, M., McCallion, P., Reilly, E. et al. (2014) A prospective 14-year longitudinal follow-up of dementia in persons with Down syndrome. *Journal of Intellectual Disability Research,* 58, 61–70.

Marshall, M. (1998) How it helps to see dementia as a disability. *Journal of Dementia Care,* 6, 15–17.

Mohan, M., Bennett, C. & Carpenter, P. K. (2009a) Memantine for dementia in people with Down syndrome. *Cochrane Database of Systematic Reviews,* (1), CD007657.

Mohan, M., Bennett, C. & Carpenter, P. K. (2009b) Galantamine for dementia in people with Down syndrome. *Cochrane Database of Systematic Reviews,* (1), CD007656.

Mohan, M., Bennett, C. & Carpenter, P. K. (2009c) Rivastigmine for dementia in people with Down syndrome. *Cochrane Database of Systematic Reviews,* (1), CD007658.

Mohan, M., Carpenter, P. K., Bennett, C. (2009d) Donepezil for dementia in people with Down syndrome. *Cochrane Database of Systematic Reviews*, (1), CD007178.

Moran, J. A., Rafii, M. S., Keller, S. M. et al. (2013) The National Task Group on Intellectual Disabilities and Dementia Practices consensus recommendations for the evaluation and management of dementia in adults with intellectual disabilities. *Mayo Clinic Proceedings*, 88, 831–40.

Nagdee, M. (2011) Dementia in intellectual disability: A review of diagnostic challenges. *African Journal of Psychiatry*, 14, 194–9.

NICE [National Institute of Health and Care Excellence] (2006) [webpage] Dementia: Supporting people with dementia and their carers in health and social care. clinical guidelines. CG42. Available at: www.nice.org.uk/CG42 [accessed 11 August 2018]

Nieuwenhuis-Mark, R. (2009) Diagnosing Alzheimer's dementia in Down syndrome: Problems and possible solutions. *Research in Developmental Disabilities*, 30, 827–38.

Oliver, C. & Holland, A. J. (1986) Down's syndrome and Alzheimer's disease: A review. *Psychological Medicine*, 16, 307–22.

Prasher, V. P. (1995) Age specific prevalence, thyroid dysfunction and depressive symptomatology in adults with down syndrome and dementia. *International Journal of Geriatric Psychiatry*, 10, 25–31.

Prasher, V. P. (2005) *Alzheimer's Disease, Dementia, Down Syndrome and Intellectual Disabilities*. Radcliffe Press.

Prasher, V. P. (2014) *Practical Dementia Care for Adults with Down Syndrome or with Intellectual Disabilities*. Nova Science.

Prasher, V. P. & Corbett, J. A. (1993) Onset of seizures as a poor indicator of longevity in people with Down syndrome and dementia. *International Journal of Geriatric Psychiatry*, 8, 922–7.

Prasher, V. P., Cumella, S., Natarajan, K. et al. (2003) Magnetic resonance imaging, Down's syndrome and Alzheimer's disease: research and clinical implications. *Journal of Intellectual Disability Research*, 47 (part 2), 90–100.

Prasher, V. P., Mahmood, H. & Mitra, M. (2016) Challenges faced in managing dementia in Alzheimer's disease in patients with Down syndrome. *Degenerative Neurological and Neuromuscular Disease*, 6, 85–94.

Prasher, V. P., Sachdeva, N., Adams, C. et al. (2013) Rivastigmine transdermal patches in the treatment of dementia in Alzheimer's disease in adults with Down syndrome: Pilot study. *International Journal of Geriatric Psychiatry*, 28, 219–20.

Prasher, V. P., Sachdeva, N. & Tarrant, N. (2015) Diagnosing dementia in adults with Down's syndrome. *Neurodegenerative Disease Management*, 5, 249–56.

Pueschel, S. M., Louis, S. & McKnight, P. (1991) Seizure disorders in Down syndrome. *Archives of Neurology*, 48, 318–20.

Strydom, A., Chan, T., King, M. et al. (2013) Incidence of dementia in older adults with intellectual disabilities. *Research in Developmental Disabilities*, 34, 1881–5.

Strydom, A., Hassoitis, A., King, M. et al. (2009) The relationship of dementia prevalence in older adults with intellectual disability (ID) to age and severity of ID. *Psychological Medicine*, 39, 13–21.

Tsiouris, J. A., Patti, P. J. & Flory, M. J. (2014) Effects of antidepressants on longevity and dementia onset among adults with Down syndrome: A retrospective study. *Degenerative Neurological and Neuromuscular Disease*, 75, 731–7.

Wark, S., Hussain, R. & Parmenter, T. (2014) Down syndrome and dementia: Is depression a confounder for accurate diagnosis and treatment? *Journal of Intellect Disabilities*, 18, 305–14.

World Health Organization (1992) *The ICD-10 Classification of Mental and Behavioural Disorders: Clinical Descriptions and Diagnostic Guidelines*.

Zeilinger, E. L., Stiehl, K. A. & Weber, G. (2013) A systematic review on assessment instruments for dementia in persons with intellectual disabilities. *Research in Developmental Disabilities*, 34, 3962–77.

Zigman, W. B., Schupf, N., Devenny, D. A. et al. (2004) Incidence and prevalence of dementia in elderly adults with mental retardation without Down syndrome. *American Journal on Mental Retardation*, 109, 126–41.

Chapter 12

Forensic Psychiatry and Intellectual Disability

Harm Boer and Liz Beber

12.1 Background

Historically, intellectual disability (ID) was believed to be associated with offending behaviour. People with ID, mental illness and epilepsy were often seen as a single, homogeneous mass along with those who engaged in prostitution or other criminal activity. During the latter part of the nineteenth and earlier part of the twentieth centuries, there was a view that ID was a social problem which needed to be dealt with. Henry Goddard, a US psychologist and eugenicist, proposed that people with ID were kept in institutions: 'Such colonies would save an annual loss in property and life, due to the actions of these irresponsible people, sufficient to nearly, or quite, offset the expense of the new plant' (1912). Like many of his contemporaries, Goddard believed that much criminal activity could be attributed to this group and their incarceration would be a reasonably cost-effective solution. Although a number of early surveys supported the opinion that criminality was rife among those of low intelligence, these were mainly methodologically flawed, not least because definition and measurement of supposed ID were absent. Following the introduction of standardised IQ (intelligence quotient) testing a different picture began to emerge: Sutherland (1931) showed that the distribution of IQ in the criminal population was broadly similar to that of the US general population.

Since this time the debate has gone on with some protagonists arguing for a link between offending and ID, others against. Whatever the truth, the reality remains that some people with ID do find themselves accused of criminal behaviour and therefore subject to the criminal justice system (CJS).

Before the high secure hospitals came into being, care for mentally disordered offenders had traditionally taken place within secure wings of the county asylums. The 1856 Tenth Report of the Commissioners in Lunacy criticised the conditions in the male 'criminal' wing of Bethlem Hospital and paved the way for the construction of Broadmoor Special Hospital in Berkshire which opened in 1863. As the demand for beds increased, further provision was made at Parkhurst Prison until a second secure hospital, Rampton in Nottinghamshire was built in 1912. It was not until the 1913 Mental Deficiency Act was implemented following the First World War that a board of control was established and required to provide specific facilities for *mental defectives* (the contemporaneous term for people with ID) who were 'violent or dangerous'. The Act equipped the courts with the necessary powers to direct intellectually disabled offenders to specialist psychiatric services rather than sending them to prison.

Since this time the development of specialist secure services and successive revisions of the Mental Health Act and various criminal acts have resulted in complex but useful legislation which allows for a range of disposal options for people with ID who find themselves in the grasp of the long arm of the law.

12.2 Prevalence

People with ID make up a small but significant subpopulation of those finding their way into the CJS. Although having a below average intellectual ability appears to be predictive of future offending behaviour (West & Farrington, 1973), it is far less clear whether those who have a significant ID are over-represented in the CJS (Holland et al., 2002). Prevalence rates of offenders in the CJS show huge variations, possibly due to issues such as geographical differences and disparities in the definition and ascertainment of ID. It is possible that people with ID have increased recorded offending rates due to a lower ability to avoid arrest but it is also possible that actual offending is underestimated because of a higher tolerance of disturbed behaviour by both care staff and the police and prosecution or reluctance to involve the police (see Barron et al., 2002).

Studies of the prevalence of ID in the CJS are inherently difficult to conduct. In one of the largest studies of its kind, looking at ten prison surveys across four countries involving almost 12,000 inmates, Fazel et al. (2008) found substantial heterogeneity and hence did not undertake a summary estimate of prevalence. The results suggested that typically 0.5–1.5% of prisoners were diagnosed with ID (range 0–2.8% across studies). A recent study from Norway (Søndenaa et al., 2008) suggested that up to 10% of sentenced prisoners had ID.

In the UK, figures from No One Knows (Talbot, 2008) suggest that assuming a prison population of 82,000, there will be around 5,740 people with an IQ less than 70 (7%) and about 20,500 with an IQ between 71 and 80 (25%). Elsewhere, it has been suggested that up to 11% of remand and 5–7% of sentenced prisoners have ID, although there appears to be a problem with reliably identifying this group because of insufficient screening (Singleton et al., 1998). It is therefore likely that people with ID are at risk of receiving insufficient support and treatment despite this population being known to present with multiple co-morbid problems (including mental illness, physical problems, autism, ADHD and substance misuse) more often than the general population.

12.3 Offending

In English law (England and Wales), *actus reus* is defined as the act of crime and *mens rea* as the intent to commit that crime. The latter can be difficult to elicit in people with moderate to profound ID and is a key issue when it comes to legal perception of the difference between challenging behaviour and criminal behaviour (Royal College of Psychiatrists, 2014). Similarly, these factors influence police decisions to caution or to arrest and convict an individual with ID. A person with moderate-to-severe ID is unlikely to be dealt with through the CJS unless the criminal act is very serious. However, the issue becomes far less clear-cut for those with milder degrees of cognitive impairment.

It has been argued that the involvement of the CJS in cases of offending by those with ID is punitive. A review by McBrien and Murphy (2006) confirmed that care staff were reluctant to report incidents by people with ID to the police. However, if challenging behaviour remains unchallenged, this may lead to individuals believing that such behaviour is acceptable, leading to further and potentially more serious acts, which then in turn may lead to more serious consequences both for society and the perpetrator (Royal College of Psychiatrists, 2014).

Given a general reluctance to seek prosecution against people with ID, little is known about what sort of behaviours are more likely to trigger a referral into forensic services. Lindsay et al. (2010) looked at people who had committed offences or displayed offending behaviour who had been referred to community and secure inpatient services for people with ID, and found that physical and verbal aggression, and contact or non-contact sexual offences were common index behaviours. They found relatively low levels of referrals for fire-setting and theft. However, Lindsay et al. (2010) noted that 40% of those referred to secure forensic services had previous offending type behaviours relating to contact sexual offences, and fire setting was recorded in more than 30%. Perhaps not surprisingly, very few were charged with road traffic offences.

ID is not in itself a mental illness, but many people with the condition, particularly those who come into contact with the CJS, have additional mental health problems including pervasive developmental disorders, mental illness or substance misuse disorders (Alexander et al., 2011). When a person in police custody appears to be suffering from a mental disorder including ID or appear as if they may need clinical attention, then appropriate help must be sought as soon as possible.

12.4 Criminal Justice System

For people with ID, the often-convoluted processes which make up our CJS can be both daunting and confusing. They may have little long-term perspective and limited ability to understand the consequences of their actions. They may be easily manipulated. They often make no attempt to disguise what they have done. In trying hard to please authority figures, or as a response to questions which are too complex they may confess to what they have not done (Finlay & Lyons 2002; Royal College of Psychiatrists, 2014).

All people in police custody have to be assessed in order to highlight whether they are likely to present any particular risks either to themselves or other people. This role is undertaken by the custody officer. Recent research has suggested that the screening processes used in police custody may not always detect that a person has an ID (McKinnon & Grubin, 2013). It is usually the police surgeon who assesses whether the detainee is 'fit to be interviewed' although sometimes a psychiatrist might be asked to provide an opinion.

In England and Wales, the Police and Criminal Evidence Act (PACE) (1984) helps to provide special protection to people at police stations who could be mentally disordered or mentally vulnerable. Section 76(2) of PACE requires the judge to exclude confession evidence if the prosecution cannot prove beyond reasonable doubt that it was not obtained by oppression or in consequence of something said or done which was likely to have made it unreliable, notwithstanding that it may be true (Ventress et al., 2008). An appropriate adult may be required to attend the interview as it is fundamental to a just and fair interview about an alleged criminal offence that the detainee should understand the nature and purpose of the interview as people with ID do not always understand the caution.

In England and Wales, people with ID can also come into contact with the police if they are detained on section 136 (removal of a person suffering from mental disorder in immediate need of care or control found in a public place to a place of safety) of the Mental Health Act 1983 (England and Wales) for a mental health assessment. On assessment, professionals sometimes express the view that nothing can be done under mental health legislation because the person is not 'mentally ill'. This can happen particularly when the assessing professionals do not have expertise or experience in working with people who have ID. It is important to note that ID associated with abnormally aggressive or seriously irresponsible behaviour can be seen as a mental disorder which needs treatment under the Mental Health Act, even if the person does not have an additional mental illness (Royal College of Psychiatrists, 2014).

A court appearance can be a daunting experience for offenders or suspected offenders with ID. In England and Wales this has been recognised by the CJS in the criminal procedure rule (2005, amended 2010) which set out provisions for those people classified as 'Vulnerable Defendants'. This group includes people with ID.

In order to assist a vulnerable defendant to understand and participate in court proceedings, all possible steps should be taken to help vulnerable defendants to understand and to participate in court proceedings and the court process should be adapted where necessary. Such adaptations include the defendant having a chance to visit the court out of hours to familiarise him or herself with the environment, having the proceedings and possible outcomes explained in advance in understandable language, being free to sit with family or a supporting adult during the proceedings, having frequent breaks to aid concentration and having the trial (including cross examination) conducted in simple, clear language. There is also provision for evidence to be given by video link and for restrictions to be put in place on who can be in attendance in the court room.

Court diversion schemes play an important role in the recognition of mental disorder in defendants but there is often little expertise in ID in these teams. Nacro (2005) noted that most diversion schemes were focused on offenders with mental illness and that there were only three such schemes in England and Wales that had either ID practitioners or links with ID services. This is despite the recommendations of the Reed Report (Department of Health & Home Office, 1992) that 'court diversion and assessment schemes should develop effective links with local Intellectual Disability teams, and where possible, team members should be encouraged to contribute to teams'. Not all the courts in England and Wales are served by a diversion scheme, let alone for people with ID, and many of these schemes work only a limited number of days per week (Royal College of Psychiatrists, 2014).

The Bradley Report (Department of Health, 2009) recognised the difficulties inherent in the diversion schemes and the problems resulting from the non-recognition of ID at the court stage. It was recognised that the most likely people to have contact with people with ID were professionals working in the CJS and the Bradley Report recommended that the Probation Service and the judiciary should receive mental health and ID awareness training. In response the Department of Health (2009 produced a booklet aimed at professionals working in the CJS that highlights the needs of people with ID. The booklet 'Positive Practice – Positive Outcomes' contains a section for court professionals and includes advice on communication and rights and responsibilities when dealing with people with ID.

A further area of concern highlighted in this report was the difficulties courts faced in obtaining timely and good quality psychiatric reports. It was noted that the courts relied on a limited number of psychiatrists who were willing to undertake such work outside of their NHS duties. There are only a limited number of ID psychiatrists who have experience in forensic psychiatry across England and Wales, compounding the problem in this particular area. This situation may have been further worsened by the ruling that expert witnesses would no longer be immune from suit (*Jones* v. *Kaney* [2011] UKSC 13). Assessment of people with ID by practitioners with little or no experience of working with this group can lead to problems with diagnosis or assessment of fitness to plead and there may be confusion about how the Mental Health Act applies to them. Conversely, generic ID psychiatrists may feel that they do not possess the necessary skills to undertake forensic assessments.

12.5 The Mental Health Act (England and Wales)

In the England and Wales Mental Health Act of 1983 (amended in 2007) learning disability is defined as a mental disorder, but a person with a learning disability can only be considered to have a mental disorder for the purposes of the provisions specified in section 1(2B) of the Act, without another concomitant mental disorder, where the learning disability is associated with abnormally aggressive behaviour or seriously irresponsible conduct. Unless very urgent action is required, it would not be good practice to diagnose a person as having a learning disability associated with abnormally aggressive behaviour or seriously irresponsible conduct (or both) without an assessment by a consultant psychiatrist in learning disabilities and a formal specialist psychological assessment (Department of Health, 2015).

Although 'forensic' patients can be admitted to hospital under part 2 of the Mental Health Act (e.g. sections 2 or 3) or given a guardianship order, most patients are admitted to secure services under part 3 of the Act, which describes the provisions for those who are involved with the CJS), for instance under section 37 of the Mental Health Act (Hospital Order), with or without restriction (section 41). Section 38 allows the Crown Court to make an interim hospital order, which allows the hospital to assess treatability prior to a possible hospital order. Admitting patients to hospital under Section 38 can have, apart from being able to avoid admitting a patient who is not 'treatable', an additional advantage, in that it can allow the patient to make a positive decision as to whether he or she wants to participate in treatment or whether to face the consequences in court if he or she does not, thus allowing the patient to have some degree of choice. Sections 35 and 36 are rarely used but may be useful in certain circumstances.

Section 48 allows for patients on remand to be transferred to hospital for treatment, and section 47 allows sentenced prisoners to be transferred for treatment. Both are nearly always accompanied by additional restrictions (section 49).

Scotland and Northern Ireland have similar arrangements in their respective Mental Health Acts. Other parts of the British Isles (e.g. Isle of Man, Channel Islands) also make use of mainland forensic services through individual pieces of legislation.

When dealing with any aspects of the Mental Health Act, for instance when writing a court or tribunal report, it is useful to consult books such as the *Code of Practice* (Department of Health, 2015), the *Mental Health Act Manual* (Jones, 2016) and Zigmond and Brindle (2016).

12.6 Fitness to Plead

People with ID may not be able to sufficiently understand the court process for a trial to take place. Fitness to plead has been roughly described as an understanding of the charge and its meaning, the ability to distinguish between a plea of guilty and not guilty, and to follow court proceedings. Fitness to plead may be compromised in cases of mental disorder and should be assessed carefully in all cases where the defendant has not yet pleaded (Humphreys, 2000). If a person is found unfit to plead, the court can make a hospital order (with or without restriction order) or a supervision and treatment order (including supervision by probation or social services, and if appropriate, medical treatment as directed by a specified medical practitioner).

12.7 Forensic Patients in the Community

There needs to be a balance between appropriately diverting people with significant mental health problems from the CJS and ensuring the public are protected.

For mentally disordered offenders with ID, a number of factors determine whether a community disposal is appropriate. These not only include the nature of the offence, history of offending, the presence of mental illness, co-morbid substance misuse, capacity to consent and the need for public protection but also issues of vulnerability in prison settings and the availability of adapted treatment programmes.

A guardianship order can help in establishing boundaries and can include a requirement for the person to allow access to professionals and to attend for specific activities such as medical treatment, and in the right case can prevent more restrictive options being used. However, guardianship does not provide legal authority to detain a person physically in accommodation or to remove them against their wishes, and should never be used solely for the purposes of transferring any unwilling person into residential care. Nor does it allow for force to be used to secure attendance at specified places for medical treatment to be administered without the person's consent. Even if granted an absolute discharge, appropriate follow-up by specialist services should be organised with use of the CPA structure (Royal College of Psychiatrists, 2014).

Khanom et al. (2009) argue in 'A Missed Opportunity?' that the option of a community order in conjunction with mental health treatment requirement option (MHTR) should be used more often. In order for psychiatrists and psychologists to make such recommendations to the court requires early identification of those offenders with an ID and professionals with the appropriate expertise to assess these individuals and make recommendations for treatment. Community forensic teams for people with ID are ideally placed to assess and treat such patients, and can potentially reduce the number of people who would otherwise have risked being given a prison sentence (Benton & Roy, 2008; Devapriam et al., 2012; Dinani et al., 2010). However, community forensic ID teams are still very rare in the UK. A bailed offender who, following an alleged offence, is assessed and who accepts active treatment by a learning disability community forensic team is far less likely to face a prison sentence or even admission to secure hospital than an offender for whom, as often happens, a court report from the local forensic psychiatrist is commissioned only a few weeks before sentencing.

The NHS England document Building the Right Support (2015) set out to reduce the number of inpatients with neurodevelopmental disorders in secure services, both in the NHS as the independent sector. In order to achieve this reduction in beds, the document anticipated that community forensic services would be commissioned to support people to be discharged who are currently out of area and enhance the support locally to avoid future admissions

12.8 Inpatient Services

Currently in the UK, there are forensic ID hospital beds at three levels of security – high, medium and low. Reliable information about the number of these beds and the occupancy rates is lacking although some projections could be made using data from the Count me in Censuses (Care Quality Commission, 2005) and the Ministry of Justice (MoJ) data on restricted patients (Ministry of Justice, 2010). In addition, there are also an unknown number of locked units for offenders with ID with names such as mental impairment unit, locked rehabilitation unit and step-down unit that are not formally classified as secure units. In England, whereas patients in low, medium and high secure units are generally funded directly by NHS England, those in locked units are currently funded by local clinical commissioning groups (CCGs).

An earlier survey of forensic ID beds estimated that there were 48 high, 414 medium and 1,356 low secure beds for people with ID in 2009 within the ten strategic health authority regions of England (Alexander et al., 2011). In a recent report, people with ID and mental health, behavioural or forensic problems: the role of inpatient services, the Royal College of Psychiatrists (2013) identified six categories of inpatient bed categories within a four-tiered model of service provision.

Both these surveys showed a very uneven distribution of beds with some regions not having any medium or low secure unit within their borders. It is this uneven distribution that has led to some offenders with ID often being placed in units far away from their families because suitable local units are not available (Yacoub et al., 2008). On the other hand, some authors (Barron et al., 2002) have discussed the economies of scale and commented about how it is unrealistic to have very specialised services of this nature in every district. It is accepted that offenders with ID should be treated as near as possible to their home area.

There are few services specifically for women offenders with ID, although high secure hospitals, where women make up about 10% of the population, have always operated strict segregation policies (Beber & Boer, 2004). This group of patients have high levels of mental illness, are more likely to have suffered from sexual abuse, and may be more challenging to manage.

Patients referred or admitted to secure units have a high rate of psychiatric and developmental morbidities. Most have histories of early deprivation and abuse, about half have personality disorders, the same proportion have substance misuse as part of their presentation, a third have mental illnesses and about one-third to one-quarter have disorders within the autistic spectrum (Alexander & Cooray, 2003; Hogue et al., 2006). They also have extensive histories of offending behaviour with risk profiles that are as serious as those detained in generic forensic units (Hogue et al., 2006).

Although the usual definition of a learning disability would require a person's IQ to be below 70, sometimes the courts have accepted evidence that those with an intellectual ability equivalent to an IQ of up to about 74 (and therefore falling within what has been called 'borderline learning disability') may be classified as suffering from mental impairment due to their adaptive functioning. This is important as people who fall into this slightly higher range may still struggle to cope with standard prison offender treatment programmes. Some NHS and independent ID secure units will accept patients with borderline ID, particularly if they have additional disabilities such as genetic abnormalities, autism, cerebral palsy or brain injury. These services often have specialist skills in treating those with borderline ID and, unless this population have additional diagnoses such as mental illness, they are not generally accepted for treatment in non-ID facilities.

Through the Transforming Care programme, the government have pledged that people with ID and/or autism who are in hospital who could be supported elsewhere should be discharged to the community as soon as possible (NHS England, 2015). Those admitted to secure care are not exempt from this process. It is anticipated that the programme will lead to the closure of a proportion of the secure estate with a reciprocal increase in community-based ID forensic services.

12.9 Treatment

A substantial number of offenders with ID have additional psychiatric disorders such as schizophrenia, bipolar disorder or depression requiring specific treatment including psychotropic medication as appropriate. However, as a significant number of inpatients are diagnosed with a personality disorder, the mainstay of treatment for this group consists of relational and psychotherapeutic treatment. Many patients present with additional psychosocial disadvantages (Holland, 2004) and benefit from a period of stability in a stable environment, allowing for trusting relationships to develop with members of staff prior to active psychological treatment. Motivational work with patients can be both formal (e.g. psychology-led) or informal (e.g. by qualified and experienced unqualified nursing staff).

A number of specific treatments are available, including cognitive treatment (thinking skills), and offence-specific therapies such as anger management and sex offender work.

Several studies have described in detail the process and outcome of specific psychological, offence-focused therapies such as anger (Taylor & Novaco, 2005) and sexual offending (Lindsay, 2004). Other mainstream treatments have been successfully adapted for use in the ID population such as dialectical behaviour therapy (Morrissey & Ingamells, 2011).

The length of treatment may be important. Day (1988) noted in a study of offenders with ID that those with more than two years' inpatient care had a better longer-term outcome, and Lindsay and Smith (1998 found that sex offenders treated in the community on probation orders for two years had better outcomes than those with a one-year order.

12.10 Court Reports

When writing a report for the court it is important to be aware that this is a time-consuming process. The practitioner should use plain English, be prepared to explain medical terms, avoid ambivalence (such as 'yesterday she told me she stole an apple'). The conclusion should be supported by the body of the report. When writing reports for people with ID it essential that the writer has access to all the documentation (depositions) and other background information such as general practitioner records or inmate medical records (prison medical file) and to listen to recordings of the police interviews.

An appropriate adult should always have been present at police interviews with people with ID, it is their role to facilitate communication between the police and the person and to provide support (see Rix, 2011).

The Witness Intermediary Scheme was introduced in 2004 to help vulnerable witnesses give evidence in court. These registered intermediaries are professionals from a number of different backgrounds who have experience in working with people with communication difficulties and have received specialist training from the MoJ.

When asked to prepare a court report it is important for the writer to ensure that there are clear instructions and not to be tempted to comment on issues outside his or her area of expertise.

12.11 Risk Assessment

There is evidence that some of the commonly used standardised, structured risk assessment instruments have good predictive validity for future violence and/or sexual offending. They also provide a good framework for the meticulous collection of data. However, the clinician needs to be aware of their limitations: difficulty in translating group norms to the individual;

generalisability, little ability to take day-to-day factors into account and the difficulty inherent in attempting to predict rare events. This is particularly true when using such instruments in the ID population. Forensic ID services generally use the mainstream instruments as the people using these services tend to have mild degrees of impairment. Lindsay et al. (2008) looked at the Violence Risk Appraisal Guide (VRAG), Historical Clinical Risk Management-20 (HCR 20), Risk Matrix 2000 C and the Short Dynamic Risk Scale (SDRS) in men in high, medium and low secure services and found them to have predictive validity for violence in the ID population.

12.12 Conclusion

Although only a small proportion of people with ID offend, this group of people often have disadvantaged background and present with poor social skills and impulse control difficulties. They may not be recognised as suffering from ID, may be more difficult to assess, and treatment may not be always available. After a period of expansion of inpatient beds in the 1990s and the early years of the twenty-first century recently there has been a call for a reduction of beds and more community-based services. If this strategy is to be successful, it is essential that mechanisms are available to ensure that people with ID in the CJS are recognised, and that when they are, appropriate placement and treatment is sought.

References

Alexander, R. et al. (2011) Evaluation of treatment outcomes from a medium secure unit for people with intellectual disability. *Advances in Mental Health and Intellectual Disabilities*, 5 (1), 22–32. Available at: www.emeraldinsight.com/10.5042/amhid.2011.0013 [accessed 11 August 2018]

Alexander, R. & Cooray, S. (2003) Diagnosis of personality disorders in learning disability. *British Journal of Psychiatry*, 182 (suppl. 44).

Barron, P., Hassiotis, A. & Banes, J. (2002) Offenders with intellectual disability: The size of the problem and therapeutic outcomes. *Journal of Intellectual Disability Research*, 46 (6), 454–63.

Benton, C. & Roy, A. (2008) The first three years of a community forensic service for people with a learning disability. *British Journal of Forensic Practice*, 10, 4–12.

Beber, E. & Boer, H. (2004) Development of a specialised forensic service for women with learning disability: The first three years. *British Journal of Forensic Practice*, 6(4), 10–20. Available at: http://dx.doi.org/10.1108/14636646200400022 [accessed 11 August 2018]

Care Quality Commission (2005) Count me in Census 2005: Results of the national census of inpatients in mental health hospitals and facilities in England and Wales. Available at: www.cqc.org.uk [accessed 11 August 2018]

Day, K. (1988) A hospital based treatment programme for male mentally disordered handicapped offenders. *British Journal of Psychiatry*, 153, 636–44.

Department of Health (2009) *Lord Bradley's Review of People with Mental Health Problems or Learning Disabilities in the Criminal Justice System*. Stationery Office.

Department of Health (2015) *Mental Health Act 1983: Code of Practice*. Stationery Office, pp. 1–459. Available at: www.gov.uk/government/uploads/system/uploads/attachment_data/file/435512/MHA_Code_of_Practice.PDF [accessed 11 August 2018]

Department of Health & Home Office (1992) *Review of Health and Social Services for Mentally Disordered Offenders and Others Requiring Similar Services*. Stationery Office.

Devapriam, J. et al. (2012) Tiered model of learning disability forensic service provision. Available at: www.researchgate.net/publication/264533409_Tiered_model_of_learning_disability_forensic_service_provision [accessed 11 August 2018]

Dinani, S. et al. (2010) Providing forensic community services for people with learning disabilities. Available at: www.emeraldinsight.com/doi/abs/10.5042/jldob.2010.0179 [accessed 11 August 2018]

Fazel, S., Xenitidis, K. & Powell, J. (2008) The prevalence of intellectual disabilities among 12000 prisoners – A systematic review. *International Journal of Law and Psychiatry*, 31 (4), 369–73. Available at: http://linkinghub.elsevier.com/retrieve/pii/S0160252708000903 [accessed 11 August 2018]

Finlay, W. M. L. & Lyons, E. (2002) Acquiescence in interviews with people who have mental retardation. *Mental Retardation*, 40 (1), 14–29.

Goddard, H. H. (1912) *The Kallikak Family: A Study in Feeble-Mindedness*. Macmillan.

Hogue, T., Steptoe, L., Taylor, J., Lindsay, W., Mooney, P., Pinkney, L. et al. (2006) A comparison of offenders with intellectual disability across three levels of security. *Criminal Behavior and Mental Health*, 16, 13–28.

Holland, A. (2004) Criminal behavior and developmental disability: An epidemiological perspective. In *Offenders with Developmental Disabilities* (eds. W. Lindsay, J. Taylor & P. Sturmey). Wiley.

Holland, T., Clare, I. C. H. & Mukhopadhyay, T. (2002) Prevalence of 'criminal offending' by men and women with intellectual disability and the characteristics of 'offenders': Implications for research and service development. *Endocrine-Related Cancer*, 9 (suppl. 1), 6–20.

Humphreys, M. (2000) Aspects of basic management of offenders with mental disorders. *The Law*, 6, 22–32.

Jones, R. (2016) *Mental Health Act Manual*. Thomson Reuters.

Khanom, H., Samele, C. & Rutherford, M. (2009) Report: A Missed Opportunity? Sainsbury Centre for Mental Health. Available at: http://citeseerx.ist.psu.edu/viewdoc/download?doi=10.1.1.627.1651&rep=rep1&type=pdf [accessed 11 August 2018]

Lindsay, W. R. (2004) Sex offenders: Conceptualisation of the issues, services, treatment and management. In *Offenders with Developmental Disabilities* (eds. W. Lindsay, J. Taylor & P. Sturmey), pp. 163–85. Wiley.

Lindsay, W. R. et al. (2008) Risk assessment in offenders with intellectual disability: A comparison across three levels of security. *International Journal of Offender Therapy and Comparative Criminology*, 52(1), 90–111. Available at: http://ijo.sagepub.com/cgi/content/abstract/52/1/90 [accessed 11 August 2018]

Lindsay, W. R. et al. (2010) Pathways into services for offenders with intellectual disabilities: Childhood experiences, diagnostic information, and offense variables. *Criminal Justice and Behavior*, 37(6), 678–94. Available at: http://cjb.sagepub.com/cgi/doi/10.1177/0093854810363725 [accessed 11 August 2018]

Lindsay, W. & Smith, A. (1998). Responses to treatment for sex offenders with intellectual disability: A comparison of men with 1- and 2-year probation sentences. *Journal Of Intellectual Disability Research*, 42(5), 346–53.

McBrien, J. & Murphy, G. (2006) Police and carers' views on reporting alleged offences by people with intellectual disabilities. *Psychology, Crime & Law*, 12(2), 127–44. Available at: http://dx.doi.org/10.1080/10683160512331316262 [accessed 11 August 2018]

McKinnon, I. G. & Grubin, D. (2013) Health screening of people in police custody – Evaluation of current police screening procedures in London, UK. *European Journal of Public Health*, 23(3), 399–405. Available at: http://eurpub.oxfordjournals.org/cgi/doi/10.1093/eurpub/cks027 [accessed 11 August 2018]

Ministry of Justice (2010) *Breaking the Cycle: Effective Punishment, Rehabilitation and Sentencing of Offenders*. Available at: www.justice.gov.uk/consultations/docs/breaking-the-cycle.pdf [accessed 11 August 2018]

Morrissey, C. & Ingamells, B. (2011) Adapted dialectical behaviour therapy for male offenders with learning disabilities in a high secure environment: Six years on, *Journal of Learning Disabilities and Offending Behaviour*, 2(1), 8–15.

Murphy, G. & Mason, J. (2007) People with intellectual disabilities who are at risk of offending. In *Psychiatric and Behavioural Disorders in Intellectual and Developmental Disabilities* (eds. N. Bouras & G. Holt), pp. 173–201. Cambridge University Press.

Nacro (2005) Findings of the 2004 survey of Court Diversion/Criminal Justice Mental Health Liaison Schemes for mentally disordered offenders in England and Wales. Available at: www.ohrn.nhs.uk/resource/policy/CourtDiversion.pdf [accessed 11 August 2018]

NHS England (2015) *Building the Right Support*. Stationery Office.

Rix, K. (2011) *Expert Psychiatric Evidence*. Royal College of Psychiatrists.

Royal College of Psychiatrists (2013) *People with Intellectual Disability and Mental Health, Behavioural or Forensic Problems: The Role of In-Patient Services*.

Royal College of Psychiatrists' Faculty of Psychiatry of Intellectual Disability (2014) *Forensic Care Pathways for Adults with Intellectual Disability Involved with the Criminal Justice System*.

Singleton, N., Meltzer, H. & Gatward, R. (1998) *Psychiatric Morbidity among Prisoners in England and Wales*. Stationery Office.

Søndenaa, E., Rasmussen, K., Palmstierna, T. & Nøttestad, J. (2008) The prevalence and nature of intellectual disability in Norwegian prisons. *Journal of intellectual disability research*, 52(12), 1129–37.

Sutherland, E. H. (1931) *Mental Deficiency and Crime in Social Attitudes* (ed. Kimball Young). Rinehart & Wilson.

Talbot, J. (2008) *No One Knows: Offenders with Learning Difficulties and Learning Disabilities*. Prison Reform Trust.

Taylor, J. L., Novaco, R. W., Gillmer, B. T., Robertson, A. & Thorne, I. (2005) Individual cognitive-behavioural anger treatment for people with mild-borderline intellectual disabilities and histories of aggression: A controlled trial. *British Journal of Clinical Psychology*, 44(3), 367–82.

Ventress, M., Rix, K. J. B. & Kent, J. H. (2008) Keeping PACE: fitness to be interviewed by the police. *Advances in Psychiatric Treatment*, 14, 369–81.

Yacoub, E., Hall, I. & Bernall, J., 2008) Secure in-patient services for people with learning disability: Is the market serving the user well? *Psychiatric Bulletin*, 32(6), 205–7. Available at: http://pb.rcpsych.org/cgi/doi/10.1192/pb.bp.107.018523 [accessed 11 August 2018]

West, D. J. & Farrington, D. P. (1973) *Who Becomes Delinquent?* Heinemann.

Zigmond, T. & Brindle, N. (2016) *A Clinician's Brief Guide to the Mental Health Act*. Royal College of Psychiatrists.

Further Reading

Jones, R. (2017) *Mental Health Act Manual* (20th edn). Sweet & Maxwell.

Lindsay, W. R., Taylor, J. L. & Sturmey, P. (2004) *Offenders with Developmental Disabilities*. Wiley.

Rix, K. (2011) *Expert Psychiatric Evidence*. Royal College of Psychiatrists.

Royal College of Psychiatrists (2013) *People with Intellectual Disability and Mental Health, Behavioural or Forensic Problems: The Role of In-Patient Services*.

Royal College of Psychiatrists' Faculty of Psychiatry of Intellectual Disability (2014) *Forensic Care Pathways for Adults with Intellectual Disability Involved with the Criminal Justice System*.

Chapter 13

Psychotherapy in People with Intellectual Disabilities

Rajnish Attavar and Kuljit Bhogal

13.1 Introduction

Psychological approaches to the treatment of mental disorder are well established in all psychiatric specialities.[1] Psychotherapy is a broad discipline that can help the patient and practitioner to find a way through distress or trauma using a combination of skilled communication and reflection. Different modalities have come in and out of fashion and provision for people with intellectual disability (ID) will vary widely from locality to locality. This chapter will highlight some of the general issues to consider when providing psychotherapy to people with ID.

Therapy will evoke feelings in the patient towards their therapist (transference) and feelings in the therapist towards their patient (countertransference). These feelings will be used actively in psychoanalytic or psychodynamic therapies, and may be less important in more behavioural or skills-based therapies.

Psychotherapy is most effective when there is the right fit between the patient, the therapist and the approach being provided. It is essential that professionals providing therapy have the theoretical knowledge required to structure their approach and receive the appropriate amount of supervision to support their therapy.

13.2 The Context

People with ID will have been exposed to multiple challenges during their childhood and will continue to be at risk of adversity as adults. Complex communication issues and limited control over their environment may increase their vulnerability to stress and anxiety. Although it is well known that individuals with ID are at higher risk of developing mental health problems (Whitaker & Read, 2006) they often do not have the same access to psychological therapies as people without ID. The reasons for this are complex but will be in part due to historic assumptions that people with ID will not benefit from talking therapies, diagnostic overshadowing and under-resourced or under-commissioned specialist psychotherapy services.

The presence of ID does not preclude a patient from accessing psychotherapy, but some therapists may feel understandable apprehension or anxiety about how to adapt their technique for a patient with ID. In their review of the literature, Brown et al. (2011) found that the existing research base for psychological interventions still remains small and provision is patchy or non-existent. This is despite literature suggesting that people with

---

[1] The patient names and accounts in this chapter are fictional, but are based on the clinical experience of the authors.

> **Box 13.1** An account from 'Psychological disturbance associated with sexual abuse in people with learning disabilities' (Sequeira et al., 2003)
>
> When the self-locking door had slammed behind me and I stood in the ward, I was both appalled and terrified. It was a very chastening experience, exposing fears and prejudices which until then I would have furiously denied. The ward consisted of three huge bare rooms, like community halls rather than places in which to live. Some of the 20 men were sitting rocking in padded metal chairs that were bolted to the floor. Others ran round in circles, some shouting and/or whooping. One sat, naked, roaring loudly. Gradually these emotions faded. The better I got to know the men in the long periods of the day and night that I spent with them, the more moved I was by their individuality, their desperate desire to communicate, and the extent of their individual physical and emotional suffering.

ID would value the experience (Macdonald et al., 2003) or may show improvements in their symptoms (Royal College of Psychiatrists, 2004).

13.3 Labelling and Stigma

A diagnosis of ID can carry stigma and therapists should be aware of this when planning and delivering psychotherapy. Without the diagnosis individuals may not be able to access support or services that they need, but with it they are marked out as different to many people that they interact with on a daily basis. It is important to try to understand what the diagnosis means for each individual and to be aware that some may be more comfortable with it than others.

Labelling has a mixed history and social response. The terms used for ID have changed over time and this may be in part an effort to shed the stigma that the labels accumulate over time (Sinason, 1992). People with ID may have well-developed defence mechanisms that help them cope with the challenges of having an ID.

13.4 Communication

In their qualitative study of the subjective experiences of adults with ID who have mental health problems, Robinson et al. (2016) found that most of the participants experienced difficulties expressing themselves and feeling heard. They also had a limited understanding of their diagnoses and symptoms.

Some people will show skill in their expressive language and struggle with receptive language. Some will need extra time to process verbal information or for information to be provided in other modalities.

People with ID will have varying difficulties with their communication and the therapist will have to make an ongoing effort to understand the communication needs of the person they are working with.

Having access to any communication assessments before the start of the therapy can be immensely useful in ensuring that the therapist takes into account the person's strengths and weaknesses from the beginning.

13.5 Life Stages and Identity

In the UK it was not long ago that people with ID were segregated in large institutions and isolated from most aspects of life. You may work with individuals who experienced this life

> **Case Study 13.1**
>
> Eileen often recounted that the reason she would not go out was that she felt people would notice that she had a learning disability. She incessantly asked what it meant to have a 'mild learning disability', consoling herself that 'mild' meant only 'a little bit'. In session thirty, she said that staff told her she should make the most of the fact that she did not look like someone with a learning disability.
>
> (O'Conner 2001)

first-hand. Although people with ID are generally better integrated within wider society, they will still be vulnerable to discrimination and exclusion. It is important to note that people with severe and enduring mental illness will also be subject to similar levels of exclusion and discrimination.

All families cope with the news that their child has an ID differently. The usual life stages that a parent will expect for their child may be delayed or absent and the normal process of individuation that takes place as the child becomes an adult can be disrupted. Families may experience grief at the loss of the child that they expected, and this grief may continue throughout the individual's life.

Most people define themselves by their occupation or relationships and people with ID may struggle with their identity as individuals and their self-esteem.

For some patients a more systemic approach may help understand the complex pattern of family interactions that may need to be understood before attempts at an intervention can be made (Rhodes et al., 2011). The psychological formulation is important in identifying a suitable approach.

13.6 Challenging Behaviour and Psychotherapy

At a basic level challenging behaviour can be seen as a form of communication. A person may feel a strong emotion and be unable to articulate this emotion. This emotion may then be translated into an action. Despite the current focus on positive behaviour support, psychotherapy might also be important in offering a space for individuals to explore their emotional needs, develop a safe, therapeutic relationship and explore what is needed to change things and improve their quality of life and emotional well-being.

13.7 Mainstream or Specialist Services

The current political driver is that people with ID should be treated within mainstream mental health services where possible (National Development Team for Inclusion (NDTI), 2012) to ensure that people with disabilities are not discriminated against. In saying this, there is limited research into what is most effective and what people with learning disID want for themselves. Without appropriate thought and planning, the risk is that people with ID end up experiencing the same stigma and marginalisation within services that they may be subject to in society as a whole.

A survey of practitioners who have provided therapy to people with ID (Shankland & Dagnan, 2015) found that memory, understanding emotions, and problems with using supporting materials were significant challenges. In saying this, in general they felt that people

> **Case Study 13.2**
>
> Amanda is a middle-aged lady with a mild-to-moderate learning disability. She has displayed challenging behaviour during most of her adult life. She spent her adolescent years in an institution and her parents feel that this is when she started to show aggression towards her caregivers. She does not talk about this time in her life.
>
> It was recently discovered that another resident who had been at the same institution may have been subject to physical abuse. Amanda was referred to art therapy to consider whether she had an unresolved trauma. It took her time to trust the therapist but as the course progressed the pictures that she drew became less preoccupied with the past. The challenging behaviour reduced in frequency.

> **Case Study 13.3**
>
> Tomasz is a 23-year-old man with Down syndrome and a mild ID. He usually works in an office canteen and lives in supported living. He was referred to the local primary care psychotherapy service by his GP as she become increasingly anxious about getting on buses. The problem started after he was on a bus that was involved in a crash.
>
> He met with a CBT therapist who adapted her approach to use fewer words and more pictures when explaining the main points of the therapy. She was also able to extend the length of the therapy to give Tomasz more time to understand and reflect on the strategies needed to treat his anxiety. The therapist used tick lists that could be completed with support staff to support the therapy.

with ID should access mainstream therapies but that more support and supervision was needed.

13.8 Choosing the Right Psychotherapeutic Modality

In their 2016 report the British Psychological Society published their joint review with the Royal College of Psychiatrists *Psychological Therapies and People Who Have Intellectual Disabilities*. Nine different psychotherapies are considered, and suggestions made for how they can be adapted to be used in people with ID. Table 13.1 summarises five of these approaches. There is no clear outcome data suggesting that one therapy is more effective than the other and although expanding, the evidence base remains relatively limited.

13.9 Opportunities for Developing Skills in Psychotherapy

Higher trainees in ID psychiatry are required to 'demonstrate the ability to conduct a range of individual, group and family therapies using standard accepted models and to integrate these psychotherapies into everyday treatment'. In practice opportunities for the development of these skills will be dependent on the local skill mix of psychologists, psychotherapists and psychiatrists.

Complex communication and autism can make the delivery of psychotherapy to people with ID very challenging and trainees should start by identifying a suitable supervisor who

Table 13.1 Countertransference: an emotional reaction

Modality	Approach	Techniques used	Potential adaptations for people with ID
Psychodynamic psychotherapy	Making links between earlier life experiences and conscious expectations of relationships in the present day	Listening, observation, interpretation of transference and countertransference	For those with limited verbal ability pay more attention to the words that are used and any non-verbal behaviour. Interpretation should be done in short sentences. Be aware that the patient may act out during therapy
Cognitive behavioural therapy	Beliefs and thinking styles can contribute to significant emotional problems and patterns of behaviour. Interventions are targeted at cognitive, emotional and behavioural levels	Identifying negative or maladaptive thoughts or behaviours and challenging them using discussion and behavioural experiments	Using visual aids to support sessions and more abstract concepts. Recognise that the rate of therapeutic change may be slower, and more sessions may be needed. Consider the use of technology such as Dictaphones to support homework tasks
Cognitive analytic therapy	A time-limited, relational therapy that looks at the patient's difficulties in the context of their relating to others	Mapping out the interpersonal patterns/difficulties and using a narrative and pictorial process to recognise and reformulate these patterns	Lloyd and Clayton (2014) have adapted the CAT tools and process for use in people with ID
Mindfulness and acceptance-based therapies	A behavioural therapy that aims to change the way people relate to mental events by cultivating a non-judgemental awareness of the present moment	A broad group of therapies which use meditation to increase the individual's awareness of the present moment	Offering additional sessions to support the processing of ideas, practice and the refinement of exercises. Breaks may need to be scheduled. Abstract language should be minimised
Dialectical behaviour therapy	It assumes that there are personal and environmental factors that prevent an individual acting in the most effective or skilful way. It was developed for people with borderline personality disorder	A structured approach that uses individual work, group skills teaching, and telephone skill coaching	Care needs to be taken to check that people fully understand the concepts and to take into account cognitive deficits such as poor memory, lack of a concept of time and limited capacity for abstract thinking

will help them select a case and modality. Trainees who want to develop advanced skills in psychotherapy can consider undertaking further education in psychotherapy.

13.10 Conclusion

Psychotherapy should be offered to people with ID and where possible patients should access mainstream services. For those whose disability causes them significant difficulty with accessing mainstream services, the intervention should be offered by an ID specialist. Although the evidence base for psychotherapy in people with ID has not been extensive (British Psychological Society, 2016), the evidence base is growing, and studies generally report that people with ID benefit from interventions.

Providing psychotherapy to people with ID requires us to be mindful of our own limitations and defences. The psychological needs of people with ID are as diverse as those without ID, but challenges in communication can mask these needs or make them more difficult to access. Although it can be daunting to deliver psychotherapy to a person with significantly different communication needs to yours, remaining flexible and responsive to the flow of information between you and the patient can help ensure that the intervention is meaningful.

Choosing the therapeutic modality will be dependent on the needs of the patient, the skills of the therapist and their supervisor and for some patients the modality may need to be changed during the course of the therapy. The evidence base for which modality will work best needs further development, but as for people without an ID, it is likely that the relationship and rapport will be just as important as or more important than the modality employed.

References

British Psychological Society (2016) *Psychological Therapies and People Who Have Intellectual Disabilities.*

Brown, M., Duff, H., Karatzias, T. & Horsburgh, D. (2011) A review of the literature relating to psychological interventions and people with intellectual disabilities: Issues for research, policy, education and clinical practice. *Journal of Intellectual Disability*, **15**(1), 31–45. doi: 10.1177/1744629511401166

Hubert, J. & Hollins, S. (2006) Men with severe learning disabilities and challenging behaviour in long-stay hospital care: Qualitative study. *British Journal of Psychiatry*, **188**(1), 70–4. doi:10.1192/bjp.bp.105.010223

Lloyd, J. & Clayton, P. (2014) *Cognitive Analytic Therapy for People with Learning Disabilities and their Carers.* Jessica Kingsley.

MacDonald, J., Sinason, V. & Hollins, S. (2003) An interview study of people with learning disabilities' experience of, and satisfaction with, group analytic therapy.

Psychology and Psychotherapy Research, **76**(4), 433–53. PMID: 14670190 DOI: 10.1348/147608303770584764

National Development Team for Inclusion (2012) *Reasonably Adjusted? Mental Health Services for People with Autism and People with Learning Disabilities.*

O'Connor, Hester (2001) Will we grow out of it? A psychotherapy group for people with learning disabilities. *Psychodynamic Counselling*, 7(3), 297–314.

Robinson, L. et al. (2016) The subjective experience of adults with intellectual disabilities who have mental health problems within community settings. *Advances in Mental Health and Intellectual Disabilities*, **10**(2), 106–15.

Royal College of Psychiatrists (2004) *Psychotherapy and Learning Disability (Report CR116).*

Sequeira, H. Howlin, P. & Hollins, S. (2003) Psychological disturbance associated with sexual abuse in people with learning disabilities. *British Journal of Psychiatry.* Available at: www.cambridge.org/core/journals/the-british-journal-of-psychiatry/article/psychological-disturbance-associated-with-sexual-abuse-in-people-with-learning-disabilities/F9FC04B9A9B23E115F69FE2AD128CCBD [accessed 11 August 2018]

Sinason, V. (1992) *Mental Handicap and the Human Condition*. Free Association Books.

Whitaker, S. & Read, S. (2006) The prevalence of psychotic disorders among people with intellectual disabilities: An analysis of the literature. *Journal of Applied Research in Intellectual Disabilities*, **19**(4), 330–46.

Further Reading

British Psychological Society (2016) *Psychological Therapies and People Who Have Intellectual Disabilities*.

Foundation for People with Learning Disabilities (2015) *Learning Disabilities Positive Practice Guide*.

Rhodes, P. Whatson, L. Mora, L. Hasson, A. Brearly, K. & Dikian, J. (2013) Systemic hypothesising for challenging behaviour in intellectual disabilities: A reflecting team approach. *Australian and New Zealand Journal of Family Therapy*, **32**(1), 70–82.

Royal College of Psychiatrists (2017) *A Competency Based Curriculum for Specialist Training in Psychiatry*.

Shankland, J. & Dagnan, D. (2015) IAPT practitioners' experiences of providing therapy to people with intellectual disabilities. *Advances in Mental Health and Intellectual Disabilities*, **9**(4), 206–14.

Chapter 14

Psychological Treatment of Common Behavioural Disorders

Audrey Espie and Andrew Jahoda

14.1 Introduction

Behaviour problems are commonly referred to as challenging behaviour or behaviour that challenges. The aim of using the term 'challenging behaviour' is to try to place emphasis on how services can respond most appropriately or effectively to behavioural challenges rather than blaming the individual for their behavioural problems. In 2015 NICE published their quality standards titled 'Challenging Behaviour and Learning Disabilities: Prevention and Interventions for People with Learning Disabilities Whose Behaviour Challenges'. These standards apply to the care of people across the lifespan, including those with a dual diagnosis such as autistic spectrum disorder and learning disabilities or intellectual disabilities (ID). The guidelines use Emerson et al.'s (1995) definition of challenging behaviour which remains relevant today: 'culturally abnormal behaviour(s) of such an intensity, frequency or duration that the physical safety of the person or others is likely to be placed in serious jeopardy, or behaviour which is likely to seriously limit use of, or result in the person being denied access to, ordinary community facilities'. Thus, they described behavioural problems in social terms, as having an impact on people's relationships and the quality of their lives. Sadly, significantly challenging behaviour continues to have potentially devastating consequences on the lives of people with ID. The horrific abuse of adults with ID at Winterbourne View hospital highlighted the vulnerability of these individuals and the need for local services to provide effective help, rather than being sent to remote institutional services (NHS England, 2014).

Historically, psychological treatments in the ID field have tended to focus on behavioural paradigms with interventions originating from the wealth of applied and experimental work in this field (for a comprehensive review, see Emerson, 1995). However, there has been a growing number of other approaches which aim to help support staff work more effectively or work directly with the individuals concerned to reduce their challenging behaviour. Singh (2006) found that mindfulness techniques reduced the use of restrictive practices by staff working with people presenting challenging behaviour. Anger management, drawing on cognitive behavioural principles, has also been successfully used with clients with more mild-to-moderate levels of ID and problems of anger and aggression (Willner et al., 2013). However, intervention techniques built on applied behavioural analysis remain core strategies for tackling challenging behaviour.

Challenging behaviour is not a diagnostic term but is a descriptor for a range of behaviours occurring in a range of contexts with many possible causes. The term is adopted in relation to stereotypy or self-stimulatory movements defined as 'frequent, idiosyncratic, repetitive movements and/or vocalisations that can be self-injurious, exhibiting little variation, often constant across settings and having no unequivocal function' (Paul, 1997).

Challenging behaviour also includes verbal and physical aggression to others and inanimate objects, which on occasion may result in contact with the criminal justice system for those with mild learning disabilities. The 2015 NICE guidelines highlight the most effective interventions for challenging behaviour, and point to the support and care required to help the individuals concerned maintain a good quality of life. In reality, there is considerable variability in service provision for individuals with problems in different parts of the UK even though this remains a major issue for a substantial minority of people with ID.

Recent data on prevalence rates of challenging behaviour has suggested lower figures than in the past (Lowe et al., 2007) from around 10% of this population, to 10–15% (Emerson et al., 2001) and 18.7% (Lundqvist et al., 2013). Studies in the 1980s and 1990s indicated higher rates in institutional settings (Dura et al., 1987; Matson & Rojahn, 1986; Volkmar, 1997). The downward trend could possibly be related to the decommissioning of hospital services resulting in either a true decline in the behaviours, or less of a focus on their prevalence. In many cases, people have moved to significantly smaller group living situations and others have returned from out of area placements to more local person-centred services, in keeping with the recommendations of the Mansell Report (revised 2007). In some areas, more specialist multidisciplinary teams have developed to support carers in these circumstances and the range and types of interventions has expanded. There is still contention about the use of hospital assessment and treatment units, where there can be an absence of psychological treatments. However, the efficacy of the shift to community-based services will only become apparent by obtaining evidence about whether the pattern of incidence changes (McClintock et al., 2003). Looking forward, there are significant challenges on the horizon as we have a rapidly ageing population. In this context, we need to consider the risks and needs of adults with ID who develop dementia and associated psychological symptoms, as well as other age-related physical complications. The Alzheimer's Society estimates that by 2025, one million people in the UK will have dementia and dementia is around three to four times more common in people with ID than in the general population (Strydom et al., 2007). We need to continue to work towards a more proactive approach to managing the presenting symptoms of psychological decline amongst those with ID.

Crocker et al. (2006) categorised aggressive behaviour displayed by people with ID using the Modified Overt Aggression Scale. They identified five typologies comprising property damage, verbal, self-oriented, physical and sexual. They then recorded prevalence and severity over a twelve-month period in 3,165 adults with learning disabilities. Their results indicated that only 4.9% of those individuals observed displayed aggressive behaviour resulting in injury to others. Although their study found no significant gender differences, there is a perception that these behaviours tend to be more prevalent in men and peak when they are between their mid-teens and mid-thirties (Tsiouris et al., 2011). Increasing levels of aggressive behaviour are positively correlated with degree of ID. Whatever the nature of the presentation, all challenging behaviour requires to be fully assessed before intervening, particularly as the efficacy of antipsychotics for treatment remains controversial (Willner, 2015).

14.2 Differential Diagnosis and Diagnostic Overshadowing: Starting with a Real Understanding of the Person

Behavioural problems have a range of potential contributory causes: genetic, physical, emotional, communicative, interpersonal and environmental. Before embarking on any psychological intervention a key first step is to carry out a thorough assessment to help determine the best way to intervene and careful steps need to be taken to rule out a range of other factors. Consequently, the assessment is likely to be multidisciplinary, involving a wide range of professionals such as psychiatry, clinical psychology, speech and language therapy and learning disability nursing. There is still a risk that important factors can be overlooked with people who have ID because their problems are simply attributed to having a disability. This is known as diagnostic overshadowing and both the Royal College of Psychiatrists (2016) and the BPS Faculty for People with Intellectual Disabilities (2011) urge caution in this area and the need for clinicians to be careful to remain open to different underlying causes of behavioural difficulties. For example, despite the frequency of motor disorders such as Tourette's syndrome, Parkinson's disease and other tremor or dystonic type conditions in the general population, they are rarely diagnosed in people with ID. When carrying out a differential diagnosis of challenging behaviour it is vitally important to be aware of a range of possible contributory factors. Epilepsy is present in around 30% of all people with profound ID and can be overlooked as a possible cause of self-harm (Bowley & Kerr, 2000). It may be difficult to determine why a person with a severe to profound ID flaps their arms, swings their arms back and forth, slaps their face and slaps flat surfaces while simultaneously vocalising loudly. Repetitive, complex motor behaviours or vocalisations can be symptomatic of complex partial seizures. Equally, the drugs for the treatment of seizures may cause side effects and these side effects may be communicated through a change in behaviour.

A systematic review by Robertson et al. (2015) concluded that prevalence rates for all people with ID are at least 22%, yet the external manifestation of a seizure may be so subtle that it is difficult to differentiate from a routine motor movement. The symptoms may simply comprise the blinking of eyes or a brief jerking of a limb. Carers may be unclear as to whether the behaviour is a stereotypy or a possible seizure event and recordings in client records will differ. In this instance, circumstances may necessitate further professional support in the form of neurological investigation. Standard assessment procedures for epilepsy comprise sound history-taking, eyewitness report (if possible) and finally an electroencephalogram (EEG). The picture is further complicated by the fact that we know epilepsy can be difficult to differentiate from syncope or conversion disorder for example. EEG is also not conclusive in many cases and not all clients with ID are willing to tolerate an EEG assessment. From the data obtained from their systematic review of studies from 1998 to 2008, Chapman et al. (2011) concluded that epilepsy may be misdiagnosed in approximately 25% of this population. Their rationale for this conclusion lay in the fact that they believed symptom presentation was misinterpreted by professionals and lay carers alike. Commonly, this misinterpretation was not only prevalent in behavioural type symptoms observed in people with challenging behaviour but also applied to confusion over physiological symptoms, behaviours related to drug side effects, the impact of psychological events and syndrome-specific behaviours.

Other physical problems like pain need to be considered (Gore et al., 2013). A recent study by Poppes et al. (2016) conducted univariate analysis on identified risk factors and challenging behaviour in almost 200 people with profound ID and challenging behaviour. They found that the strongest predictive factors were not related to the environment but to biopsychological factors such as sleep problems and auditory difficulties. The implications of this study are that those working with people who have severe and multiple disabilities need to eliminate physical causes before conducting full psychological assessment.

Another challenge can be differentiating between behavioural problems and mental health problems, an issue of considerable controversy. Jopp and Keys (2001) reported that clinicians who are more open to exploring presenting symptoms in a 'multidimensional fashion' were more likely to detect co-morbidities. Moss et al. (2000) used the PASSAD checklist to identify psychiatric symptoms in 320 people with ID, both with and without challenging behaviour. They concluded that those with severe challenging behaviour had over double the prevalence of psychiatric symptoms than those who displayed no challenging behaviour. Therefore, care has to be taken to ensure that emotional problems are not ignored or overlooked, particularly when the individual may be unable to self-report their own emotional state.

Understanding syndrome-specific behaviours, or what are commonly referred to as behavioural phenotypes, can be of help to the individuals themselves and their carers. For example, if family or carers of someone with Tourette's syndrome become aware that an individual's complex motor movements and involuntary vocalisations are outwith the individual's control then they are likely to be more accepting and compassionate. Although autism is not a syndrome per se, carers report that obtaining a diagnosis of autism can help to aid understanding and tolerance of the more challenging aspects of a person's presentation such as their obsessive behaviour. Similarly, there is an awareness of the extreme self-injurious behaviour displayed by adults with a diagnosis of Smith–Magenis syndrome or Lesch–Nyhan syndrome. The self-injury of those with Cornelia de Lange syndrome is thought to be related to the discomfort caused by gastrointestinal reflux, which has significant implications for their management and support (Hall et al., 2008). Unfortunately, knowing that certain behavioural difficulties are linked to certain behavioural problems does not necessarily mean that clinicians know what they can do to intervene. Nevertheless, being able to anticipate challenges and ensure that sensitive and timely input is provided will help to sustain support. Again, the efficacy of psychopharmacological interventions for these behaviours remains questionable (McQuire et al., 2015) and psychological interventions are regarded as the treatment of choice in many cases, with NICE recommending antipsychotic medication only when 'psychological or other interventions alone do not produce change within an agreed time' and only in combination with psychological or other interventions.

14.3 Functional Analysis

Behavioural interventions should always start with sound behavioural assessment encompassing the principles of functional analysis. There are a range of assessment manuals to assist with the assessment process (LaVigna & Donnellan, 1986; Sturmey, 2001).

Functional analysis is based on the principles of operant conditioning (Skinner, 1957), which concerns how people's behaviour is shaped and maintained by environmental contingencies. The analysis begins with the premise that all behaviour serves a function. For example, presenting challenging behaviour may serve the purpose of demand avoidance. Carers may quickly respond to someone throwing crockery by removing them from the dining room. Throwing crockery could prove to be a very effective way of escaping from an anxiety-provoking situation if the person is unable to communicate their distress in any other way. Therefore, if the challenging behaviour results in the individual being removed from a situation they find aversive, then their behaviour will be reinforced. Lack of control, an unstimulating environment and a high level of dependency on others can all be reasons for presenting challenges.

In others, the functional basis of their challenging behaviour has been described as residing within a neurobiological model. Self-injurious or extreme motor movement is believed to lead to dopamine excretion which may increase tolerance to self-injury and an increased dependence or enjoyment of the biofeedback apparent in engaging in this behaviour. Psychologists have also considered hypotheses around sensory feedback in an attempt to better understand the presentation of some of the more self-stimulatory and self-injurious behaviours. These hypotheses seem ever more relevant now that DSM 5 encompasses a diagnostic component related to hypo or hyper-reactivity to sensory input in adults and children with autism spectrum disorder (ASD). For some people with this dual diagnosis, their challenging behaviour might be in response to simple environmental stimuli such as the colour of the walls, the level of noise in the room or other factors leading to sensory overload and subsequent anxiety. Thus, a detailed exploration of presentation and context may serve to identify precipitating and perpetuating factors.

Carers' responses can play a powerful role in shaping and maintaining people's behaviour (Griffith & Hastings, 2014). However, carers' responses are also shaped by their views about the challenging behaviour and the emotional impact of dealing with challenges (Dagnan & Cairns, 2005). Very understandably, this can make it difficult for carers to step back and take a more objective view of the person's behaviour and its function. At times carers will describe challenging behaviours as originating from a desire for attention. This can be a critical and somewhat simplistic interpretation, with the carer viewing the person as deliberately behaving 'badly' to gain attention. Even if it is an accurate view, seeking attention is not maladaptive and is part of being human. Neonates quickly learn ways of gaining the attention of the primary caregiver, such as crying, to ensure their needs are met. Sometimes, the psychologist's work to reframe a carer's negative statement such as 'his behaviour is just attention seeking' is the first stage in building a cooperative intervention plan with staff.

A range of methods can be used to gather data for a functional analysis and many of these are well described in a text by Jones et al. (1995). The methods of gathering data include time sampling and interval recording. Time sampling involves observing an individual for a specified amount of time then recording whether a behaviour has occurred within that time period. Event recording is adopted when behaviour has a discrete beginning and end such as screaming out. Observation sessions can be split into particular periods such as fifteen minutes and a tally mark is made each time the behaviour occurs. Interval recording can be either whole interval or partial. Whole interval pertains to whether the behaviour being recorded has been present throughout the entire observation period (in this example, fifteen minutes) and is helpful for exploring long-lasting behaviours such as excessive rocking. Partial asks whether it has occurred at any point in the entire observation interval. Partial interval recording is better used when the behaviour in question typically doesn't last for as long as the recording interval, again in this case, fifteen minutes.

Antecedent, behaviour and consequence (ABC) charts are often given to staff or family members to help gain insight into the function of the behaviour and the maintaining factors. However, without careful explanation and training, staff or families can find these apparently straightforward forms difficult to complete in an objective fashion. This is not surprising, as they are usually used to record highly emotive events. For example, recording that 'John was in a bad mood when he entered the lounge' as the 'antecedent' to an incident of challenging behaviour does not provide the information that is required. Thus, staff and family members usually need training and careful guidance about how to complete ABC charts.

An alternative approach is the STAR form which covers four key areas: setting, trigger, action and response. Similar to the ABC methodology, there are sections to record details about the behaviour, the setting event(s) and the outcome. In this particular case, however, the person recording the information is encouraged to consider both intrinsic and extrinsic factors relating to the setting conditions, ranging from medication taken, general mental health, the individual's arousal level as well as environmental factors such as time of day, number of people in the room, etc. The trigger should be recorded as the event(s) immediately prior to the behaviour occurring and again, detail is important. The action is the target behaviour and the result is what occurred after the event. Detailed recordings such as these, if completed over a specified time period, can provide useful information for both carers and the psychologist on frequency of the behaviour, intensity, possible key time periods when the behaviour occurs, etc.

Charting challenging behaviour can be an onerous task and so it is perhaps unsurprising that carers struggle to maintain good records. Thus, a helpful adjunct to such recordings is the Motivation Assessment Scale (MAS), which can be completed by interview when obtaining an initial history of a behavioural presentation from the carer. There are only four subscales: attention, escape, tangibles and sensory consequences.

There are also analogue measures, which are easy to complete, provide a helpful visual representation of the carer's perception of the severity of the behaviour and are readily adapted to the specific circumstances. Analogue scales can be drawn up to include a diverse range of behaviours such as irritability, attention span, lethargy, etc. Usually the scales comprise 10-cm horizontal lines anchored with word descriptions at the end points e.g. from 'not a problem' to 'multiple times per day'. For a comprehensive review of analogues measures, see Wewers and Lowe (1990).

By the end of the assessment, the clinician should have carried out a thorough investigation of the function of the behaviour and set out their hypotheses about the function of the behaviour, providing a framework for the intervention.

14.4 Interventions

The recent NICE guidelines (2015) recommended a number of evidence-based interventions for challenging behaviour. The main interventions with a convincing evidence base are behavioural interventions that draw on a functional assessment, anger management based on cognitive behavioural therapy (CBT) principles and offering structured daytime activity (NICE, 2015). Although not a psychological intervention as such, there was also a recommendation that there should be a behavioural plan for people presenting challenging behaviour. Interestingly, the cumulative impact of the above approaches is not merely to reduce challenging behaviour but also to increase the quality of life of those presenting challenging behaviour.

14.5 Positive Behavioural Support

Although not mentioned by name, the key ingredients of positive behavioural support (PBS) were included in the NICE guidelines. PBS is currently the most widely used framework for addressing challenging behaviour in the UK. It emerged from an applied behaviour analysis conceptual framework, having at its core a functional analysis as described above and a concern with the communicative function of challenging behaviour (Gore et al., 2013). However, in line with the NICE guidelines, a set of positive values are also at the heart of the approach, with respect for the individual and the aim of promoting activity and a more purposeful life. There is a rejection of negative or punitive approaches. This means applying the principles of learning theory in order to reduce challenging behaviour in the longer term and includes addressing contextual factors which increase the likelihood of challenging behaviour occurring, teaching the person functionally equivalent ways of communicating their needs, and teaching other skills and ways of coping that make challenging behaviour less likely. This is a data-based approach, using the data collected from the functional analysis to develop the intervention and continuing to collect data in order to evaluate the outcomes and reshape the intervention in relation to changing circumstances or evidence.

PBS is not new. Psychologists have used positive behavioural programmes for a considerable period of time. However, PBS presents a broader framework that includes an explicit attempt to promote a better quality of life for individuals presenting challenging behaviour, which chimes with the philosophy of providing person-centred care in community settings. The PBS model has also garnered the support of professional bodies who have published authoritative guidance in the area, including the joint 'Clinical and Service Guidelines for Supporting People with Learning Disabilities Who Are at Risk of Receiving Abusive or Restrictive Practices'. This guideline, entitled 'Challenging Behaviour: A Unified Approach' was produced by the Royal College of Psychiatrists, British Psychological Society and Royal College of Speech and Language Therapists (2007). Voluntary and third sector organisations such as the Challenging Behaviour Foundation have also embraced this philosophy by offering staff development and training opportunities in PBS.

These guidelines are helpful but it remains vital to ensure there are professionals with the necessary skills, know-how and experience to implement a PBS framework. Specialist behavioural therapy teams have been found to work more effectively with people presenting challenging behaviour than generic community learning disability teams (Hassiotis et al., 2009). The stepped care model, where the least intensive psychological interventions are offered first, allows psychologists or other specialist clinicians to both screen clients and develop support mechanisms in keeping with the severity of the problem. Research in delivery of psychological therapy has indicated that we can adopt a more efficient use of scant resources by training others to deliver more minimal interventions for less significant psychological problems. Routinely using research findings to influence our healthcare delivery (what we refer to as implementation science) should be paramount. First-level interventions in a stepped care model initially comprise reading materials and e-learning which can be distributed in a range of settings and do not require skilled psychological practitioners. If more support is required, then low-level interventions can be appropriately supported by psychological practitioners, learning disability nurses and other allied health professionals. This model in turn frees up the clinical psychologists to deliver more highly specialist interventions necessary for more complex and multifaceted presentations. Challenging behaviours more readily fall within this latter category of complex, multifaceted problems requiring detailed formulation and intervention.

Table 14.1 Types of differential reinforcement schedules

Type	Description
Differential reinforcement of other behaviours (DRO)	Present a reinforcer only when the target behaviour has not been exhibited for a predetermined period of time
Differential reinforcement of alternative behaviour (DRA)	Present a reinforcer only when an alternative appropriate behaviour is exhibited
Differential reinforcement of incompatible behaviour (DRI)	Present a reinforcer only when an appropriate behaviour which is incompatible with the target behaviour, has been exhibited
Differential reinforcement of low rate of behaviour (DRL)	Present a reinforcer only when the inappropriate behaviour occurs at a sufficiently low rate

14.6 Principles of Differential Reinforcement

Social learning theory provides a range of differential reinforcement strategies that can be used to help reduce challenging behaviour and teach functionally equivalent ways of behaving. Each of these schedules is described in turn in Table 14.1.

Decision-making on the most appropriate technique to apply in a particular context should be informed by the data gathered at the stage of functional analysis. In addition, given the challenges in developing an appropriate and applicable behavioural support plan, assessment of risk should be integral to this process. There exist numerous risk assessments and risk management plans for adaption and application across a variety of care context. Determining which risk assessment tool to select is a very individualised process and is best undertaken in a multidisciplinary fashion. In addition, health, social care and voluntary sector alike often have their own risk assessment tools pertinent to their services. While PBS also includes reactive strategies to help carers cope with challenging behaviour when it occurs (Gore et al., 2013) as well as offering an important framework for working with individuals presenting challenging behaviour, it does not rule out other psychological interventions which might be of value to the individuals concerned. It would be rare for challenging behaviour to be the person's only presenting difficulties. For example, in Willner et al.'s (2013) anger management trial, almost one-third of the participants had clinically significant problems of depression and two thirds had clinically significant anxiety problems. Thus, these individuals may also have benefited from psychological interventions for anxiety or depression.

14.7 Anger Management

People with ID are a heterogeneous group. The aggressive actions of someone with a profound ID and no expressive language are not the same as someone who has a mild-to-moderate ID and has a tendency to react aggressively when they feel unfairly treated. Anger management is a NICE guideline recommended psychological intervention for people with mild-to-moderate ID who present with problems of aggression. The approach is based on CBT principles and rather than emphasising environmental contingencies, the aim is to increase people's own ability to remain in control when faced with perceived threats.

Anger management places emphasis on the regulation of anger as a key factor in determining how people respond in situations of conflict or potential conflict, with uncontrolled anger making aggressive responses more likely. In turn, anger is mediated by cognitive factors and in particular by how people perceive and appraise interpersonal situations. For example, if people display an attributional bias of hostile intent then they are more likely to think that others are behaving in a deliberately hostile fashion, causing them to be frequently angry (Larkin et al., 2013). The interpersonal nature of conflict is also emphasised, as anger is seen as a social emotion and the impact of the person's broader social environment and relationships are taken into account. The goals of the intervention is not to prevent people from becoming angry, but to help reduce the frequency and intensity of their anger, thereby allowing them to cope more constructively with anger-provoking situations.

Just as in behavioural work, a thorough assessment and formulation of the person's anger and aggression is required in order to tailor the intervention to individual difficulties (Richardson et al., 2016; Taylor, 2002). The assessment examines the cognitive, behavioural, emotional, somatic and environmental factors underlying the person's anger and aggression. Cognitive and emotional factors are examined in terms of both process and content. Assessment of process considers areas of social-cognitive functioning where the person might have deficits, such as problem-solving ability and emotion recognition. Regarding cognitive content, it is important to know what individuals become angry about and the nature of their appraisals and evaluations of events. In other words, how people perceive events and the resulting inferences about self and others. Consequently, someone might have a heightened sensitivity to being put down by others, leading them to have anger outbursts when someone makes a mildly critical comment. This may lead them to think that the other person is treating them like 'a piece of rubbish' and that 'nobody really cares about me'.

In practice, anger management consists of a package of interventions, with group and individual treatment formats used. It can be argued that there are advantages in using a group approach to tackle an interpersonal problem like aggression. There are a number of excellent anger management group manuals available Willner et al. (2013) and a comprehensive guide to individual formulation-driven interventions for anger management (Taylor & Novako, 2005).

Broadly speaking, the three phases of an anger management intervention are education, skill acquisition and practice of new skills. The education phase is largely concerned with teaching about the role of anger and both its positive and negative uses. Presenting anger as a normal feeling helps to examine how different situations evoke different emotions, introducing the link between a person's perceptions of events, feelings and behaviour. Moreover, there is the accompanying somatic arousal associated with anger. In order to gain greater self-control in situations of actual and potential conflict, a person has to learn to recognise the early signs of this arousal. Psychologists would describe socialising someone into a particular treatment model in the first stages of an intervention. As part of this process, it may be necessary to teach or negotiate a shared language to describe thoughts and feelings more fully during treatment. When working with individuals with a ID, a greater period of time might be required to achieve this goal and the therapist needs to tailor the approach and materials to the individual concerned.

After the learning phase and the raising of awareness, the individual receives coaching in a range of methods of controlling or modifying their anger. This includes relaxation training, in order to help individuals lower their level of arousal in anger-provoking situations. Being calmer makes it less likely that individuals will 'shoot from the hip' or act without thinking, and more likely they will be able to work out a non-aggressive response. Cognitive work carried out as part of group anger management interventions still tends to focus on cognitive processes and skills. Self-instruction and positive self-statements are used to cue individuals' coping strategies in stressful situations. Individual, formulation-based approaches will have a greater emphasis on tackling cognitive distortions or a tendency to perceive threat where none is intended or beliefs that aggression is a helpful way of dealing with problems.

In the final phase of treatment, individuals are encouraged to practise their new skills, both within sessions and between sessions. This might involve bringing records or reporting verbally on situations of potential conflict they have experienced between sessions and how they have coped. Role play can prove an effective way of practising how to deal with particular situations that they find most anger provoking.

Of course there are good reasons why people may become angry and those with an ID, who are often socially marginalised, are likely to have more reasons than most. However, being aggressive and having anger outbursts can have a negative effect on people's quality of life, making it difficult for them to sustain relationships and lead to exclusion from activities they may enjoy. Consequently, when using an anger management approach the aim is not to deny the real ill treatment someone may face, but to help them recognise that being able to control their anger may allow them to feel more in control and enjoy better life opportunities.

14.8 Achieving and Maintaining Change: A Systemic Task

If the drive for change originates primarily from others in a person's life, then the psychologist should explain from the outset that the involvement of those others will be important in consistently applying an individualised psychological intervention. Systemic involvement is vital, particularly given that the majority of people with ID do not live in isolation but are surrounded by a range of services and supports. Studies indicate that behavioural principles can be applied successfully for short term improvements (Jones 1999; Lindsay & Walker 1999) but unless carers continue to follow the devised programme then there is longitudinal evidence to suggest these gains are not maintained.

14.9 Measuring Outcomes

Treatment efficacy not only relies on the responses of the client but also the responses of the environment in which they function. As referred to previously, in our changing landscape of multidisciplinary teams (MDTs) we are increasingly working with third and voluntary sector staff in managing challenging behaviours within community facilities. McHugh and Barlow (2012) have identified what they believe to be three main barriers to implementation of an intervention in a mental health context. First, the degree to which practitioners are actually motivated to apply new interventions; second, factors related to the organisation itself and the setting in which it functions and finally, the degree to which priority is given to both the training and supervising of individual practitioners.

In addition, health professionals attempting to support and advise external agencies should give due consideration to the core belief systems of those agencies. Otherwise, practitioners may find their recommendations for psychological intervention in conflict with the values and goals of an organisation, subsequently reducing the probability of a successful outcome.

The Division of Clinical Psychology Faculty of Intellectual Disabilities has run a project entitled *Outcome Measures for Challenging Behaviour Interventions* (Morris et al., 2012). They piloted a range of tools measuring: quality of life, frequency and intensity of the challenging behaviour, adaptive behaviour and generic mental well-being. Ten specialist services adopted these scales pre and post intervention for challenging behaviour. Four main measures proved statistically significant in differentiating pre and post intervention groups and thus were recommended for future use. These included the Behavior Problems Inventory-01 (Rojahn et al., 2001), the Challenging Behaviour Interview (Oliver et al., 2003), the Health of the Nation Outcome Scales – Learning Disability version (Roy et al., 2002) and the Maslow Assessment of Needs Scales – Learning Disability (Skirrow & Perry, 2009).

14.10 Conclusion

This chapter aimed to provide an overview of current thinking and practice in the area of psychological assessment and interventions for challenging behaviour. The recent Winterbourne View investigation and the drive towards decommissioning the remaining long-stay institutions has led to a renewed focus on a community-based network of services. These community resources are placing an emphasis on PBS and improving the quality of life of individuals who present challenging behaviour, as well as having the longer-term goal of reducing individuals' behavioural problems. For those with problems of aggression and moderate-to-mild ID, CBT-based anger management approaches are recommended. A growing interest in mindfulness and cognitive-based paradigms is in keeping with developments in other specialist populations. As therapeutic models develop and are applied, it is important that we build evidence-based models of service delivery in order to reflect the drive towards an inclusive service for all.

References

Bowley, C. & Kerr, M. (2000) Epilepsy and intellectual disability: A review. *Journal of Intellectual Disability Research*, **44**, 529–43.

British Psychological Society, Division of Clinical Psychology, Faculty for People with Learning Disabilities (2011) *Commissioning Clinical Psychology Services for Adults with Learning Disabilities*.

Chapman, M., Iddon, K., Atkinson, K. et al. (2011) The misdiagnosis of epilepsy in people with intellectual disabilities: A systematic review. *Seizure, European Journal of Epilepsy*, **20**, 101–6.

Clarke, D. J. (1998) Psychopharmacology of severe self-injury associated with learning disabilities. *British Journal of Psychiatry*, **172**, 389–94.

Crocker, A. G. et al. (2006) Prevalence and types of aggressive behaviour among adults with intellectual disabilities. *Journal of Intellectual Disability Research*, **50**(9), 652–61.

Dagnan, D. & Cairns, M. (2005) Staff judgements of responsibility for the challenging behaviour of adults with intellectual disabilities. *Journal of Intellectual Disability Research*, **49**, 95–101.

Dura, J. R., Mulick, J. A. & Rasnake, L. K. (1987) Prevalence of stereotypy among institutionalised non-ambulatory mentally retarded people. *American Journal of Mental Deficiency*, **91**, 548–9.

Emerson, E. (1995) *Challenging Behaviour: Analysis and Intervention in People with Learning Disabilities*. Cambridge University Press.

Emerson, E. (1998) Working with people with challenging behaviour. In *Clinical Psychology and People with Intellectual Disabilities* (eds. E. Emerson, C. Hatton, J. Bromley et al.), pp. 127–53. Wiley.

Emerson, E. & Bromley, J. (1995) The form and function of challenging behaviours. *Journal of Intellectual Disability Research*, 39, 388–98.

Emerson, E., Kiernan, C., Alborz, A. et al. (2001) The prevalence of challenging behaviors: A total population study. *Research in Developmental Disabilities*, 22(1), 77–93.

Gore, N., McGill, P., Toogood, S. et al. (2013) Definition and scope for positive behavioural support. *International Journal of Positive Behavioural Support*, 3(2), 14–23.

Griffith, G. M. and Hastings, R. P. (2014) 'He's hard work, but he's worth it'. The experience of caregivers of individuals with intellectual disabilities and challenging behaviour: A meta-synthesis of qualitative research. *Journal of Applied Research in Intellectual Disabilities*, 27, 401–19.

Hall, S. S., Arron, K., Sloneem, J. & Oliver, C. (2008) Health and sleep problems in Cornelia de Lange Syndrome: A case control study. *Journal of Intellectual Disability Research*, 52(5), 458–68.

Hassiotis, A., Robotham, D., Canagasabey, A. et al. (2009) Randomised, single-blind, controlled trial of a specialist behaviour therapy team for challenging behaviour in adults with intellectual disabilities. *American Journal of Psychiatry*, 166(11), 278–1285.

Jones, R., Walsh, G. & Sturmey, P. (1995) *Stereotyped Movement Disorders*. Wiley.

Jones, R. S. P. (1999) A 10 year follow-up of stereotypic behaviour with eight participants. *Behavioural Interventions*, 14, 45–54.

Jopp, D. & Keys, C. (2001) Diagnostic overshadowing reviewed and reconsidered. *American Journal on Mental Retardation*, 106(5), 416–79.

Larkin, A., Jahoda, A. & MacMahon, K. (2013) The social information processing model as a framework for explaining frequent aggression in adults with mild to moderate intellectual disabilities: A systematic review of the evidence.

Journal of Applied Research in Intellectual Disabilities 26, 447–65.

LaVigna, G. W. & Donnellan, A. M. (1986) *Alternatives to punishment: Solving behavior problems with nonaversive strategies*. Irvington.

Lindsay, W. R. & Walker, B. (1999) Advances in behavioural methods in intellectual disability. *Current Opinion in Psychiatry*, 12, 561–5.

Lowe, K. et al. (2007) Challenging behaviours: Prevalence and topographies. *Journal of Intellectual Disability Research*, 51, 625–36.

Lundqvist, L. (2013) Prevalence and risk markers of behaviour problems among adults with intellectual disabilities: A total population study in Orebro County, Sweden. *Research in Developmental Disabilities*, 34, 1346–56.

McHugh, R. K. & Barlow, D. H. (2012) *Dissemination and Implementation of Evidence-Based Psychological Treatments*. Oxford University Press.

McQuire, C., Hassiotis, A., Harrison, B. & Pilling, S. (2015) Pharmacological interventions for challenging behaviour in children with intellectual disabilities: A systematic review and meta-analysis. *BMC Psychiatry*, 16, 2.

Mansell, J. (2007) *Services for People with learning Disabilities and Challenging Behaviour or mental Health Needs: Report of a Project Group*. Department of Health.

Matson, J. L. & Volkmar, F. A. (1997) Autism in children and adults: Etiology, assessment and intervention. *Contemporary Psychology*, 42, 932.

Morris, J., Bush, A. & Joyce, T. (2012) *Outcome Measures for Challenging Behaviour Interventions*. British Psychological Society.

Moss, S., Emerson, E., Kiernan, C., Turner, S., Hatton, C., Alborz, A. (2000) Psychiatric symptoms in adults with learning disability and challenging behaviour. *British Journal of Psychiatry*, 177(5), 452–6.

NHS England (2014) *Winterbourne View – Time for Change*.

NICE (2015) *Challenging Behaviour and Learning Disabilities: Prevention and Interventions for People with Learning Disabilities Whose Behaviour Challenges*. NICE Guideline (NG11).

NICE (2016) *Mental Health Problems in People with Learning Disabilities: Prevention, Assessment and Management. NICE Guideline (NG 54)*.

Oliver, C., McClintock, K., Hall, S., Smith, M., Dagnan, D. & Stenfert-Kroese, B. (2003) Assessing the severity of challenging behaviour: Psychometric properties of the challenging behaviour interview. *Journal of Applied Research in Intellectual Disabilities*, **16**, 53–61.

Paul, A. (1997) An investigation of epilepsy and stereotyped behaviours in people with learning disabilities using EEG spectral analysis and behavioural methodologies. PhD thesis, University of Strathclyde, UK.

Poppes, P., van der Putten, A., Post, W. & Vlaskamp, C. (2016) Risk factors associated with challenging behaviour in people with profound intellectual and multiple disabilities. *Journal of Intellectual Disability Research*, **60**, 537–52.

Richardson, C., Killeen, S., Jahoda, A. & Willner, P. (2016) Assessment of anger-related cognitions of people with intellectual disabilities. *Behavioural and Cognitive Psychotherapy*, **44**, 580–600.

Robertson, J., Hatton, C., Emerson, E. & Baines, S. (2015) Prevalence of epilepsy among people with intellectual disabilities: A systematic review. *Seizure: European Journal of Epilepsy*, **29**, 46–62.

Rojahn, J. (1986) Self-injurious and stereotypic behaviour of non-institutionalized mentally retarded people: Prevalence and classification. *American Journal of Mental Deficiency*, **91**, 268–276.

Rojahn, J., Matson, J. L., Lott, D., Esbensen, A. J. & Small, Y. (2001) The Behavior Problems Inventory: An instrument for the assessment of self-injury, stereotyped behavior, and aggression/destruction in individuals with developmental disabilities. *Journal of Autism and Developmental Disorders*, **31**(6), 577–88.

Rojahn, J., Rowe, E. W., Sharber, A. C. et al. (2012) The Behavior Problems Inventory-Short Form for individuals with intellectual disabilities: Part II: Reliability and validity. *Journal of Intellectual Disability Research*, **56**(5), 546–65.

Roy, A., Matthews, H., Clifford, P., Fowler, V. & Martin, D. (2002) Health of the Nation Outcome Scales for People with Learning Disabilities (HoNOS-LD) 180, 61–6.

Royal College of Psychiatrists (2016) *Psychiatric Services for Young People with Intellectual Disabilities. CR200*.

Royal College of Psychiatrists, British Psychological Society & Royal College of Speech and Language Therapists (2007) Challenging Behaviour: A Unified Approach – College Report CR144. *Psychiatric Bulletin*, **31**(10), 400. doi:10.1192/pb.31.10.400

Singh, N. N., Lancioni, G. E., Winton, A .S. W. et al. (2006) Mindful staff increase learning and reduce aggression in adults with developmental disabilities. *Research in Developmental Disabilities*, **27**, 545–58.

Skinner, B. F. (1957) *Verbal Learning*. Appleton-Century-Crofts.

Skirrow, P. & Perry, E. (2009) *The Maslow Assessment of Needs Scales*. Mersey Care NHS Trust.

Strydom, A., Livingston, G., King, M. & Hassiotis, A. (2007) Prevalence of dementia in intellectual ability using different diagnostic criteria. *British Journal of Psychiatry*, **191**, 150–7.

Sturmey, P. (2001) The functional analysis checklist: Inter-rater and test–retest reliability. *Journal of Applied Research in Intellectual Disabilities*, **14**(3), 141–6.

Taylor, J. L. (2002) A review of assessment and treatment of anger and aggression in offenders with intellectual disability. *Journal of Intellectual Disability Research*, **46** (suppl. 1), 57–73.

Taylor, J. L. & Novaco, R. W. (2005) *Anger Treatment for People with Developmental Disabilities: A Theory, Evidence and Manual Based Approach*. Wiley.

Tsiouris, J. A., Kim, S. Y., Brown, W. T. & Cohen, I. L. (2011) Association of aggressive behaviours with psychiatric disorders, age, sex and degree of intellectual disability: A large scale survey. *Journal of Intellectual Disability Research*, **55**, 636–49.

Wewers, M. E. & Lowe, N. K. (1990) A critical review of visual analogue scales in the measurement of clinical phenomenon. *Research in Nursing and Health*, **13**, 227–36.

Willner, P. (2015) The neurobiology of aggression: Implications for the pharmacotherapy of aggressive challenging behaviour by people with intellectual disabilities. *Journal of Intellectual Disability Research*, **59**(1), 82–92.

Willner, P., Rose, J., Jahoda, A. et al. (2013) Group-based cognitive-behavioural anger management for people with mild to moderate intellectual disabilities: Cluster randomised controlled trial. *British Journal of Psychiatry*, **203** (4), 288–96.

Chapter 15

Challenging Behaviour and the Use of Pharmacological Interventions

John Devapriam and Regi T. Alexander

15.1 Introduction

Behaviour can be described as challenging when it is of such intensity, frequency or duration as to threaten the quality of life and/or the physical safety of the individual or others and is likely to lead to responses that are restrictive, aversive or result in exclusion (Royal College of Psychiatrists, British Psychological Society & Royal College of Speech and Language Therapists, 2007). Significant proportions of people with intellectual disability (ID) develop challenging behaviour and these are more common in people with a more severe degree of ID. Prevalence rates are around 5–15% in educational, health or social care and are higher at 30–40% in hospital settings (NICE, 2015). The broad definition of challenging behaviour means that while everyone who presents with it may not necessarily have a mental illness or disorder (Bowring et al., 2017), almost anyone with a mental health problem that reaches the threshold of needing attention from primary or secondary care services would have one of the presenting features. It is therefore very important to tease out any underlying causal and/or associated factors before making decisions about interventions.

Most people with ID and mental health or challenging behaviour access mainstream and primary care services (Devapriam et al., 2015). There have been concerns that psychotropic drugs are used inappropriately in people with ID to merely deal with challenging behaviour (Brylewski & Duggan, 2004; Department of Health 2012a, 2012b; Glover et al., 2014; Matson et al., 2000; Molyneux et al., 1999; Tsiouris, 2010) and that the proportion of people with ID treated with psychotropic drugs exceed the proportion with recorded mental illness (Sheehan et al., 2015). Primary care data in England show that about 30,000–35,000 adults with ID are on antipsychotics or antidepressants or both without appropriate indications (Public Health England, 2015) and as part of transforming the care of people with ID, NHS England (2015) has announced a 'call to action' to stop over-medication of people with ID (STOMP). However, data from secondary care mental health services suggests that antipsychotics are not widely used outside of evidence-based indications in people with ID (Paton et al., 2016) and that previous studies may have overestimated prevalence rates of psychotropic medication use in adults with ID (Bowring et al., 2017). In fact, a survey of psychiatrists working in secondary care suggested that non-pharmacological interventions are the first choice treatment for aggression where no psychiatric condition is diagnosed (Unwin, 2008) unless other interventions are unsuccessful and the frequency and/or severity of the aggressive behaviour poses a serious risk to self or others.

Several evidence and consensus-informed prescribing guidelines have been in use for many years (Bhaumik et al., 2015; Deb et al., 2006), with NICE (2015) providing the most up-to-date guideline on the management of challenging behaviour.

15.2 A Conceptual Framework for Understanding Challenging Behaviour

Challenging behaviour is a socially constructed descriptive concept that has no diagnostic significance and makes no inferences about the aetiology of the behaviour. It may serve a 'purpose' or 'function' for the person with an ID such as stimulation, attention from others, access to 'tangibles', avoidance of demands and pain reduction (Carr, 1977; Hastings et al., 2013; Matson et al., 2012). The behaviour itself can range from 'aggression towards self' (in the form of self-injurious behaviour) to 'outward aggression' (towards objects and other persons), which, in severe circumstances, and depending on context, may bring the person into contact with the criminal justice system. The presence of communication difficulties, autism, sensory impairments, sensory processing difficulties and physical or mental health problems (including dementia) increases the likelihood of challenging behaviour in people with ID (NICE, 2015). Challenging behaviour may be unrelated to psychiatric disorder but can also be a primary or secondary manifestation of it (Xeneditis, 2001); the association is strongest in those with severe ID (Felce et al., 2009).

To be able to inform the type(s) of interventions (pharmacological and non-pharmacological), it is important to have a conceptual framework to understand challenging behaviour. Hastings (2013) describes a conceptual framework based on social effects, vulnerability and maintaining factors all of which have to be taken into account to support rational prescribing where appropriate.

(1) Challenging behaviours are defined in terms of their social effects, i.e. exclusion from typical community life in some way, (risk of) harm to self and (risk of) harm to others. These can occur at a frequency, severity or duration at a level that has serious social consequences and as a result come into contact with primary or secondary care services.
(2) Vulnerability factors for challenging behaviour include some biological, psychological and social risks relating to life situations and inequalities experienced by people with learning disabilities. This can range from any physical illness, mental illness and sensory problems, behavioural phenotypes related to several genetic syndromes associated with ID, negative life events, lack of communication skills, impoverished social networks and lack of meaningful activity.
(3) Social contextual processes are primarily responsible for maintaining challenging behaviours. The basis of this hypothesis is that the behaviour serves an important function or purpose for the individual. Stimulation, attention from others, access to tangibles, avoidance of demands and pain reduction as functions have been relevant to a good understanding of the vast majority of challenging behaviour (Carr, 1977).

The above framework can form the theoretical basis which informs formulation and intervention plans. In order to decide on the best pharmacological treatment option as part of a wider intervention plan, it is important to undertake the exercise of formulation – identifying the presenting behaviour, establishing the contributory factors, formulating the needs and planning interventions in a holistic and multidisciplinary manner.

15.3 The Role of Formulation-Informed Intervention Plans

Formulation is a task that is core to psychiatric practice; it is a synthesis of knowledge about an individual and his or her circumstances, which in turn sets out a proposed course of action (Holland, 2011). In the context of challenging behaviour, formulation sets the

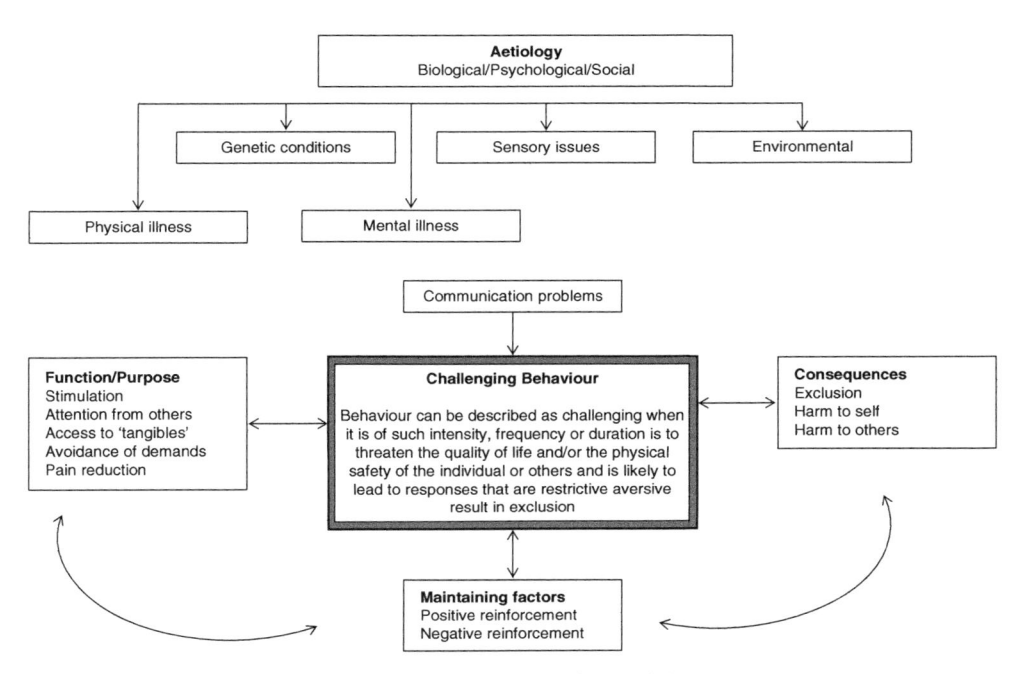

Figure 15.1 Biopsychosocial framework for understanding challenging behaviour

understanding of the behaviour within the context of established conceptual theory (see Figure 15.1). Due to the heterogeneity of the needs of the population with ID, no one professional discipline has the full breadth of knowledge necessary to fully understand and to intervene in an informed and evidence-based manner and therefore multidisciplinary and interagency work including families and support providers is vital.

The role of a psychiatrist in the process of formulation of challenging behaviour should be to:

(1) bring a medical and psychiatric perspective to understanding the behaviour;
(2) tease out the knowledge of the person and behaviour that is most relevant in the current context; and
(3) influence the team's understanding of the person and behaviour in the context of research evidence and sound conceptual frameworks that exist about the aetiology and treatment of both physical and mental illness, challenging behaviour, etc. and making the relevant diagnoses where applicable.

Diagnoses (where applicable) of mental illnesses are a crucial element of any multidisciplinary formulation especially where prescribing of psychotropic drugs is to be one of the interventions. The recording of diagnoses can be particularly problematic in those patients with ID who are unable to give a clear verbal account of their psychopathology. Even in those who do have expressive speech, many find it difficult to describe precisely their psychopathology and the clinician may have difficulty making the subtle distinction between hallucinations and pseudo-hallucinations or between overvalued ideas, obsessions or delusions. Thus, in clinical practice, it can happen that a psychiatric diagnosis is recorded

```
┌─────────────────────┐     ┌─────────────────────┐     ┌─────────────────────┐
│ Assessment of need  │     │ Multidisciplinary   │     │ Multidisciplinary   │
│ Mental health       │────▶│ Formulation of need │────▶│ (overarching)       │
│ Physical health     │     │ Mental health       │     │ Intervention plan   │
│ Social need         │     │ Physical health     │     │ Mental health       │
└─────────────────────┘     │ Social need         │     │ Physical health     │
                            └─────────────────────┘     │ Social need         │
                                                        └─────────────────────┘
                                                                   │
                                                                   ▼
                                                        ┌─────────────────────┐
                                                        │ Individual Care     │
                                                        │ Delivery plans      │
                                                        └─────────────────────┘
                                                            ↙         ↘
                                              ┌──────────────────┐  ┌──────────────────┐
                                              │ Pharmacological  │  │ Non-pharmacological│
                                              │ interventions    │  │ interventions    │
                                              └──────────────────┘  └──────────────────┘
                                                      │
                                                      ▼
                                              ┌──────────────────────────┐
                                              │ Undertake cycle of       │
                                              │ prescribing              │
                                              │ See Figure 15.3          │
                                              └──────────────────────────┘
```

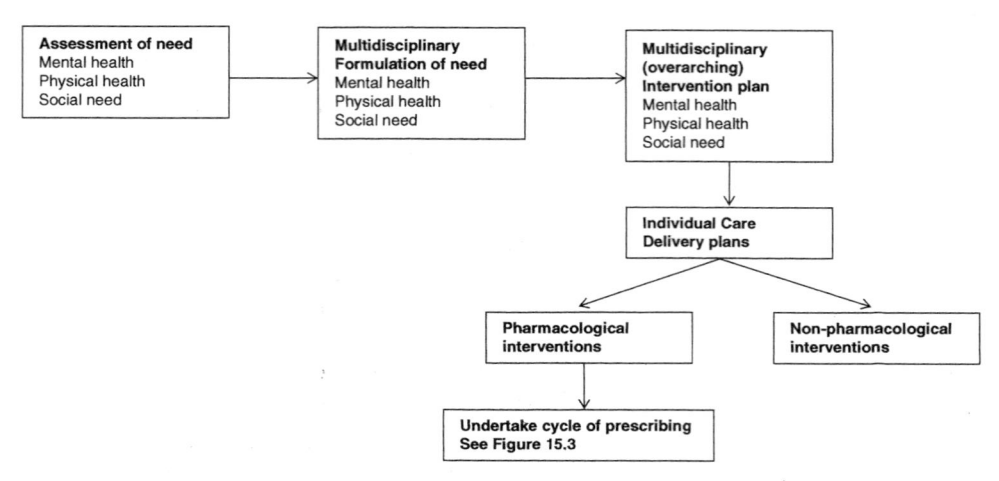

Figure 15.2 Formulation of a treatment/care plan and role of pharmacological intervention

only when the main syndromes are present (e.g. schizophrenia or bipolar disorder), while the narrative account of psychopathology (e.g. transient psychotic symptoms and affective lability in someone with mild ID and a personality disorder) is omitted. This clearly contributes to the problem of under-recording of psychiatric diagnoses and the inability to adequately monitor prescribing practices. It is clear that this is a problem not just in ID, but also in mainstream mental health services (Sheehan et al., 2015). This dynamic means that in rationalising prescribing practice, one has to carefully balance the need to stop unnecessary treatment with the risk of under-treatment (NICE 2016; Royal College of Psychiatrists, 2016).

Previous guidance (Bhaumik et al., 2015; Deb et al., 2006, 2009; Kalachnick et al., 1998; NICE, 2015; Rush & Frances, 2000) suggests that the most important part of psychotropic drug prescribing for this group is the need for a clear assessment and formulation before the prescribing, followed by regular review and monitoring of the drug and its effects (positive and negative). The formulation is underpinned by the clinician's awareness that while challenging behaviour may be the presenting symptom, it may be the result of conditions that have no need for medication at all as well as conditions that will improve only with medication. This process should include a full recording of the diagnostic or needs formulation that covers all the below across three domains – mental (including psychological) health, physical health and social as well identifying any predisposing, precipitating, perpetuating and protective factors.

In this structure, challenging behaviour is not treated as a diagnosis per se, but as a presenting symptom that should be placed in the context of a range of mental (psychological), physical and social factors. As a result of this assessment and formulation, the prescriber generates what is essentially a multi-axial diagnosis/needs formulation and a treatment/care plan (Figure 15.2) which in turn are associated with detailed care delivery plans (NICE, 2016; Royal College of Psychiatrists, 2016).

(a) If the formulation shows that there are no mental illnesses or other mental disorders and the presentation with challenging behaviour is purely the result of physical or social factors, then there may be no role for prescribing other than in the very short term to alleviate a serious risk to the safety of the patient or others while other non-drug programmes are implemented to manage the behaviours.

(b) If an independent mental illness or mental disorder is diagnosed, then treatment should follow established guidelines for that condition.

(c) Because presentations are rarely straightforward in clinical practice, there is often a combination of several symptoms and this may not be captured by categorical diagnoses. Therefore, there should be clear identification of the psychotic, affective and behavioural symptoms including clusters of symptoms that are the target of treatment. All psychotropic drug prescribing should target specific symptoms and if the specific symptoms are not improving satisfactorily within three months, then that drug should be tapered or stopped and other options considered (Royal College of Psychiatrists, 2016).

It is important therefore to acknowledge that the term 'challenging behaviour' is not precise enough as a recorded indication for prescribing. One should record all diagnoses systematically and more importantly, the narrative that underpins them as part of a wider formulation that includes mental (including psychological), physical and social factors. This will allow the prescriber to record target symptoms or syndromes, have professional time frames for evaluation and communicate that to all concerned.

15.4 Good Prescribing Practice for Challenging Behaviour

The standards for good prescribing are described by the Royal College of Psychiatrists (2016) as follows (see also Figure 15.3).

- The indication(s) and rationale for prescribing the psychotropic drug should be clearly stated, including whether the prescribing is off-label, polypharmacy or high dose.
- Consent-to-treatment procedures (or best-interests decision-making processes) should be followed and documented.
- There should be regular monitoring of treatment response and side effects (preferably every three months or less, at a minimum every six months).
- Review and evaluation of the need for continuation or discontinuation of the psychotropic drug should be undertaken on a regular basis (preferably every three months or less, at a minimum every six months) or whenever there is a request from patients, carers or other professionals.

For people with an ID and challenging behaviour who come into contact with services, there are three broad prescribing circumstances (Royal College of Psychiatrists, 2016):

(1) The presence of challenging behaviour that is associated with symptoms which *fulfil* the diagnostic criteria for mental illness.
(2) The presence of challenging behaviour that is associated with some psychiatric symptoms, but the latter *not quite fulfilling* the diagnostic criteria for mental illness.
(3) The presence of challenging behaviour that is *not associated* with mental illness.

In the absence of a clear-cut diagnosis of mental illness, clinicians sometimes arrive at a working diagnosis as part of formulation based on assessment and investigations. This may lead to a therapeutic trial with a careful monitoring of the impact of drugs prescribed on target symptoms and side effects. The fundamental principle in such a trial is to consider

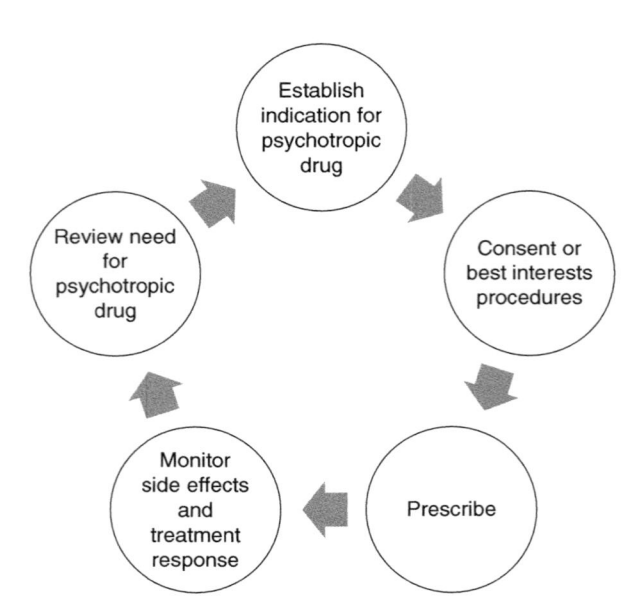

Figure 15.3 Cycle of good prescribing practice

stoppage of the drugs prescribed if the clinical response is not satisfactory within a reasonable time scale or if alternative non-drug management strategies are deemed to improve behaviour or if unacceptable side effects emerge. In this scenario, in the UK, General Medical Council guidance (2013) on off-label use of medicines applies. In this case prescribers are expected to assure themselves about the evidence, take responsibility for overseeing all aspects of treatment, record usage carefully and inform patients and carers fully (Glover et al., 2014).

NICE (2015) offers the most comprehensive and up-to-date guidance on prescribing of psychotropic drugs in challenging behaviour. It recommends that antipsychotic drugs be considered to manage challenging behaviour only if:

- psychological or other interventions alone do not produce change within an agreed time; or
- treatment for any coexisting mental or physical health problem has not led to a reduction in the behaviour; or
- the risk to the person or others is very severe (for example, because of violence, aggression or self-injury).

However, due to the lack of good-quality evidence, National Institute of Health and Care Excellence (NICE) does not mention the use of other psychotropic drugs in the management of challenging behaviour which then relies on professional diligence on off-label prescribing. To this effect, consensus guidelines guide the clinician in choosing the most appropriate psychotropic drug which can be used as a last resort as well as in combination with other non-pharmacological interventions. The choice of drug for the two most common outcomes of challenging behaviour – harm to self and harm to others are as set out in the following sections.

15.4.1 Harm to Self (Self-injurious Behaviour)

There is evidence for the role of dysregulation of biological systems in self-injurious behaviour involving the three neurotransmitters – dopamine, opioids and serotonin. The evidence base is best available for antipsychotics such as risperidone, aripiprazole, olanzapine, ziprasidone and quetiapine; antidepressants such as SSRIs (sertraline) and clomipramine and opioid antagonists such as naltrexone.

The subtype of self-injurious behaviour and drug selection are described in Biswas and Bhaumik (2015).

15.4.2 Harm to Others (Violence and Aggression)

NICE (2005) provides guidance on the use of psychotropic drugs in the management of violence in the short term. There is no evidence of efficacy of antipsychotics for managing aggressive behaviour (Tyrer, 2009). However, some studies have found some efficacy (Gagiano, 2005) especially for risperidone in children with autism spectrum disorder and ID (National Collaborating Centre for Mental Health, 2012; Unwin, 2011).

NICE also recommends that:

- antipsychotic drugs should be offered only in combination with psychological or other interventions;
- they should be initially prescribed and monitored by a specialist who should identify the target behaviour, set timelines for assessment, discuss widely with a patient and the family and taper off the drug based on its effectiveness.

This emphasises the need for meaningful follow-up, the purpose of which may be for continuation or discontinuation of drugs. In doing that, narrative accounts of improvement (or lack of) in target symptoms or syndromes may not be enough. These narrative accounts need to be supplemented by standardised measures. The Clinical Global Impression (CGI) scale may be a very useful choice for this. It is freely available online, can be administered in a matter of minutes by a clinician who knows the patient well and generates a summary score of improvement as well as the efficacy index. Other options for monitoring change over time which are well established in NHS- and NHS-funded services in the UK include tools like the Health of the Nation Outcome Scale (HoNOS). Although the CGI rates the balance between therapeutic benefit and side effects, clinicians may want to consider using additional objective measures like the Liverpool University Neuroleptic Side Effect Rating Scale (LUNSERS) to record side effects. Using both narrative accounts and standardised measures in this way will help the prescriber determine objectively which drugs are ineffective and aid the process of stopping them in consultation with patients and their carers (see Figure 15.4).

15.5 Conclusion

Challenging behaviour is a socially constructed descriptive concept that has no diagnostic significance and makes no inferences about the aetiology of the behaviour. The presence of communication difficulties, autism, sensory impairments, sensory processing difficulties and physical or mental health problems (including dementia) increases the likelihood of challenging behaviour in people with ID (NICE, 2015).

To be able to inform the type(s) of interventions (pharmacological and non-pharmacological), it is important to have a conceptual framework to understand

Standards	Key lines of enquiry	1	2	3	4	5	6	7	8	9	10	Overall
The indication(s) and rationale for prescribing the psychotropic drug should be clearly stated including whether the prescribing is off-label, polypharmacy or high dose	Is the prescribing part of a wider multidisciplinary care plan?											
	Is there documentation of indication for prescribing (this can include the diagnoses as well as the narrative account of the target symptoms)?											
	If the prescription is only for behaviour that challenges, are the NICE guidelines being followed? (i.e. psychological interventions have not produced a change within an agreed time period or treatment of coexisting mental and physical conditions have not led to a reduction or risk to the person or others is very severe *and* drugs is offered only with psychological or other interventions)											
	Is there off-label prescribing? And if so is the rationale explained											
	Is there polypharmacy and if so is the rationale explained?											
	Is there prescribing over BNF maximum limits and if so the rationale is explained?											
Consent (or best interests decision-making process) to treatment procedures should be followed and documented	Is there evidence of a capacity assessment?											
	If the patient is deemed to lack capacity, is the best-interests process followed?											
	Is there evidence of recording the patient's views about the drug treatment?											
	Is there evidence of recording the carers' or family members' views about the drug treatment?											

	If patient is detained (e.g., under the Mental Health Act (1983)) are the legal requirements around consent to treatment satisfied?
There should be regular *monitoring* of treatment response and side effects (preferably every 3 months or less, minimum of every 6 months)	Is there documentation about progress on the target symptoms for treatment?
	Is there evidence of objective evaluation of treatment response (e.g. use of standardised instruments)?
	Is there evidence of objective evaluation of side effects (e.g. use of standardised instruments)?
Review and evaluation of the need for continuation or discontinuation of the psychotropic drug should be undertaken on a regular basis (preferably every 3 months or less, minimum of every 6 months) or whenever there is a request from patients, carers or other professionals	Is there evidence of objective evaluation of treatment response (e.g. use of standardised instruments)?
	Is there evidence of objective evaluation of side effects (e.g. use of standardised instruments)?
	Is there evidence of regular review of the need for continuation or discontinuation of the drug? (This includes discussion of risks/benefits with patient/carer).

Figure 15.4 Clinician's self-evaluation/audit template

challenging behaviour to support rational prescribing where appropriate. This framework can form the theoretical basis which informs formulation and intervention plans. Diagnoses (where applicable) of mental illnesses are a crucial element of any multidisciplinary formulation especially where prescribing of psychotropic drugs is to be one of the interventions. The recording of diagnoses can be particularly problematic in those patients with ID who are unable to give a clear verbal account of their psychopathology. This dynamic means that in rationalising prescribing practice, one has to carefully balance the need to stop unnecessary treatment with the risk of under-treatment (NICE, 2016; Royal College of Psychiatrists, 2016). Where medication is prescribed this should be done in keeping with Royal College of Psychiatrists good prescribing guidelines (2016).

References

Bhaumik, S., Branford, D., Barrett, M. & Gangadharan, S. K. (2015) *The Frith Prescribing Guidelines for People with Intellectual Disability* (3rd edn). Wiley-Blackwell.

Biswas, A. & Bhaumik, S. (2015) Self-injurious behaviour. In *The Frith Prescribing Guidelines for People with Intellectual Disability* (eds. S. Bhaumik et al.) (3rd edn), pp. 153–60. Wiley-Blackwell.

Bowring, D., Totsika V., Hastings, R., Toogood, S. & McMahon, M. (2017) Prevalence of psychotropic medication use and association with challenging behaviour in adults with an intellectual disability: A total population study. *Journal of Intellectual Disability Research*, **61**(6), 604–17.

Brylewski, J. & Duggan, L. (2004) Antipsychotic medication for challenging behaviour in people with learning disability. *Cochrane Database of Systematic Reviews*, **3**: CD000377.

Carr, E. G. (1977) The motivation of self-injurious behaviour: a review of some hypothesis. *Psychological Bulletin*, **84**(4), 800–16

Deb, S., Clarke, D. & Unwin, G. (2006) Using medications to manage behavioural problems among adults with a learning disability. *DATABID*. Available at: www.LD-Medication .bham.ac.uk [accessed 2 September 2018]

Deb, S., Kwork, H., Bertelli, M. et al. (2009) International guide to prescribing psychotropic medication for the management of problem behaviours in adults with intellectual disabilities. *World Psychiatry*, **8**, 181–6.

Devapriam, J., Rosenbach, A. & Alexander, R. (2015) In-patient services for people with intellectual disability and mental health or behavioural difficulties. *BJPsych Advances*, **21** (2), 116–23.

Department of Health (2012a) *Department of Health Review: Winterbourne View Hospital Interim Report*. Department of Health.

Department of Health (2012b) *Transforming Care: A National Response to Winterbourne View Hospital: Department of Health Review Final Report*. Department of Health.

Felce, D., Kerr, M. & Hastings, R. P. (2009) A general practice based study of the relationship between indicators of mental illness and challenging behaviour among adults with intellectual disabilities. *Journal of Intellectual Disability Research*, **53**(3), 243–54.

Gagiano, C., Read, S., Thorpe, L., Eerdekens, M. & Van Hove, I. (2005) Short- and long-term efficacy and safety of risperidone in adults with disruptive behaviour disorders. *Psychopharmacology*, **179**(3), 629–36.

General Medical Council (2013) *Good Practice in Prescribing and Managing Medicines and Devices*. General Medical Council.

Glover, G. Bernard, S. Branford, D. et al. (2014) Use of medication for challenging behaviour in people with intellectual disability. *British Journal of Psychiatry*, **205**: 6–7.

Hastings, R. P., Allen, A., Baker, P. et al. (2013) A conceptual framework for understanding why challenging behaviours occur in people with developmental disabilities. *International Journal of Positive Behavioural Support*, **3** (2), 5–13.

Holland, T. (2011) The art of formulation. *Learning Disability Psychiatry – Newsletter of the Faculty of Learning Disability, RCPsych*, **13**(2).

Kalachnik, J. E., Leventhal, B. L., James, D. H. et al. (1998) Guidelines for the Use of psychotropic medication. In *Psychotropic Medication and Developmental Disabilities: The International Consensus Handbook* (eds. S. Reiss & M. Aman), pp. 45–72. Ohio State University.

Matson, J. L., Bamburg, J., Mayville, E. A. et al. (2000) Psychopharmacology and mental retardation – A 10 year review (1992–1999). *Research in Developmental Disabilities*, **21**: 263–96.

Matson, J. L., Tureck, K. & Riske, R. (2012) The Questions About Behavioural Function (QABF): Current status as a method of functional assessment. *Research in Developmental Disabilities*, **33**(2), 630–4.

Molyneux, B., Emerson, E. & Caine, A. (1999) Prescription of psychotropic medication to people with intellectual disabilities in primary healthcare settings. *Journal of Applied Research in Intellectual Disability*, **12**: 46–57.

National Collaborating Centre for Mental Health (2012) *Autism: The NICE Guideline on Recognition, Referral, Diagnosis and Management of Adults on the Autism Spectrum (National Clinical Guideline Number 142)*. British Psychological Society & Royal College of Psychiatrists

NHS England (2015) *The Use of Medications in People with Learning Disabilities*. NHS England. Available at: www.england.nhs.uk/2015/07/14/urgent-pledge [accessed 2 September 2018]

NICE (2015) *Challenging Behaviour and Learning Disabilities: Prevention and interventions for People with Learning Disabilities Whose Behaviour Challenges (NG11)*. NICE. Available at: www.nice.org.uk/guidance/ng11 [accessed 2 September 2018]

NICE (2016) *Mental Health Problems in People with Learning Disabilities: Prevention, Assessment and Management (NG54)*. NICE. Available at: www.nice.org.uk/Guidance/NG54 [accessed 2 September 2018]

Paton, C., Bhatti, S., Purandare, K., Roy, A. & Barnes, T. (2016) Quality of prescribing of antipsychotic medication for people with intellectual disability under the care of UK mental health services: A cross-sectional audit of clinical practice. *British Medical Journal Open*, **6** (12), e013116.

Public Health England (2015) *Prescribing of Psychotropic Drugs to People with Learning Disabilities and or Autism by General Practitioners in England*. Public Health England.

Royal College of Psychiatrists (2016) *Psychotropic Drug Prescribing for People with Intellectual Disability, Mental Health Problems and/or Behaviours That Challenge: Practice Guidelines. FR/ID/09*. Royal College of Psychiatrists. Available at: www.rcpsych.ac.uk/pdf/FR_ID_09_for_website.pdf [accessed 2 September 2018]

Royal College of Psychiatrists, British Psychological Society, Royal College of Speech and Language Therapists (2007) *Challenging Behaviour: A Unified Approach (CR144)*. Royal College of Psychiatrists. Available at: www.rcpsych.ac.uk/files/pdfversion/cr144.pdf [accessed 2 September 2018]

Rush, A. J. & Frances, A. (2000) Expert Consensus Guidelines Series: treatment of psychiatric and behavioural problems in mental retardation. *American Journal of Mental Retardation*, **105**, 159–227.

Sheehan, R., Hassiotis, A., Walters, K., Osborn, D., Strydom, A. & Horsfall, L. (2015) Mental illness, challenging behaviour, and psychotropic drug prescribing in people with intellectual disability: UK population based cohort study. *British Medical Journal*, **351**, h4326.

Tsiouris, J. A. (2010) Pharmacotherapy for aggressive behaviours in persons with intellectual disabilities – Treatment or mistreatment? *Journal of Intellectual Disability Research*, **54**, 1–16.

Tyrer, P., Oliver-Africano, P.., Romeo, R. et al. (2009) Neuroleptics in the treatment of aggressive challenging behaviour that challenges for people with intellectual disabilities: a randomised controlled trial (NACHBID). *Health Technology Assessment*, **13**: iii–iv, ix–xi, 1–54.

Unwin, G. L. & Deb, S. (2008) The use of medication for the management of behaviour problems among adults with intellectual disability: A clinician's consensus survey.

American Journal on Mental Retardation, **113**, 19–31.

Unwin, G. L. & Deb, S. (2011) Efficacy of atypical antipsychotic medication in the management of behaviour problems in children with intellectual disabilities and borderline intelligence: A systematic review. *Research in Developmental Disabilities*, **32**, 2121–33.

Xeniditis, K., Russell, A. & Murphy, D. (2001) Management of people with challenging behaviour. *Advances in Psychiatric Treatment*, **7**, 109–16.

Section 4 Delivering High-Quality Care

Chapter 16
History of Services for People with Disorders of Intellectual Development

Peter Carpenter

Any history of the services for people with disorders of intellectual development (DID) has first to deal with the people who is being discussed. The naming convention of the people being discussed has changed frequently and as the names have changed over the years so has the group to whom it refers. In order to try to follow the progression, this chapter will use the contemporary terms of the time discussed (however objectionable the term has become), as the group so labelled was not necessarily the same as modern patients with Intellectual Disability (ID). The newest term, 'people with disorders of intellectual development', for example, excludes many of those who filled the *mental deficiency* colonies in the early twentieth century, who were then labelled *feeble-minded*. An additional consideration is that those people now covered by the term 'intellectual disability' (ID) include many people who would have died in infancy in earlier times and so would not have been included in the terminology used then (for example people with cardiac lesions or severe epilepsy). The population to be discussed here is therefore a fluid group of people that have had many names and definitions. The medieval terms *natural fools, idiots and innocents* gave way to an increasing plethora of names, both as groups and as individuals splintered off with their own names (such as *cripples* becoming *spastics* and now *physically disabled*) or have been excluded altogether (such as those once called *feeble-minded* or *moral defectives*). The core has had difficulty gaining social status, and in the last fifty years the treadmill of euphemism powered by stigma has forced a flow of new 'non-stigmatising' terms to be invented, only for these in turn to become used in a pejorative way.

16.1 Pre-Specialist Care

Prior to 1600 there is little documentation in Britain and Ireland specifically about the care of those who were considered *natural fools* or *idiots* as almost all were in the community. Isolated documents suggest they commonly had a short life, and were probably cared for in a similar way to *non-violent 'lunatics'* (the collective term used for those with mental illness and other conditions such as epilepsy). The medieval property laws (De Praerogativa Regis, 1324) show that the property of *lunatics* was treated differently from that of the *fatuus naturalis* who were assumed to never be able to gain the ability to manage their affairs. The medieval hospitals that developed in the 1100's across Europe generally excluded lepers, epileptics, lunatics, the pregnant and it is presumed *idiots* (included within *lunatics*) (Orme & Webster, 1995). *Idiots* would have had to have been looked after by their families, as we have no evidence of hospitals for *idiots* other than their possible inclusion in Bethlem. With

> **Box 16.1** A Tudor definition of an idiot, from a legal textbook
>
> And he who shall be said to be a *Sot and Idiot* from his Birth, is such a Person who cannot accompt or number Twenty-pence, nor can tell who was his Father or Mother, nor how old he is &c. so as it may appear that he hath no understanding of Reason what shall be for his Profit, or what for his Loss.
>
> (Judge Fitzherbert *Natura Brevium* 1534)

the disappearance of leprosy in the 1400's, some leper hospitals were probably repurposed for the previously excluded groups: in Bath one came to admit *idiots* (Carpenter, 1998)

By the English Poor Law of 1601 the term *innocent* was often used in lay society to refer to *idiots* to separate them from *lunatics*. The new Poor Law systematised care for the 'deserving poor' and was principally one of 'outdoor relief' – keeping care in the community by paying families to look after their disabled children and adults if they could not afford to do so without help, and so avoiding admission to the poorhouse – and as such, provided care that resembled that based at Gheel in Belgium, which is celebrated as a town specifically providing care for *lunatics* since medieval times. The care of *innocents* then was just that – simple supportive care of the helpless. It was only those considered *dangerous idiots* that could be 'locked up'. *Innocents* were deemed incurable and most died young. It is worth noting that, prior to the nineteenth century, 45% of all infants died by age 5; it is therefore not surprising that few of the *intellectually disabled* children survived. A few orphanages and poorhouses were available, but due to overcrowding and insanitary conditions, these were death traps as the chances of emerging alive at age 16 for any child was less than 5% and often only 1%.

What were the common causes of ID at this time is unknown. It is presumed that many were due to childhood infections or injuries, or epilepsy syndromes. Disorders seen less frequently in more modern times were probably much more prevalent; such as neonatal infections associated with ID or congenital hypothyroidism. Many may have suffered the effects of foetal alcohol syndrome, given the quantity of alcohol drunk before the supply of safe water in the late nineteenth century.

Prior to the Industrial Revolution most people lived in the countryside in relatively stable, small communities. In a rural setting, it was perhaps easier to find work for local *innocents*. However this village life was not necessarily an idyll for them – most of the literature of the nineteenth century relates the poor lives and ill treatment of many with disability as the justification for setting up institutions for their welfare in the first place (Carpenter, 1997 & 2000; Twining, 1843; Wright, 2001).

In England after 1740 and with the onset of industrialisation, what can best be described as a trade in *lunacy* developed, with the growth of a profusion of private madhouses servicing the poorhouses. Some of these entrepreneurial institutions claimed to be able to cure *idiots*, but probably few were admitted to such places other than potentially those needing containment due to violence.

Medical interest first developed around 1800, following the development of successful teaching systems for the blind and deaf. Itard used these techniques to train the feral boy 'Victor', but though he trained the (possibly autistic) child, he declared it a failure as he was not 'cured' (Lane, 1979). Other doctors advocated education for *idiots* and Belhomme started classes at the Salpêtrière in Paris and Guggenbuhl followed with teaching *cretins* at the Abendberg in

Switzerland, where many English travellers on the grand tour admired his methods. As Twining wrote after visiting the Abendberg, 'The *Idiot* can be cured' (Twining, 1843). There was now also talk of a less disabled group even more amenable to training – the *imbecile*.

The English Poor Law of 1834 attempted to cut care costs by making admission to a workhouse the only means of state care. Though this never occurred in practice and outdoor relief remained more common, the New Poor Law Commissioners also started to publish statistics for the national system – they estimated in 1842 that there were 8,012 *idiots* chargeable to the rates in England and Wales and 7,902 *lunatics* (Poor Law Commissioners, 1843). They emphasised that many *lunatics* should be in asylums though '*mere idiots*' could be held in workhouses. However, people who did not respond to 'discipline' became a bigger problem in the new larger workhouses. Eventually, the Lunacy Act of 1845 created county *lunatic* asylums where the workhouse could send its *lunatics* and dangerous *idiots* for management and cure.

16.2 The Developmental of Specialist Care

The development of specialist care in Victorian Britain starts with the *Bath Idiot and Imbecile Institution*, started in April 1846 by the Miss Whites as a school, supported principally by female benefactors, and using teachers from the nearby deaf and blind institution (Carpenter, 2000). In London, Reverend Andrew Reed was the force behind Park House, which evolved into Earlswood asylum (Wright, 2001). The Baldovan Institution for *Imbecile Children* opened in 1855 in Scotland and the Stewart Institution for *Idiotic and Imbecile Children* in 1869 in Ireland. The intention of these asylums was to train their residents in order for them to be more useful within society but how far they succeeded is unclear – one of the 'star' children at the Bath Institution still ended up in the workhouse and then *lunatic* asylum after leaving (Stewart, 2016).

By the 1880s the care of *idiots and imbeciles*, as they were now identified, occurred in a variety of settings. The majority remained in the community, with state-funded 'outdoor relief' or private family wealth enabling their care. There were probably a large number of unregistered families being privately paid to look after an individual, this never needed official acknowledgement as they cared for only one person. Then there were a few big charitable subscription asylums or schools, such as Starcross in Devon and the Royal Albert in Lancashire, and the large private asylum, Normansfield in Twickenham, set up by Dr Langdon Down following his work at the Royal Earlswood.

In addition, there were also the vast public institution system run by the local authorities – the workhouse now cared for what were considered the *harmless idiots* and epileptics (often in dedicated wards) while *lunatic* asylums looked after what were considered the *dangerous idiot*. By the 1870s, the Metropolitan Asylums Board in London, finding a large number of *idiot and imbecile* children in their new asylums and workhouses, built Darenth School by Dartford in Kent. Very quickly, as life expectancy improved, these *idiot* asylums (both charitable and state) realised that they would need to provide for an adult population. The 1886 Idiots Act in England set out to give 'facilities for the care, education, and training of *Idiots and Imbeciles*' and legally recognised these *idiot* asylums as providing 'training' rather than 'treatment' with the focus on trying to ensure their usefulness within society (Idiots Act, 1886)

By 1900 some areas had developed special schools for the deaf and epileptic and the *mentally defective*, and their admission was usually determined by the local medical officers.

The problem of having special schools was that it highlighted the lack of services when the child left the school. The special schools, census returns and enlarging asylums led to an increasing number of identified *mentally defectives* within society. This fuelled a eugenics movement with mounting public concern, described by various witnesses to the Royal Commission. One response was the growth of 'preventative missions' and laundry homes for the new category of *feeble-minded* women (most of whom did not have ID), to learn to become virtuous servants (Carpenter, 2001). Another was a campaign for sterilisation, with sterilisation of *mental retards* starting in the United States in 1907, culminating in England with the recommendation of the 1934 Brock Committee for the voluntary sterilisation of '*defectives* and the *mentally disordered*' and only fading in the aftermath of the Second World War and horror at the Nazi eugenic programme.

16.3 The Great Incarceration

The Victorian concerns culminated in a Royal Commission on the Care and Control of the *Feeble-Minded* that after four years reported in 1908 that:

> ... our ... investigations compel the conclusion that there are numbers of *mentally defective* persons whose training is neglected, over whom no sufficient control is exercised, and whose wayward and irresponsible lives are productive of crime and misery, of much injury and mischief to themselves and others, and of much continuous expenditure wasteful to the community and to individual families.

The Commission estimated that 0.46% of the population were *mental defectives* and recommended 'care' and 'protection' that would be supervised by a Board of Control. The recommendations covered England, Wales, Scotland and Ireland and described how to put this into law. Importantly, it provided a definition and classification of *mental defectives* that effectively *became* the medical definition for the next fifty years. The English 1913 Mental Deficiency Act (see Box 16.2) was only modified in 1927 to clarify that *defectiveness* did not have to occur from birth, and to talk of therapy rather than control. The 1913 Act required local authorities to set up institutions to accommodate *mental defectives* inadequately controlled or cared for in the community. Scotland's equivalent Act came in 1914 but that of Ireland never arose.

The term *mental defective* included patients with ID but more commonly children and youths with criminal convictions, or epilepsy or physical disabilities. As the test of *mental deficiency* at the time was the ability to live independently and out of trouble, independent of IQ; the definition of *mental defectives* also included habitual drunkards and unmarried women who were pregnant and on state benefits.

The Mental Deficiency Act led to the development, by local authorities, of a vast number of beds in *mental deficiency* colonies, often reusing old workhouses. These colonies operated like *lunatic* asylums, but were designed for long-term care and used the inmates to reduce costs, with the more able, often providing colony labour and care for the less able. A villa design soon became popular but as the government ordered the costs to be reduced, wards become more crowded and care less individual: dormitories for over one hundred patients are known to have existed and a ratio of one qualified and one unqualified staff for sixty patients was relatively standard (Carpenter, 2002).

Some patients lived in the colonies until they died, but the more able were often discharged, usually by first going out 'on licence' either back to their family or to work.

> **Box 16.2** Definition of a mental defective in Mental Deficiency Act 1913 [with changes of 1927 Amendment Act in strikeout/italic]
>
> The following classes of persons who are mentally defective shall be deemed to be defectives within the meaning of this Act:
>
> *Mental Defectiveness means a condition of arrested of incomplete development of mind existing before the age of 18 years, whether arising from inherent causes or induced by injury or disease.*
>
> (a) **Idiots**; that is to say, persons so deeply defective in mind from birth or from an early age as to be **unable to guard themselves against common physical dangers.**
>
> (b) **Imbeciles**; that is to say, persons in whose case there exists from birth or from an early age mental defectiveness not amounting to idiocy, yet so pronounced that they are **incapable of managing themselves or their affairs**, or in the case of children, of being taught to do so.
>
> (c) **Feeble-minded persons**; that is to say, persons in whose case there exists from birth or from an early age mental defectiveness not amounting to imbecility, yet so pronounced that they **require care, supervision, and control for their own protection or for the protection of others**, or in the case of children, that they by reason of such defectiveness appear to be permanently **incapable of receiving proper benefit from the instruction in ordinary schools.**
>
> (d) **Moral imbeciles**; that is to say, persons who from an early age display some **permanent mental defect coupled with strong vicious or criminal propensities** on which punishment has had little or no deterrent effect. *and who require care, supervision and control for the protection of others.*

Work was most commonly as a female servant or a male labourer, though with some men working in the colony as carpenters, tailors and cobblers, more skilled trades were sometimes possible. In some colonies patients could have a degree of autonomy – in Brentry in the 1930s two wards were each run by a committee of three patients, with the minutes of their weekly meetings sent to the medical superintendent with nurses only visiting intermittently, leaving the patients to keep themselves and the ward in order (Carpenter, 2002).

In the Free State of Ireland (1922), the fledgling state had few resources and a strong Catholic identity. The relationship between the two became enmeshed and most of the support for those with disabilities, epilepsy, mental illness and unmarried mothers was devolved to the Church (Barrington, 1987). A number of religious orders including the Daughters of Charity (1922), the Sisters of Charity of St Vincent de Paul (1926), the St John of God order (1931) and Brothers of Charity (1937) all opened institutions for *mental defectives* which dominated the model of care up to the 1970s (Robins, 1992).

When the NHS was formed, it took over the *mental deficiency* colonies in 1948; the money spent on care was removed from the local authorities and given to the central government as colonies became 'hospitals', like the new mental illness hospitals. With this change from a 'social' to a 'medical' model, there was once again a change in nomenclature with, for example, colony work becoming industrial therapy. It was now even easier to confuse *mental deficiency* with *mental illness* in the popular imagination. The medical superintendents of these new hospitals may have been psychiatrists and the care staff *mental deficiency* nurses, but these were not psychiatric hospitals but training and care settings – the nurses' training manual did not discuss mental illness (RMPA, 1931) and even

> **Box 16.3** Definition of mental subnormality in Mental Health Act 1959
>
> **Severe subnormality:** a state of arrested or incomplete development of mind which includes subnormality of intelligence and is of such a nature or degree that the patient is incapable of leading an independent life or of guarding himself against serious exploitation, or will be so incapable when of an age to do so.
>
> **Subnormality:** a state of arrested or incomplete development of mind (not amounting to severe subnormality) which includes subnormality of intelligence and is of a nature or degree which requires or is susceptible to medical treatment or other special care or training of the patient.
>
> **Psychopathic personality:** a persistent disorder or disability of mind (whether or not including subnormality of intelligence) which results in abnormally aggressive or seriously irresponsible conduct on the part of the patient, and requires or is susceptible to medical treatment [or care or training under medical supervision].

in the 1960s if an inmate became mentally ill then they would be transferred to a 'mainstream' mental hospital for treatment.

With free care under the NHS, informal admission became more common and the new 1959 Mental Health Act reversed the assumptions of the 1913 Mental Deficiency Act by assuming most patients were voluntary inmates for treatment and not compulsorily in hospital for control (see Box 16.3). The new Mental Health Act was also renamed *mental deficiency* as *subnormality* and excluded *moral defectives* by relabelling them *psychopathic personalities*. The result of these legal changes was an exodus of a group of patients, mainly the previously *feeble-minded*, from the renamed *subnormality* hospitals, most of whom never used their services again. The hospitals refilled with *subnormals* queuing for admission from the community (mainly from the workhouses), due to the lack of community facilities (Heaton-Ward, 2011).

Most people with *mental subnormality* continued to live in the community. Local authorities, it seems, paid this community group little attention until the NHS removed their access to the old colonies (that had become hospitals) and only started to develop day centres and respite hostels for community clients in the 1960s.

From the outset of the NHS in 1948, money was diverted from the *subnormality* and psychiatric hospitals to bolster the acute care hospitals (Webster, 1988). The result worsened both care and overcrowding in the former. In 1952 the average cost for England and Wales of *Mental Deficiency* Hospitals was £3 14s 3d per patient per week (about £100 a week in 2017 prices) (Ministry of Health, 1953). Relatives were rarely allowed to see the wards where their loved ones lived, but were reassured they were in the best place, so when the *mental handicap* hospitals were eventually hit by a succession of scandals the public were shocked. Public enquiries into ill treatment in *mental handicap* hospitals became an annual event sparing no part of the country: 1969 at Ely in Cardiff, 1971 Farleigh in Bristol, 1973 Coldharbour in Sherborne, 1974 South Ockenden in Essex, 1975 Brockhall in Lancashire, 1976 St Ebba's in Epsom, 1977 Mary Dendy in Cheshire and 1978 Normansfield in London. The media became interested in these repeated enquiries and, in 1972, Stoke Park in Bristol allowed a horrifying film of life on its slum wards to be broadcast on prime-time television (Heaton-Ward, 2011). This, in part, contributed to the 'deinstitutionalisation' that followed.

16.4 The Return to Community Care

In 1971 the Government published the White Paper: *Better Services for the Mentally Handicapped*. Most of the money spent by public authorities to support people with disabilities was still used by the NHS for those living in the newly named *mental handicap* hospital. Like the psychiatric hospitals these were usually large campus sites located out of town, with those converted from old Victorian workhouses being particularly dilapidated. The hospitals were still behind high walls with the pubic excluded. The White Paper promulgated a move from hospital-based care to new community services, with multidisciplinary assessments and a new attendance allowance for family carers. However in retrospect its vision was still conservative with new 'homely' local authority hostels of 'only' twenty-five residents and only halving the number of hospital beds and confining them to treatment only. However the fact that there were 59,000 beds made even discharging 30,000 seem optimistic. At the same time the 1970 Education Act (and equivalents in Scotland in 1975 and Northern Ireland in 1987) brought all children into education and transformed the previous 'junior training centres' into schools, once again, under the control of local authorities. *Mental handicap* was now the medically preferred term used in the UK; however the World Health Organization's International Classification of Diseases (ICD) and the American Psychiatric Association's Diagnostic and Statistical Manual (DSM) used the term *mental retardation* and introduced the distinction between mild, moderate, severe and profoundly affected individuals based upon IQ ranges.

The closure of the hospitals affected the roles of psychiatrists, nurses and other clinicians working in the *mental handicap* hospitals. The *Mental Deficiency* section of the new Royal College of Psychiatrists averted its demise by specialising in the psychiatry (and neuropsychiatry) of *mental handicap* and the first books dedicated to the psychiatry of *mental handicap* soon followed in the 1970s. Specialist community *mental handicap* teams started to appear in the 1970s. These were staffed by clinicians from the hospitals, so specialist GPs or physicians were rarely employed and the specialist physician never emerged in the British Isles, though they did in the Netherlands where there were no specialist psychiatrists. In the 1970's *mental handicap* nurses were advised to transform from hospital carers into community carers or social workers and many retrained or left to run community homes. Nurse training reduced, but nurses continued as a mainstay of the community teams, often specialising in conditions such as dementia, epilepsy, mental illness and challenging behaviour.

The original plan of the 1970s was for a move to hostels and smaller hospitals – there was a burst of twenty-four bedded hospitals built in Wessex and elsewhere. These twenty-four bedded units became the new hospital ward size. The local authorities though did not have the money to build a large number of hostels and private finance became the norm with many large old houses turned into new community homes. However, as hospitals closed in the 1980's and 1990's many of the sites were sold to release capital to fund the new homes that had to be built or purchased.

The plan for community care was modified in the 1980's by the normalisation movement. This movement started in Denmark in the 1960's and spread to Sweden and the United States – the pressure was to 'allow the *Mentally Retarded* to obtain an existence as close to normal as possible' (Wolfensberger, 1972), with the view that a person with *mental handicap* would not want to live next to another similar person on a campus site. By the early 1980's there was a campaign for the patient to move into the community and live 'An Ordinary Life' in 'normal' houses (King's Fund, 1980). The five accomplishments of John O'Brien, published in 1987, recommended that all proposed services should strive for five things:

(1) community presence;
(2) relationships;
(3) choice;
(4) competence; and
(5) respect.

These accomplishments became the five principles used in planning many of the health and social services for patients with ID in England over the next fifteen years, though the move to smaller homes was sometimes modified by the economics of closure. Many hospital staff moved with their patients into the new community homes, often after training to instil the new principles of normalisation and respect in the new homes, and by 2000 these formed half the NHS-managed beds. There was also a development of service user groups such as People First who demanded involvement in planning. Their demands were strengthened by the Human Rights Act and the Disability Discrimination Act.

The 1983 Mental Health Act abandoned the term *mental subnormality* and used the new term *mental impairment*. It further stated that a person with *mental impairment* (or *severe mental impairment*) could not be detained for more than a month unless they had seriously irresponsible or abnormally aggressive behaviour. Having *mental impairment* alone was not to be seen as grounds for prolonged detention.

The move to the community had initially relied on private capital to develop new homes with new state benefits paying for board and lodgings, irrespective of support needs. The system was revised following the 1988 Griffiths Report and care management was introduced to limit these costs. In addition, the existing community home inspection system was found wanting in the 1994 Longcare scandal in Buckinghamshire, and so a central inspection system was introduced. The term *mental handicap* was now considered pejorative but the term *learning difficulties*, liked by service user groups, was felt to be too vague as it was an education term relating to children, so a new term *'learning disability'* was launched by Mr Dorrell in a speech on 25 June 1991, and took over as the British medical term for the international term mental retardation.

For all these financial difficulties, the 1990s saw a progressive closure of the old hospitals and transfer of patients from the responsibility of the NHS back to local authorities and by the year 2000 the service bore little resemblance to that of 1971 or that planned by the 1971 white paper (see Table 16.1).

The White Papers of the millennium (*The Same as You* (2000) in Scotland; *Valuing People* (2001) in England, *Fulfilling the Promises* (2001) in Wales) had to face the practicalities of people with *'learning disability'* living in a stigmatising community. All emphasised that mainstream services should provide for all, with a very small specialist *'learning disability'* service supporting this process by facilitating access to mainstream services. They also emphasised the involvement of service users within the planning processes – using People First's slogan 'Nothing About Us without Us'. The new emphasis was on rights, independence, choice and inclusion. The government soon became committed to individual budgets and supported living, where a person became a tenant or houseowner like anyone else, funded through the state. The English Mental Capacity Act of 2005 and Deprivation of

Table 16.1 Services in 1969 and 2000 in England

1969	2000
58,850 patients (adults and children) in NHS hospitals or units	Nearly 10,000 places in NHS facilities:
	1,550 NHS specialist places
	1,570 NHS long-stay places
	1,520 NHS campus places
	5,100 places in residential accommodation managed by the NHS
4,900 places in residential care homes	53,400 places in residential care
24,500 places in adult training centres	84,000 adults receiving community-based services (day care, home help, meals, etc.), of whom
	49,600 are in receipt of social services day services
	6,630 patients using NHS day care facilities

(source Valuing People, 2001)

Liberty Safeguards in 2007 made carers clearer about their responsibilities and duties and in addition the English Autism Act of 2009 forced the state to look at the needs of people with autism and the quality of the services they received. The 2006 enquiry into poor care in Cornwall put an end to NHS Trusts managing residential care homes (Commission for Healthcare Audit and Inspection, 2006).

Concerns now shifted to the deficiencies in care provided by mainstream health and care services. All acute hospital trusts were encouraged to appoint specialist liaison nurses to facilitate good care for patients with ID. GPs were encouraged to develop registers of their patients with ID and to provide annual health checks. A 'greenlight toolkit' was developed for mental health services to audit their services for people with ID (Foundation for People with Learning Disabilities, 2004) and reissued in 2013. Mencap led a campaign with *Death by Indifference* and its follow-up documents publicising the shocking care of people with ID in mainstream services (Mencap, 2007). A later confidential inquiry into the deaths of people with ID estimated that 42% died prematurely (Heslop, 2013).

The next major change of policy followed the *BBC Panorama* 2011 television broadcast of abuse within the private hospital, Winterbourne View. The Care Quality Commission immediately surveyed all hospital assessment units for patients with ID and the government recommended closure of many of the beds through the 'Transforming Care' project. The use of medication was to be reviewed and reduced. A survey of the time estimated there were fewer than 4,000 beds in operation as shown in Table 16.2.

Now in Great Britain most people with ID live in the community, mainly supported by their families funded through the benefit system. Those who need additional support are care managed by their local authority using the now preferred 'supported living', though recent austerity has increased pressure to use care homes or care homes subdivided into 'supported living' places. Day care, if provided, is now commonly provided on an individual

Table 16.2 Estimate of specialist ID inpatient beds in 2012

	NHS operated	Private operated
Forensic beds	1,011	1,727
'Acute admission' beds	646	168
Continuing care beds	104	173
Other specialist beds	125	0
Total	1,886	2,068

(source Faculty of Intellectual Disabilities, 2013)

basis rather than in day care centres. However, despite the targets of the White Papers to increase access to employment, CareEngland claimed in 2016 that only 17% of people with ID were in employment (CareEngland, 2016).

Now the main provider of healthcare is the primary care health service. The specialist community ID teams seem to have split into two parallel roles – first of supporting GPs, local authority workers or direct carers over physical health and challenging behaviour and second the provision of a specialist mental health service either from a base within the mainstream mental health services, or from a team based with the rest of the ID team. The team still does not include specialist physicians but usually includes specialist psychiatrists, psychologists, learning disability nurses and occupational therapists and sometimes speech and language therapists, physiotherapists and specialist psychotherapists.

With the revision of medical classification in ICD11 and DSM5 there was a strong call to remove *mental retardation* as a medical disorder but to reclassify it as a disability. This has not occurred but another new 'non-stigmatising' medical term of 'disorders of intellectual development' has replaced *mental retardation*.

Like with many other groups, services have now passed from non-existence, through institutional care and development of specialist expertise to care in the community with a message of equal rights and non-discrimination. At 0.5%, the prevalence of people with ID known to services remains very similar to that estimated in 1908 by the Royal Commission for the prevalence of mental defectives, suggesting a prevalence of need that has not changed despite the changes in nomenclature and delineation. The constant change of name for this group, suggests that the group remains stigmatised by the general public and that mainstream services have had to learn not to discriminate. Whether the dissolution of specialised services will improve or worsen that position is not yet clear.

Box 16.4 Timeline of legislation and related policy documents in England

1601 Relief of the Poor Act

1834 Poor Law Amendment Act restrict poor law relief to the workhouse

1845 Lunacy Act and County Asylum Act – includes Idiots as persons of unsound mind

1846 Start of Idiot schools and asylums

1870 Elementary Education Act

Box 16.4 (cont)

1878 Darenth School started by Metropolitan Commissioners
1886 Idiots Act – recognises idiot asylums for the training of idiots and imbeciles
1890 Lunacy Act includes idiots as persons of unsound mind
1899 Elementary Education (Defective and Epileptic Children) Act – permits special schools
1908 *Report of Royal Commission on the Care and Control of the Feeble-Minded*
1908 Tredgold publishes *Amentia* (republished as *Mental Deficiency* and becomes main textbook until the 1960s)
1914 Elementary Education (Defective and Epileptic Children) Act – requires such schools
1927 Mental Deficiency Act allows deficiency to be from childhood injury
1934 Brock Report recommends sterilisation
1948 start of National Health Service – colonies become hospitals
1959 Mental Health Act – assumes detention only if justified – defines subnormality
1962 Ministry of Health report *A Hospital Plan for England & Wales* plans hostels
1970 Education Act make education universal
1967–78 Multiple enquiries into poor care
1971 White Paper *Better Services for the Mentally Handicapped* wants care in the community
1974 NHS reorganisation
1981 People with Mental Handicap get right to vote
1990 National Service and Community Care Act
2001 White Paper *Valuing People* – advocates mainstreaming and equality
2004 Greenlight toolkit published
2005 Mental Capacity Act
2006–8 Health Care Commission & Commission for Social Care Inspection publish reports on poor community care
2007 UN Convention on the Rights of Persons with Disabilities
2008 Health and Social Care Act creates Care Quality Commission to oversee both health and social care
2008 Department of Health report *Healthcare for All* – emphasises need to improve mainstream services for people with LD
2009 White Paper *Valuing People Now* – pushes for more equality of access to services
2009 Autism Act
2012 Department of Health publishes *Transforming Care*
2013 Confidential Inquiry into the Deaths of People with Learning Disabilities published
2013 DSM5 published using term 'disorders of Intellectual development'. ICD11 indicates it will use the same term and keep as a medical disorder, after debate as to whether to remove this category as a medical disorder

References

Barrington, R. (1987) *Health, Medicine and Politics in Ireland 1900–1970.* Dublin: Institute of Public Administration.

Brock, L. G. (1934) *Report of the Departmental Committee on Sterilisation.* HMSO.

CareEngland (2016) Briefing for the Care Home Parliamentary Network. Available at: www.careengland.org.uk/sites/careengland/files/5.%20LD%20Employment%20-%20July%202016.pdf [accessed February 2017]

Carpenter, P. K. (1997) The Pauper Insane of Leicester in 1844. *History of Psychiatry,* **8**, 517–38.

Carpenter, P. K. (1998) St Mary Magdalene Hospital, Bath – Its history to 1600. *Notes and Queries for Somerset and Dorset,* **34**, 226–32.

Carpenter, P. K. (2000) The Bath Idiot and Imbecile Institution. *History of Psychiatry,* **11**, 163–88.

Carpenter, P. K. (2001) The role of Victorian women in the care of 'idiots' and the 'feeble-minded'. *Journal on Developmental Disabilities,* **8**, 31–43.

Carpenter, P. K. (2002) *A History of Brentry – House, Reformatory, Colony and Hospital.* Friends of Glenside Hospital Museum.

Commission for Healthcare Audit and Inspection (2006) *Joint Investigation into the Provision of Services for People with Learning Disabilities at Cornwall Partnership Trust.* Healthcare Commission.

De Praerogativa Regis (1324) 17 Edward 2 c.9 sets out property law, but see also Bracton (1968) *De Legibus et Consuetudinibus Angliæ* attributed to Henry of Bratton c.1210–1268. Trans. Samuel E. Thorne. Harvard University Press. Available at: http://bracton.law.harvard.edu/Common/index.htm [accessed 2 September 2018], which groups 'fools' and 'idiots' with 'deaf and dumb' and 'lunatics' in many areas

Faculty of Intellectual Disabilities (2013) *People with Learning Disability and Mental Health, Behavioural or Forensic Problems: The Role of In-Patient Services.* Faculty report FR/ID/03. Royal College of Psychiatrists.

Foundation for People with Learning Disabilities (2004) Greenlight Toolkit.

Heaton-Ward, W. A. (1963) *Mental Subnormality* (2nd edn). John Wright.

(2011) *Mental Handicap, the Shifting Sands: A Collection of Papers 1950–2001.* Friends of Glenside Hospital Museum.

Heslop, P. (2013) *Confidential Inquiry into the Deaths of People with Learning Disabilities (CIPOLD).* Norah Fry Research Centre.

Idiots Act (1886) 49 Vict. cap. 25.

King's Fund (1980) *An Ordinary Life: Comprehensive Locally-Based Services for Mentally Handicapped People.* Project paper no. 24. King's Fund.

Lane, H. (1979) *The Wild Boy of Aveyron.* Harvard University Press.

Mencap (2007) *Death by Indifference.* Mencap.

Ministry of Health (1953) *National Health Service: Hospital Costings Returns year Ending 31 March 1952.* HMSO.

Orme, N. & Webster, M. (1995) *The English Hospital 1070–1570.* Yale University Press.

Poor Law Commissioners (1843) *Ninth Annual Report of the Poor Law Commissioners for England and Wales.* Clowes.

Report of the Royal Commission on the Care and Control of the Feeble-Minded (1908), vol. 8. HMSO.

RMPA [Royal Medico-Psychological Association] (1931) *Manual for Mental Deficiency Nurses.* Bailliere.

Robins, J. (1992) *From Rejection to Integration: A Centenary of Service by the Daughters of Charity to Persons with a Mental Handicap.* Gill & MacMillan.

Stewart, D. (2016) What the Dickens! Presentation at 2016 Open University Learning Disability Conference. Available at: www.open.ac.uk/health-and-social-care/research/shld/conferences/conference-2016/what-dickens [accessed 12 February 2017]

Twining, W. (1843) *Some Account of Cretinism and the Institution for Its Cure, on the Abendberg, near Interlachen, in Switzerland.* Parker.

Webster, C. (1988) *The Health Services since the War. Volume 1: Problems of Health*

Care, the National Health Service before 1957. HMSO.

Wolfensberger, W. (1972) *The Principle of Normalization in Human Services.* National Institute on Mental Retardation.

Wright, D. (2001) *Mental Disability in Victorian England: The Earlswood Asylum 1847–1901.* Clarendon Press.

Further Reading on the Web

www.historyoflearningdisability.com – a website with useful background reading and links [accessed 2 September 2018]

www.open.ac.uk/health-and-social-care/research/shld – Open University website on the social history of learning disability [accessed 2 September 2018]

Chapter 17
Inpatient Care for People with Intellectual Disability

Kiran Purandare and Shaun Gravestock

Historically, people with intellectual disability (ID) *were cared for* by their families in their own homes. The Industrial Revolution saw the development of workhouses and prisons. Interest in ID by pioneers such as Itard and Seguin in France led to the establishment of colonies and educational establishments in Europe. In Britain, the Idiots Act 1886 enabled local authorities to build asylums for the care of people with ID. The involvement of medical doctors such as Penrose led to the asylums and 'colonies' being designated as hospitals following the establishment of the National Health Service. These institutions gradually began to decline only in the 1970s with the ideas of normalisation (Wolfensberger et al., 1972) and 'social role valorisation'. Subsequent changes to legislation enabled these ideas to become enshrined in law with gradually increasing emphasis on community care.

17.1 Need for Inpatient Services

There is a well-documented recognition of the high mental health needs in people with ID (Cooper, 2007; Read, 1994) as well as problem behaviour (Emerson, 2001). Psychotic disorders are up to five times higher (Morgan, 2008) and there is a high prevalence of other mental disorders including anxiety and affective disorders (31–41%) (Cooper, 2007). For people needing admission to inpatient units, the figures are understandably higher (Alexander et al., 2001, Tajuddin 2004). Inpatient admission is to be considered within the context and legal framework of the risk and the use of the least restrictive alternative. It could be argued that a patient who is 'liable to be detained' under the Mental Health Act 1983 (as amended 2007) is not only entitled to safe and high-quality inpatient care, but it could be a form of disenfranchisement if it were not available. Given the high rates of co-morbidity, communication difficulties and vulnerability in this group of people, there is a need for a safe place with access to suitably trained staff with specialist knowledge and expertise in treatment of mental disorder in people with ID. It has been evident from two decades of reduction of inpatient psychiatric provision for people without ID, that there remains a small but definite need for inpatient treatment (King's Fund, 2015).

17.2 Generic versus Specialist Services

This has been a long-standing debate that became more relevant following the closure of the institutions (Alexander et al., 2001; Chaplin, 2004). There has been increasing emphasis in the past two decades towards using mainstream services (Hassiotis, 2000) and government policy outlined in publications such as Valuing People (2001) underlined the need for this. Early experiences were mixed, indicating that people with ID found generic

> **Box 17.1** The Royal College of Psychiatrists Faculty of Intellectual Disability's categories of types of inpatient beds for people with intellectual disability and mental disorder
>
> Category 1 High, medium and low secure forensic beds
> Category 2 Acute admission beds in specialised ID units
> Category 3 Acute admission beds in generic mental health settings
> Category 4 Forensic rehabilitation beds
> Category 5 Complex continuing care and rehabilitation beds
> Category 6 Other beds, including those for specialist neuropsychiatric conditions and short breaks
>
> Category 1 refers to beds in forensic units in conditions of high, medium or low security and caters to those patients who present with either offending behaviour or behaviour that puts themselves or others at risk that cannot be managed in less robust environments.
>
> Category 2 and 3 consists of beds in specialist ID units and general psychiatric hospitals respectively. There is inconclusive evidence for the superiority of any one of the two models. However, specialist units (Category 2) tend to look after patients who have greater disability and co-morbidity such as autism whereas patients with predominantly mental illness and lesser disability can be looked after in Category 3 beds.
>
> Category 4 (forensic rehabilitation) beds refer to those beds in locked or open community units. The patients who use these beds have ongoing risk issues but no longer need Category 1 (more secure) beds.
>
> The beds in Category 5 (complex continuing care and rehabilitation) are used for patients who no longer need acute assessment and treatment beds but nevertheless present with a degree of behaviour that needs ongoing rehabilitation in a safe structured environment. These beds are similar to those in use elsewhere in healthcare for medical and surgical rehabilitation where the individual may not yet be able to live independently in their own home.
>
> Category 6 includes specialist beds for neuropsychiatric conditions such as epilepsy and are limited to a few highly specialist national units.
>
> Inpatient care is seen as the highest tier within a tiered-care model with the levels rising from liaison work to more intensive case management in the community and finally inpatient management if needed.
>
> (source: Royal College of Psychiatrists, 2013)

adult mental health wards to be noisy and uncomfortable with inadequate staff support (Longo & Prior, 2004; Parkes, 2007; Vos, 2007). The publication of *Valuing People Now* (Department of Health, 2009) reiterated the direction of policy travel and made it a requirement for adult mental health services to be more responsive to people with ID.

A review of the literature by Chaplin (2011) concluded that there was still evidence of poor standards of care on some general psychiatric inpatient units. The length of stay for people with ID wasn't consistently longer on specialist than general psychiatric units. Nevertheless, uncontrolled comparisons and service evaluations suggested positive outcomes in specialist services. It has been shown that intensive in-reach work and collaboration with inpatient teams can result in significant improvement in the mental health of patients with ID admitted to acute general psychiatric wards (Hall, 2006). However, a more recent audit evaluated the performance of acute general and mental health services in delivering inpatient care to people with ID in nine acute general hospital trusts and six mental health services (Sheehan, 2016). Data on seven key indicators of care collected from 176 patients covering physical health/monitoring, communication and meeting needs, capacity and decision-making, discharge planning and carer involvement found that indicators of physical healthcare (body mass index, swallowing assessment, epilepsy risk assessment) were poorly recorded in both acute general and mental health inpatient settings.

The widely held clinical observation that there are differences in clinical and demographic characteristics of patients admitted to acute general psychiatric wards and specialist inpatient assessment and treatment units has been supported by a few studies (Bakken & Martinsen, 2013; Hemmings, 2009; Sandhu, 2017). Patients with moderate–severe ID, autism and behavioural problems might benefit from specialist inpatient units whereas mental health problems in patients with mild ID could be managed in more mainstream acute general psychiatric wards.

It is important to factor in the pressure on generic inpatient beds due to the programme of bed reduction and funding cuts (King's Fund, 2015). This could also potentially have an impact on the quality of inpatient care that is provided to patients with ID. The debate between mainstream and specialist provision should therefore move on to a consideration of the most appropriate setting where care can be provided in the most person-centred approach. It seems prudent to ensure that both types of care provision are available within the care pathway while planning for services locally.

Issues that need to be addressed for access to mainstream services to be successful include a clear joint-care pathway between mainstream services and the ID teams. There are various models of managing joint care in adult inpatient units with some teams handing over treatment responsibility to the inpatient team during the period of inpatient stay while others retain the overall responsibility of care.

17.3 Reduction in the Use of Specialist Inpatient Beds

17.3.1 England

In England, much of the recent change in the provision of inpatient care for people with ID has been as a reaction to a scandal in a non-NHS inpatient unit called Winterbourne View near Bristol. A BBC undercover television report in 2011 (*Panorama*; see BBC, 2012) disclosed horrendous abuse of inpatients by a few staff members in that hospital. The national outcry resulting from this served as a catalyst for a review of services for people with ID in England. The UK government published a series of reports aimed at drastically reducing the numbers of inpatient beds across the country (Transforming Care, 2014; Winterbourne View, 2012, 2014) and strengthening community care. Among a range of findings, some salient themes emerged. A shortage of locally commissioned services for people with ID resulted in patients and their families having to travel long distances for this provision. It also discouraged regular scrutiny of the placement by the local community services and commissioning bodies with the consequence that such abuse took place without detection.

These findings need to be taken into consideration while planning for local specialist inpatient services. The practice of a large number of areas jointly commissioning an inpatient unit could potentially reproduce some of the same problems (e.g. distance from home) that contributed to this situation (Purandare, 2015).

17.3.2 Care and Treatment Reviews

One of the initiatives taken by the Department of Health to reduce dependence on hospital beds and expedite discharge is the Care and Treatment Review (CTR) (NHS England, 2015). These were put in place by the Department of Health in England to address some of the issues raised by the Winterbourne reviews, namely prolonged spells of inpatient stay in hospital, variable quality of care and distance from home. The intention was to robustly challenge the care and rationale for inpatient stay in hospital and to facilitate discharge. The panel consists of an independent expert clinician, an 'expert by experience' (usually a carer or parent of a person with ID/autism) and is headed by the local commissioner of health services.

Since the inception of CTRs in 2014, NHS England has conducted an audit of their standards and outcomes (Webster & Banks, 2015). In a sample of sixty cases audited by members of NHS England's Learning Disability Programme, deficiencies such as lack of clear formulation/diagnoses, inadequate provision for physical healthcare or lack of/inadequate PBS plans were found in twenty-two of the sixty cases audited. Among their other findings, in twenty-five out of the sixty cases, they found either an 'apparent inertia or lack of pressure to move forward' or 'hospital seen as appropriate in the absence of identified alternative'. On the whole, CTRs were felt to be helpful in reviewing care and facilitating discharge. However, it has been acknowledged that the patients discharged have been replaced by new admissions rendering the overall number of inpatients relatively unchanged. This may therefore represent the core need for a proportion of inpatient beds in the care pathway.

While the objectives of CTRs are laudable, the success of this process in effecting safe and swift discharges has yet to be robustly evaluated. It may be that the initial success in discharging patients reflected the relative ease in sourcing community placements leaving behind the significant proportion for whom such provision was either lacking or deemed inappropriate due to the complexity, risks in their presentation or significant medico-legal difficulties. The process of carrying out CTRs has now been reviewed and updated by NHS England (2017).

17.3.3 Scotland

The move towards more community provision has been prominent in Scotland as well with publications like *The Same as You?* (Scottish Executive, 2000). The number of acute beds recommended in this report was to be 4 per 100,000 population with a plan to close all long-stay beds by 2005. This was reviewed in 2007 (Perera et al., 2009) and more recently in 2017 (National Statistics Publication for Scotland, 2017) which found that between 1997 and 1998 and 2005 and 2006 discharges from ID specialist beds fell from around 4,700 to around 1,700, but there hasn't been any further reduction in the last decade. The main reasons for delays in discharge remain lack of funding, accommodation, or an appropriate care provider; or a combination of these issues. There are equivalent legal frameworks in Scotland governing mental health and incapacity (Adults with Incapacity (Scotland) Act 2000) and quality and standards are overseen by the Commission through monitoring visits and are reported on annually (Mental Welfare Commission for Scotland, 2018).

17.3.4 Wales
As is to be expected, there are differences in the structure and provision of health services in the countries in the UK and Wales is no exception. The country is served by local authorities and health boards which, between them, are responsible for this provision. A report for the Welsh Assembly undertaken by the Care and Social Services Inspectorate provides a comprehensive account of the service provision in Wales (Care and Inspectorate Wales, 2016).

17.3.5 Northern Ireland
While there is limited research in this area in Northern Ireland, the trend away from inpatient hospital beds mirrors that in the other countries of the UK. A report for the Northern Ireland Assembly (Murphy, 2014) summarises the demographic and health issues of people with ID in Northern Ireland.

17.4 Treatment Issues
In England and Wales, all pharmacological treatment is subject to NICE guidelines although there are no guidelines specifically for ID prescribing. There is NICE guidance for the management of challenging behaviour (NICE, 2015), autism (NICE, 2016a) and mental illness (NICE, 2016b) that include pharmacological and non-pharmacological interventions. Similar guidance in Scotland is provided by the Scottish Intercollegiate Guideline Network (SIGN). A detailed review of treatment modalities is beyond the scope of this chapter.

17.5 Outcome Measures
These can be classified into clinician rated outcome measures, patient rated outcome measures and patient reported experience measures. The most common clinician rated outcome measure is the Health of the Nation Scale–Learning Disability (HoNoS–LD) (Roy, 2002) and is extensively used in most inpatient units both as a baseline rating scale and subsequently to measure progress. It has been found to have good psychometric properties but does not correlate with quality-of-life measures (Pearce, 2011). The Clinical Global Impression Scale (CGI) is extensively used in generic mental health settings (Guy, 1976) to measure global symptom severity and treatment response. It has good face validity and can be used in people with ID. It is freely available for use. Other clinician rated outcome measures include the Modified Overt Aggression Scale (Sorgi et al., 1991) and more specific rating scales such as those for anxiety, depression and psychoses. There are increasingly more validated and reliable patient rated outcome measures such as the Glasgow Anxiety Scale (Mindham, 2003) for use in people with ID. Measures such as the Quality of Life Scale (Cummins, 1997) could be used in addition to those tailored for individual use.

The 'Friends and Family Test' is now widely used within the NHS as a measure of patient experience (NHS England, 2015c) and can be modified into easily accessible language.

17.6 Quality Issues
The provision of high-quality care remains a high priority for all health providers and is regulated nationally by appropriate regulators in the various countries. A review of the legislation is beyond the scope of this chapter. At a local level, regular audits and quality improvement projects have been shown to improve quality of care in inpatient units (Ali et al., 2006).

National quality standards such as Commissioning for Quality and Innovation(CQUINs) (introduced by NHS England in 2009) and local key performance indicators (KPIs) are systems that make a proportion of health providers' income conditional on meeting a set of standards and can help in ensuring quality of care.

The Royal College of Psychiatrists' Accreditation for Inpatient Mental Health Services (AIMS) incorporates ID (AIMS–LD) and is a formal recognition of a service against clinical service standards using external peer review.

17.7 Planning for the Future

There has been a dramatic reduction in the number of inpatient beds for people with ID from circa 34,000 in 1987 to fewer than 3,000 in 2015. A joint report by NHS England, the Association of Director of Social Care (ADASS) and the Local Government Authority (NHS England, 2015a) has recommended 10–15 acute inpatient assessment and treatment beds per 1 million population on the basis of a national survey of bed usage (4 per 100,000 by the Scottish Executive). It is envisaged that closing further hospital beds will provide the resources to strengthen community services.

At a local level, there have been numerous initiatives either to prevent admission or to reduce the length of stay in inpatient units (Bartle et al., 2016). Devapriam et al. (2014) reported significant reduction in the length of inpatient stay using a care pathway-based approach to treatment.

17.8 Challenges for Inpatient Units

As discussed earlier, specialist inpatient units need to address potentially long stays and delays in discharge. Due to the level of specialism and training involved, small specialist inpatient units can be expensive to run. It is increasingly common practice for contiguous areas and clinical commissioning groups to pool resources in order to jointly commission an inpatient unit. This requires commitment from commissioners, from both healthcare and social care, to ensure that services remain local. In order to provide equity of outcome for people with ID, there has to be acknowledgement that inpatient care, particularly in specialist units with appropriately trained staff, resources and environment, remains a small but crucial part of the care pathway. There is a need to continue to innovate with alternative models of care such as a crisis housing (and robust provision to support discharge)and closer liaison with intensive support teams in the community to provide a seamless service for people with ID and mental health and/or problem behaviours.

References

Alexander, R., Piachaud, J. & Singh, I. (2001) Two districts, two models: In-patient care in the psychiatry of learning disability. *British Journal of Development Disabilities*, **47**, 105–10.

Ali, A., Hall, I., Taylor, C., Attard, S. & Hassiotis, A. (2006) Auditing the care programme approach for people with learning disability: A 4-year audit cycle. *Psychological Bulletin*, **30**(11), 415–18.

Bakken, T. L. & Martinsen, H. (2013) Adults with intellectual disabilities and mental illness in psychiatric in-patient units: Empirical studies of patient characteristics and psychiatric diagnoses from 1996 to 2011. *International Journal of Developmental Disability*, **59**(3), 179–90.

Bartle, J., Crossland, T. & Hewitt, O. (2016) 'Planning Live': Using a person centred intervention to reduce admissions to and length of stay in learning disability inpatient facilities. *British Journal of Learning Disability*, **44**, 277–83.

BBC News (2012) Winterbourne View: Abuse footage shocked nation. Available at: www.bbc.co.uk/news/uk-england-bristol-20084254, *Panorama* [accessed 15 September 2018]

Bouras, N. & Holt, G. (2004) Mental health services for adults with learning disabilities. *British Journal of Psychiatry*, **184**, 291–2.

Care Quality Commission (2011) Count Me in 2010. Available at: www.cqc.org.uk/sites/default/files/media/documents/count_me_in_2010_final_tagged.pdf [accessed 15 September 2018]

Care (and Social Services) Inspectorate Wales (2016) *Chief Inspector's Annual Report 2016–2017*. Available at: https://careinspectorate.wales/sites/default/files/2018-02/171102annualreporten.pdf [accessed 28 September 2018]

Chaplin, R. (2004) General psychiatric services for adults with intellectual disability and mental illness. *Journal of Intellectual Disability Research*, **48**, 1–10.

Chaplin, R. (2009) Annotation: New research into general psychiatric services for adults with intellectual disability and mental illness. *Journal of Intellectual Disability Research*, **53**(3), 189–99.

Chaplin, R. (2011) Mental health services for people with intellectual disabilities. *Current Opinion in Psychiatry*, **24**(5), 372–6.

Cooper, S.-A., Smiley, E., Morrison, J. et al. (2007) Mental ill-health in adults with intellectual disabilities: Prevalence and associated factors. *British Journal of Psychology*, **190**, 27–35.

Cummins, R. (1997) Comprehensive Quality of Life Scale – Intellectual/cognitive disability. Available at: http://www.acqol.com.au/instruments/comqol-scale/comqol-i5.pdf [accessed 15 September 2018].

Day, K. (1999) Professional training in the psychiatry of mental retardation in the United Kingdom. In *Psychiatric and Behavioural Disorders in Developmental Disabilities and Mental Retardation* (ed. N. Bouras), pp. 439–57. Cambridge University Press.

Department of Health (2001) *Valuing People: A New Strategy for Learning Disabilities in the 21st Century*. HMSO.

Department of Health (2012) *Transforming Care: A National Response to Winterbourne View Hospital Department of Health Review: Final Report*. www.gov.uk/government/uploads/system/uploads/attachment_data/file/213215/final-report.pdf [accessed 15 September 2018]

NHS England (2014) *Winterbourne View: Time for change. Transforming the commissioning for services for people with learning disabilities and/or autism. A report by the Transforming Care and Commissioning Steering Group, chaired by Sir Stephen Bubb*.

Department of Health (2015) *Winterbourne View: Transforming Care Two Years on*. Available at: www.gov.uk/government/uploads/system/uploads/attachment_data/file/399755/Winterbourne_View.pdf [accessed 15 September 2018]

Devapriam, J., Alexander, R., Gumber, R., Pither J. & Gangadharan, S. (2014) Impact of care pathway-based approach on outcomes in a specialist intellectual disability inpatient unit. *Journal of Intellectual Disabilities Research*, **18**(3), 211–20.

Devapriam, J., Rosenbach, A. & Alexander, R. (2015) Inpatient services for people with intellectual disabilities and mental health or behavioural difficulties. *British Journal of Psychiatric Advances*, **21**, 116–23, doi: 10.1192/apt.bp.113.012153.

Emerson, E., Kiernan, C., Alborz, A. et al. (2001) The prevalence of challenging behaviours: a total population study. *Research in Developmental Disabilities*, **22**(1), 77–93.

Glover, G., Brown, I. & Hatton, C. (2014) How psychiatric in-patient care for people with learning disabilities is transforming after Winterbourne View. *Tizard Learning Disability Review*, **19**(3), 146–9.

Guy, W. (ed.) (1976) *ECDEU Assessment Manual for Psychopharmacology*. US Department of Health, Education, and Welfare. Available at: www.psywellness.com.sg/docs/CGI.pdf [accessed 15 September 2018]

Hall, I., Parkes, C., Samuels, S. & Hassiotis, A. 2006. Working across boundaries: Clinical outcomes for an integrated mental health service for people with intellectual disabilities. *Journal of Intellectual Disability Research*, **50**(8), 598–607.

Hassiotis, A., Barton, P. & O'Hara, J. 2000. Mental health services for people with learning disabilities: A complete overhaul is needed with strong links to mainstream services. *British Medical Journal*, **321**(7261), 583–4.

Hemmings, C. P., O'Hara, J., McCarthy, J. et al. (2009) Comparison of adults with intellectual disabilities and mental health problems admitted to specialist and generic in-patient units. *British Journal of Intellectual Disabilities*, **37**(2); 123–8.

HSCIC (2013) Learning disabilities census report – England. Health and Social Care Information Centre, Leeds. Available at: www.hscic.gov.uk/catalogue/PUB13149 [accessed 15 September 2018]

King's Fund (2015) Mental health under pressure. Available at: www.kingsfund.org.uk/sites/files/kf/field/field_publication_file/mental-health-under-pressure-nov15_0.pdf [accessed 15 September 2018]

Longo, S. & Scior, K. (2004) Inpatient psychiatric care for individuals with intellectual disability: The service users' and carers' perspectives. *Journal of Mental Health*, **13**, 211–21.

Mansell, J. (2006) Deinstitutionalisation and community living: Progress, problems and priorities. *Journal of Intellectual & Development Disability*, **31**, 65–76.

Mental Welfare Commission for Scotland (2018) *Adults with Incapacity Act*. Available at: www.mwcscot.org.uk/the-law/adults-with-incapacity-act [accessed 28 September 2018]

Mindham, J. & Espie, C. A. (2003) Glasgow Anxiety Scale for people with an Intellectual Disability (GAS–ID): Development and psychometric properties of a new measure for use with people with mild intellectual disability. *Journal of Intellectual Disability Research*, **47**, 22–30.

Morgan, V. A., Leonard, H., Bourke, J. et al. (2008) Intellectual disability co-occurring with schizophrenia and other psychiatric illness: Population-based study. *British Journal of Psychology*, **193**, 364–72.

Murphy, E. (2014) *Statistics on People with Learning Disabilities in Northern Ireland. Northern Ireland Assembly*. Available at: www.niassembly.gov.uk/globalassets/documents/raise/publications/2014/employment_learning/5014.pdf [accessed 28 September 2018]

National Institute for Health and Care Excellence [NICE] (2015) Challenging behaviour and learning disabilities: Prevention and interventions for people with learning disabilities whose behaviour challenges. Available at: www.nice.org.uk/guidance/ng11 [accessed 15 September 2018]

National Institute for Health and Care Excellence [NICE] (2016a) Autism spectrum disorder in adults: Diagnosis and management. Available at: www.nice.org.uk/guidance/cg142 [accessed 15 September 2018]

National Institute for Health and Care Excellence [NICE] (2016b) Mental health problems in people with learning disabilities: Prevention, assessment and management. Available at: www.nice.org.uk/guidance/ng54 [accessed 15 September 2018]

National Statistics Publication for Scotland (2017) *Hospital Inpatient Care of People with Mental Health Problems in Scotland*. Available at: www.isdscotland.org/Health-Topics/Mental-Health/Publications/2017-03-14/2017-03-14-Mental-Health-Report.pdf [accessed 28 September 2018]

NHS England (2015a) *Care and Treatment Review: Policy and Guidance*. Available at: www.england.nhs.uk/wp-content/uploads/2015/10/ctr-policy-guid.pdf [accessed 15 September 2018]

NHS England (2015b) Building the right support. A national plan to develop community services and close inpatient facilities for people with a learning disability and/or autism who display behaviour that challenges, including those with a mental health condition. Available: at www.england.nhs.uk/wp-content/uploads/2015/10/ld-nat-imp-plan-oct15.pdf [accessed 15 September 2018]

NHS England (2015c) Making the Friends and Family Test inclusive. Available at: https://www.england.nhs.uk/ourwork/pe/fft/fft-inclusive [accessed 15 September 2018]

NHS England (2017) *Care and Treatment Reviews: Policy and Guidance*. Available at: www.england.nhs.uk/.../care-and-treatment-reviews-policy-and-guidance [accessed 15 September 2018].

Parkes, C., Samuels, S., Hassiotis, A. et al. (2007) Incorporating the views of service users in the development of an integrated psychiatric service for people with learning disabilities. *British Journal of Intellectual Disabilities*, **35**, 23–9.

Pearce, M. (2011) Health of the nation outcome scales in an in-patient unit. *Intellectual Disability Practice*, **14**(3), 33–8.

Perera, C., Simpson, N., Douds, F. & Campbell, M. (2009) A survey of learning disability in-patient services in Scotland in 2007. *Journal of Intellectual Disabilities*, **13**, 161–71.

Purandare, K. & Wijeratne, A. (2015) Reflections on the use of a specialist acute assessment and treatment unit for adults with intellectual disability. *Advances in Mental Health and Intellectual Disabilities*, **9**(3), 132–8.

Reid, A. H. (1994) Psychiatry and learning disability. *British Journal of Psychiatry*, **164**, 613–18.

Roy, A., Matthews, H., Clifford, P. et al. (2002) Health of the nation outcome scales for people with learning disabilities. *British Journal of Psychiatry*, **180**, 61–6.

Royal College of Psychiatrists (2012) Enabling people with mild intellectual disability and mental health problems to access healthcare services. *College Report*, CR175.

Royal College of Psychiatrists (2013) People with learning disability and mental health, behavioural or forensic problems: The role of in-patient services. FR/ID/03.

Samuels, S., Hall, I., Parkes, C. & Hassiotis, A. (2007) Professional staff and carers' views of an integrated mental health service for adults with learning disabilities. *Psychiatric Bulletin*, **31**(1), 13–16.

Sandhu, D. & Tomlins, R. (2017) Clinical needs and outcomes of adults with intellectual disabilities accessing an inpatient assessment and treatment service and the implication for development of community services. *Journal of Intellectual Disabilities*, **21**(1); 5–19.

Sheehan, R., Gandesha, A., Hassiotis A. et al. (2016) An audit of the quality of inpatient care for adults with learning disability in the UK. *BMJ Open*, **6**(4) [no pp.], art. no. 010480.

Sorgi, P., Ratey, J., Knoedler, D. W., Marker, R. J. & Reichman, M. (1991) *Journal of Neuropsychiatry and Clinical Neurosciences*, **3**(2), S52–56. Also available at https://depts.washington.edu/dbpeds/ . . . /Modified-Overt-Aggression-Scale-MOAS.pdf

Tajuddin, M., Nadkarni, S., Biswas, A. et al. (2004) A study of the use of an acute inpatient unit for adults with learning disability and mental health problems in Leicestershire, UK. *British Journal of Developmental Disabilities*, **50**, 59–68.

Taylor, J. L. (2015) Developing discharge pathways for detained patients with intellectual disabilities: Improving discharge rates and length of stay. Paper from 10th International Congress of the EAMHID, Florence, Italy. *Journal of Intellectual Disabilities Research*, **59**, 67–8.

Valuing People (2001) *A New Strategy for Learning Disability for the 21st Century*. Available at: www.gov.uk/government/publications/valuing-people-a-new-strategy-for-learning-disability-for-the-21st-century [accessed 27 September 2018]

Vos, A., Marker, N. & Bartlett, L. (2007) A survey on the learning disability service user's view of admission to an acute psychiatric ward. *British Journal of Development Disabilities*, **53**, 71–6.

Webster, A. & Banks, R. (2015) Care and treatment reviews – A national initiative for preventing unnecessary hospital admissions and facilitating discharge. *Journal of Intellectual Disability Research*, **59**, 68–9.

Xenitidis, K., Gratsa, A., Bouras, N. et al. (2004) Psychiatric inpatient care for adults with intellectual disabilities: generic or specialist units. *Journal of Intellectual Disability Research*, **48**, 11–18.

Chapter 18

Legal Provisions and Restrictive Practices

Kevin O'Shea

The essence of the care of people with intellectual disabilities (ID), either formally or informally, is that those providing care are dealing with a particularly vulnerable group. The law in all jurisdictions of the United Kingdom and in Ireland and in common law jurisdictions throughout the world focuses on the issue of consent. Although there are regional and national variations, the basic principle that any intervention, be it therapeutic or restrictive, in relation to any citizen having attained the age of majority must be with that person's valid consent, is clearly established and sustained. There is also a presumption that all persons having attained the age of majority are capable of giving valid consent unless there is credible evidence to the contrary. The issue of consent, therefore, is crucial in relation to engaging with individuals, providing support and care and also supporting those who, due to a developmental disability or intercurrent physical or mental illness, are incapable of giving valid consent.

For practitioners in the psychiatry of ID there is professional guidance available from the General Medical Council in *Good Medical Practice* (2013) and from the Royal College of Psychiatrists in *Good Psychiatric Practice* (2009). These publications provide a framework for engaging, with patients, in a therapeutic partnership to deliver care with informed decision-making and valid consent. The principles outlined in these publications provide for a code of ethics for practitioners and outline the obligations in terms of seeking consent at whatever level it may be possible and, in the alternative where valid consent is not possible, a framework for making decisions in the individual's best interests. The principles outlined in both publications are also reflected in the developing law of capacity and consent.

One of the keystones of the liberty guaranteed by domestic legislation and international conventions is that all citizens should have the right to give or withhold consent on the basis of proper information and proper support to make any treatment decision. This goes to the heart of individual autonomy and rights such as the right to privacy and bodily integrity and the right to found a family, that are enshrined in conventions such as the European Convention on Human Rights and many other international agreements. There has, however, been recognition, from earliest times in terms of the development of our legal systems, of the special status of those who cannot decide for themselves. Provisions for the protection of those whose disability means that their decision-making ability is impaired can be traced back to native Celtic laws in the Celtic regions of the United Kingdom and in Ireland and in pre-Norman laws in England. With the increasing formalisation of legal processes the development of the common law system and the codification of certain legal principles in statute law provisions have developed over the centuries to ensure that those who suffer disability and are, therefore, particularly vulnerable, should be protected from exploitation and abuse and also should be spared the full rigour of the criminal law in the event of a criminal accusation.

In the twentieth century the development of this law has moved from common law principles and the protective duties of the Crown to greater codification in statute law. The development of law in practice, particularly in the latter half of the twentieth century, has moved away from the previous paternalism in relation to those deemed to be incapable, to a system which values the inherent contributions and rights of all citizens including those with a disability. Although contained in many features of our statute law, the principal pieces of legislation which are relevant in relation to supporting those with disabilities and those who treat them, are mental health legislation, the European Convention on Human Rights, the Human Rights Act which incorporated the European Convention principles into domestic United Kingdom law, the Constitution of Ireland which again reflects the rights in the European Convention, the Equality Act in the United Kingdom, anti-discrimination legislation in other jurisdictions and legislation to deal with issues of capacity.

18.1 Mental Health Legislation

Mental health legislation in the main jurisdictions of the United Kingdom and Ireland, although differing in its technical requirements and processes, essentially provides for a system whereby people with mental disorders can receive appropriate care and treatment.[1] While this type of legislation is often seen as conferring rights and duties on statutory authorities and individual professionals in relation to such care and treatment, it is actually designed to ensure that treatment is not denied to those who lack the capacity to make a valid decision for themselves, while also protecting society from potential risks posed by those who have a qualifying disorder and require appropriate treatment. Mental health legislation usually provides a system whereby an individual may be assessed as suffering from a mental disorder, can be supported to be a full and active participant in the treatment of that disorder and where they are either incapable of being an active participant or where, having been identified as suffering from a disorder they are deemed to pose a risk to themselves or to other people, appropriate treatment can be given and risks can be safely and appropriately managed. Mental health legislation provides a system for objective assessment of an individual with a mental disorder so that any diagnosed disorder can be categorised and identified and if necessary challenged appropriately. Treatment can be given either with or without the consent of the individual involved and if the consent is either not forthcoming or cannot be given due to reasons of incapacity, then safeguards are in place to ensure that those seeking to treat make their case to a variety of independent authorities, be it a quasi-judicial authority such as a mental health tribunal or a professional second opinion such as a second opinion-approved doctor in England and Wales or other designated medical practitioners in other jurisdictions.

In the case of people with ID, while legislation recognises ID as a mental disorder for the purposes of assessment in terms of long-term management and treatment it also requires that it should be associated with behaviours which pose a risk to either the individual themselves or to other people. Prior to the enactment of legislation in relation to mental capacity and the procedures which have flowed therefrom most people with ID tended to be

---

[1] Mental Health Act 1983 – as amended (England and Wales); Mental Health (Northern Ireland) Order 1986 – as amended; Mental Health Act 2001 (Ireland); Mental Health (Care and Treatment) (Scotland) Act 2003.

treated as informal or voluntary patients where inpatient care was required; detention under the Mental Health Acts being reserved for those who were actively resisting being admitted to hospital or being otherwise supported by professional teams and those suffering from an additional diagnosed mental disorder in relation to which it was felt the individual could not give valid consent to treatment. In particular the Mental Health Acts had tended to be used in relation to patients who required a degree of restriction or deprivation of liberty such as treatment in an inpatient unit where any attempt to leave would have resulted in a form of physical restraint, either personal or environmental, or the need to use restraint in order to administer particular forms of treatment.

Mental health legislation also provides a comprehensive system of checks and balances to ensure that treatments, particularly controversial treatments such as electroconvulsive therapy (ECT), are only given with the required level of consent or the required approval by an external agency. In essence, all forms of mental health legislation are designed to ensure that people who require treatment receive the treatment that they need and to which they are appropriately entitled, that issues in relation to consent, whether by immediate consent or advanced decisions, are respected and that risks to the individual or to the public are properly managed. In order to achieve this, there is a system of specific procedures with multidisciplinary assessment in order to determine whether someone has a mental disorder, the proper development of multidisciplinary care plans which can be reviewed by tribunals or other forums in order to ensure that the right treatment is being provided, regular reviews of the patient's care by independent bodies so that the multidisciplinary team makes its case and the patients through their representatives are in a position to challenge the case if appropriate, and the guarantee that where treatment is being given against a patient's wishes that treatment is reviewed by an independent professional, with the requisite expertise, in order to give a valid second opinion.

Mental health legislation also provides an opportunity for the criminal courts to look at the cases of people with mental disorder who come before them, whether or not that disorder is a major evidential matter in the actual case, in order to ensure that persons with mental disorder can again receive appropriate treatment. This allows the courts to follow a treatment rather than a punishment path in the disposal of people convicted of offences or found to have committed acts if they are incapable of entering a plea and also imposing further restrictions for public safety if that is felt to be necessary. Independent bodies also review the institutions and the organisations which provide care for people with mental disorder and ensure that appropriate standards are maintained.

In the case of people with ID the issue of compulsory treatment under the Mental Health Acts can be a complex and difficult path to navigate. It should always be borne in mind that when relying on ID of itself for the purposes of detention or compulsion, there is a requirement for associated abnormally aggressive or seriously irresponsible conduct, in England and Wales, or its equivalent in other jurisdictions. People with ID also suffer from a significantly higher rate of other mental disorders including psychosis and affective disorder, and these disorders in their own right are qualifying disorders within the meaning of the Mental Health Acts.

Other developmental disorders are sometimes more problematic; in particular the treatment of people with attention deficit hyperactivity disorder (ADHD) and autism raises issues as to whether these are regarded as forms of persistent disability or mental disorders amenable to treatment. As of now, it is accepted that ADHD and autism do not qualify as forms of developmental disability requiring a behavioural element in order for compulsion under mental health legislation to apply, but nonetheless they are likely to be long-term developmental conditions where the treatment is principally structural and where many of the same issues in relation to nature and degree as seen in people with developmental disabilities such as global ID are particularly live issues.

All forms of mental health legislation tend to look at issues of nature and degree when determining whether or not it is acceptable to submit a patient to some form of compulsion in order to treat a condition or manage risk. The nature of the disorder being generally defined as something intrinsic to the disorder itself which poses a risk to the health and safety of the individual or to society at large; the degree being defined as the extent to which the nature of that condition presents a risk at present and whether that risk is regarded as likely or imminent. Issues of nature and degree, therefore, in a disorder such as ADHD, which can vary significantly in relation to its symptomatic presentation due to the essentially impulsive and chaotic nature of the condition, particularly in adolescents and young adults, and also issues in relation to nature and degree concerning autism, given the often very difficult issues of identifying specific or more general triggers in relation to problematic behaviour which may cause an acute exacerbation of the underlying condition, mean that unlike various forms of mental illness where the issues of nature and degree can be addressed in a relatively straightforward manner and where the potential issues in relation to degree are often more amenable to a rational and predictive scheme, in developmental disorders this can be much less certain and more dependent on individual opinion. The jurisprudence of the various tribunal mechanisms for the review of detention under various forms of mental health legislation is developing in relation to these conditions but as of now there remains considerable uncertainty as to how these disorders satisfy the criteria for detention apart from provisions such as the short-term certificate in Scotland or a section 2 detention in England and Wales to allow for a short period of assessment before moving towards a longer-term treatment order under the relevant pieces of legislation.

In summary, therefore, mental health legislation is designed to ensure that people who need treatment receive the treatment, that the treatment is provided in a safe and evidence-based manner, that the locations in which that treatment is provided whether in the community or as an inpatient meet minimum requirements, that those who can consent to their treatment are given an appropriate framework where they can be treated by valid consent and those who are unable to consent or refuse consent are only treated against their will if a compelling argument can be made under the relevant legislation as to why that should be the case.

18.2 European Convention on Human Rights

Since the end of the Second World War one of the seminal developments in terms of legislation in relation to people with disability has been the European Convention on Human Rights.[2] The Convention provides for certain enumerated rights which particularly refer to basic rights of liberty and also rights to avoid unlawful intrusion into one's private life by the state or by any other organisation. While the original statement contained in the convention has been developed with very significant jurisprudence over the decades since its original enactment, the broad principles of the Convention are usually well known, both to practitioners and to lawyers practising in the field of mental health and disability law.

---

[2] www.echr.coe.int/Documents/Convention_ENG.pdfealthHelath [accessed 18 September 2018].

In terms of the law of England and Wales one of the most significant decisions related to the so-called *Bournewood* case (2004).[3] This case involved a situation where a young man was effectively deprived of his liberty while an inpatient in a hospital for people with ID, although he was not detained under the then extant legislation, namely the Mental Health Act 1983. The finding of the courts, ultimately, was that his detention was unlawful and there needed to be a process whereby if a deprivation of liberty was required, authorised or facilitated by a government or statutory authority, then such deprivation of liberty must be subject to an appropriate process and there must be a system of review as to guarantee the individual a right of appeal. This case led ultimately to the development of the deprivation of liberty safeguards procedures under the Mental Capacity Act, which is dealt with further in section 18.4 below on capacity legislation.

While the European Convention and its associated Court, the European Court of Human Rights at Strasbourg, has delivered a considerable body of jurisprudence over the years in relation to many aspects of mental health law, from the point of view of people with ID the key issue has been that the treatment and support of people with ID where it involves a restriction or deprivation of liberty or where any form of treatment or care is provided without valid consent must be subject to some form of review and a framework which allows for any such deprivation or restriction of liberty to be challenged. The European Court of Human Rights also identified that member states should provide a statutory scheme to deal with such issues and such a statutory scheme is provided in both the capacity legislation of England and Wales and Scotland which, while differing to a degree in terms of their technical provisions and procedure nonetheless have a commonality in terms of beginning from the standpoint of a presumption of capacity, only regarding somebody as lacking capacity when that lack of capacity has been assessed according to a formal and independent process, providing for a decision-making process in relation to treatment or restrictions on liberty and providing a system for appropriate appeal and review of any such restriction.

The Human Rights Act 1998 is an act of the UK Parliament which has incorporated the provisions of the European Convention on Human Rights into domestic British law. While this is often quoted as a significant development of human rights law, in essence, it is more to do with the enforceability of the provisions of the European Convention in domestic law and how that is handled in the courts of the United Kingdom rather than a significant change or enhancement of rights. In Ireland the European Convention also applies, but the jurisprudence in relation to this area of human rights has largely been the development of the enumerated and unenumerated rights in the Constitution of Ireland 1937.

18.3 Equality Legislation

When dealing with issues in relation to the care and treatment of people with ID an area of legislation which is often overlooked is that of equality legislation. Again there is some variation in several jurisdictions in relation to this; however, there are single acts such as the Equality Act in the United Kingdom or a combination of acts in relation to non-discrimination in other jurisdictions which identify that people should not suffer discrimination due to disability and in particular that they should not be denied opportunities or services due to lack of reasonable adjustment. While this is not generally regarded as a major issue in terms of the medical treatment of people with ID in fact there is an emerging corpus

---

[3] *HL v. UK* 45508/99 [2004] ECHR 471.

of jurisprudence in relation to equality issues when it comes to treatment and support. All equality legislation essentially identifies that every citizen should be treated equally and that, at very least, all individuals providing services and support should ensure the widest range of access to such services by means of reasonable adjustment. It can be argued that progress towards mainstreaming many aspects of mental health and behavioural care for people with ID has been significantly impeded by lack of reasonable adjustment. There is a growing demand for access to all forms of mental healthcare for people with developmental disorders. Access to such care is often provided only through specific ID services which are not resourced to provide the fullest range of available treatments. A good current example is dialectic behaviour therapy. This is a readily available therapy in adult mental health services throughout most of the United Kingdom and Ireland. However, its availability to people with developmental disabilities is restricted due to the fact that adult mental health services, which tend to provide this service, lack the ability and expertise to extend this provision to people with developmental disability. This is potentially a cause of action under equality legislation insofar as it could be regarded as a form of discrimination due to lack of reasonable adjustment. Similarly, the availability of cognitive and psychological therapies to people with autism can be restricted by the lack of necessary expertise in order to deliver such treatments to people who appear to lack the 'psychological mindedness' which is often a prerequisite for engaging in such treatment. It is becoming apparent that the issue in providing many forms of therapy for people with autism is reasonable adjustment. This is likely to be an area of law which will develop in litigation over the next several years.

18.4 Capacity Legislation

One of the most significant issues in the last twenty years has been the development of capacity legislation in relation to the support of people with ID who lack the capacity to manage their own affairs. Again, while there are variations in the process and detail of legislation in various jurisdictions what is common to all such legal schemes is that they are derived from the gradual development of common law and established precedent. Common to all capacity legislation is the presumption of capacity whereby every individual having reached the age of majority, or in some cases having not yet reached the age of majority but living independently, are regarded as having capacity to make decisions in relation to their own affairs. It is only acceptable for others to interfere and take control of an individual's decision-making where there has been a clear test for capacity and the individual has been objectively found to lack capacity in accordance with an accepted statutory scheme. While this is regarded as a new development with the enactment of the capacity acts in the United Kingdom in particular, this has in fact been the case for many decades since specific legal tests were laid down in the courts.[4] The test for lack of capacity is generally an assessment as to whether the person suffers from a mental disorder, whether that mental disorder is of such a nature and degree as to impair a person's ability to receive and retain information, to weigh the information in the balance, to make a decision and to communicate that decision. Crucially all capacity legislation insists that such tests for capacity must be in relation to specific decisions which require to be made by the individual. There is no provision for

---

[4] *Sidaway* v. *Board of Governors of the Bethlem Royal Hospital and the Maudsley Hospital and Others* [1985] 1 AC 871; *Re T* [1992] 3 WLR 782.

a general presumption of incapacity based on any specific test. In relation to each decision under consideration and each course of action which is being considered the issue of capacity must be tested in relation to that specific issue. What is often most difficult in the area of care for people with ID is that statutory frameworks clearly state that if an individual makes decisions which are objectively regarded as unwise this is not of itself grounds for stating the person lacks capacity. It is also clear that the process for assessing capacity must not be retrospective in relation to an unwise decision, rather that the assessment of capacity must be prospective and objective requiring a clear assessment of the existence and extent of any mental disorder, the effect of that disorder on decision-making capacity and the consideration of any factors which may improve the individual's ability to make decisions in their own right. All legislative frameworks provide a clear duty of inclusion, facilitation and empowerment in relation to individuals, both in relation to enhancing capacity and even if the individual is determined to lack capacity and, therefore, decisions are being taken by others, to ensure that they can be as involved as possible in the process and are able to take subsidiary decisions which arise according to their assessed level of capacity.

The frameworks impose a duty of openness and a duty to provide rationale in relation to decision-making. While capacity legislation for administrative reasons and for the facility of effective decision-making in individual cases provides for local decision-making on a number of issues the principles are the same as those required previously for declaratory relief in the higher courts:

(1) Over time the codified law in relation to capacity has essentially reflected the essential precepts of good clinical practice insofar as in dealing with people whose capacity is in question it is important that all support is offered to the individual to enhance their ability to understand the issues and to make decisions where possible.

(2) Where a decision cannot be taken by the individual due to lack of capacity that the decision in their best interests is clearly and openly taken and that decision is amenable to review, either by local procedure or in the courts.

(3) That the care plan which seeks to be implemented in relation to somebody who lacks capacity is based on evidence and has clarity of purpose and is designed in such a way as to ensure that it can be reviewed at appropriate intervals in order to ensure that the course of action is still necessary.

(4) Where issues such as deprivation of liberty are involved in any care plan that an appropriate process is followed whether by a local decision-making process or through the courts and that the justification for that deprivation of liberty is clearly established and is amenable to appropriate review at intervals which are determined either by legislation or by the court making the decision.

There is increasing jurisprudence to suggest that the Mental Capacity Act offers a better system for making treatment decisions in relation to mental disorder for people with ID than the Mental Health Act; this remains a controversial area of practice and law and at present it is still regarded as appropriate that where there is a clearly identified mental disorder, that mental disorder requires treatment and the individual either is unwilling or unable to stay in hospital or unwilling or unable to consent to treatment then the provisions of the Mental Health Act are probably most appropriate. However, provisions for deprivation of liberty and for treatment of persons who lack capacity are also contained within the provisions of the Mental Capacity Act and it is now regarded as good practice that when a decision for detention under mental health legislation is being made then consideration as to whether this particular treatment plan can be carried out under mental capacity legislation should also be considered.

In relation to the law of England and Wales it is particularly important to remember that when deprivation of liberty under the Mental Capacity Act is being considered as an alternative to detention in hospital under the Mental Health Act, deprivation of liberty under the Mental Capacity Act is for the protection of the individual and not for the protection of others.

18.5 Therapeutic Restriction

In relation to people with ID, particularly those who come to the attention of services due to behavioural reasons, treatment plans often involve a restriction on liberty and a degree of control. Sometimes this is very clear and can be objectively identified but quite often it is a more subtle approach to somebody with ID whereby the extent to which the individual is truly a free agent with the liberties enjoyed by most other members of society is often severely limited.

People with ID often have limited control over their place of residence, those with whom they interact, the type of activities in which they engage in terms of day activities or employment and also have limited control over finances and very limited financial independence. While in most cases this is due to the need to provide appropriate care and support to safeguard the individual in relation to their own needs and also to avoid exploitation and abuse, nonetheless restrictions on liberty are often part and parcel of the day-to-day life of people with ID. Although it is relatively rare for such restrictions to be formalised through the appropriate legislative framework, the life of a person with ID is often characterised by the exertion of control by other people whether members of their family or members of statutory agencies, deprivation of certain rights in relation to self-determination, a degree of isolation from the world at large and a degree of restriction in terms of the social circle in which they can engage. Concern expressed by others in relation to relationships, particularly intimate relationships, due to fear of exploitation or abuse and often for the best possible reasons mean that the individual's decision-making power may be significantly curtailed. In some cases the degree of ID will render this entirely appropriate and necessary. However, it is also the case that many people with ID find themselves in a position where an assessment of their overall need is made relatively early in their lifetime, particularly as they turn from children's to adults' services and the extent of the intrusion into their lives remains the same without significant review over a protracted period and, therefore, it can be that the protective measures in place for the individual actually perpetuate a form of dependency which may mean that any progress the individual makes may not be fully taken into account in future planning.

Where significant behavioural problems emerge spontaneously or due to intercurrent mental health or neurological disturbance it is often necessary to look at forms of control, both formal and informal, in order to manage an individual either in the community or in some form of residential care, be it social care or hospital care. The prescription of medication to reduce anxiety or to treat depression may be necessary and appropriate. It should always be recognised that some restrictions on a person's liberty may be part of a best interest process, may be necessary to preserve life and limb and may be part of a process to safeguard the interests of the individual. Often restrictions are part of a process to prevent potential abuse but such restrictions do require justification, even if not part of a formal process. Practitioners in ID psychiatry should be aware of these issues and should, if appropriate, invoke formal procedures where it is felt that a person is living a very restricted lifestyle, whether as an inpatient or as an outpatient, to ensure that there is adequate oversight in relation to the necessity of the restrictions and the care plan over time. It is crucially important also that in relation to justifying restriction on the basis of the individual's behaviour, care is taken that an individual with ID is not actually being held to a higher standard in relation to appropriate and wise behaviour than the general population. The freedom to exercise our basic human rights includes the freedom to make unwise decisions. While there is an understandable impulse on the part of professionals involved in the care of people with disability to protect individuals from the consequences of their own actions and the potentially malicious intent of others, an essential part of our basic human freedom is the freedom to make mistakes. Recent jurisprudence before the United Kingdom Supreme Court (March 2014)[5] has led to the reopening of a discussion as to what amounts to deprivation of liberty in relation to people who either lack capacity or may have variable capacity. This is likely to be a major factor in development of the jurisprudence of the United Kingdom over the next decade or so and is also likely to influence issues in relation to capacity and deprivation of liberty in other common law jurisdictions.

References and Suggested Reading

General Medical Council (2013) *Good Medical Practice*. Available at: www.gmc-uk.org/-/medi a/documents/Good_medical_practice___Englis h_1215.pdf_51527435.pdf [accessed 19 September 2018]

Barber, P., Brown, R. & Martin, D. (2016) *Mental Health Law in England & Wales*. Learning Matters.

British Medical Association and the Law Society (2009) *Assessment of Mental Capacity*.

Brown, R. (2016) *The Approved Mental Health Professional's Guide to Mental Health Law*. Sage.

Jones, R. (2017) *The Mental Health Act Manual* (20th edn). Sweet & Maxwell.

Royal College of Psychiatrists (2009) *Good Psychiatric Practice – CR154* (3rd edn). Available at: www.rcpsych.ac.uk/publications/collegere ports/cr/cr154.aspx [accessed 19 September 2018]

Royal College of Psychiatrists (2013) *CR180. Vulnerable Patients, Safe Doctors: Good Practice in Our Clinical Relationships* (2nd edn). Available at: www.rcpsych.ac.uk/usefulresour ces/publications/collegereports/cr/cr180.aspx [accessed 19 September 2018]

Websites

Codes of practice in relation to mental health and mental capacity legislation available from the relevant government websites:

www.gov.scot
www.gov.uk
www.northernireland.gov.uk
www.gov.wales
www.gov.ie

---

[5] Cheshire West and Chester Council v. P. (2014) UKSC 19 (2014) MHLO 16.

Chapter 19

Leadership and Management

Paul Winterbottom

19.1 Introduction

This chapter aims to provide a brief overview of the nature and application of management and leadership in the NHS in relation to practice in the field of intellectual disability psychiatry.

Leadership and management responsibilities have been integral to the practice of psychiatry in mental health and intellectual disability (ID) fields both prior and subsequent to the creation of the NHS. The Royal College of Psychiatrists recognises the relationship through the inclusion of leadership and management as key areas for development in both core and specialist curricula (Royal College of Psychiatrists, 2010a, 2010b).

During 2016–17 there was growing evidence of the challenge posed to the NHS and social care in the UK through a combination of the impacts of a growing and ageing population, increasing demand and expectation alongside workforce shortages and austerity impacting upon resource availability. These factors combine with a planned programme of significant service redesign and focus on the delivery of services in communities and homes while maximising opportunities for personalisation, health promotion and disease prevention. Transformation in the design and delivery of service requires effective leadership and management if it is to be a success (King's Fund, 2011).

19.2 Background

Thirty years passed between the publication of *Better Services for the Mentally Handicapped* (Department of Health, 1971) and *Valuing People* (2001) then shortly followed by *Valuing People Now* (Department of Health, 2009) and *Fulfilling Potential – Making It Happen* (Department of Work and Pensions, 2013). There have been similar strategies progressed in each of the administrative areas of the UK. The *All Wales Strategy for the Development of Services for Mentally Handicapped People* appeared first (1983) followed by *Fulfilling the Promises* (Welsh Assembly Government, 2001), Statement on Policy and Practice for Adults with a Learning Disability (Welsh Assembly Government, 2007) and the Social Services and Well-being (Wales) Act 2014.

In Northern Ireland, the Bamford Review (2002) and a continuing process to the Bamford Action Plan 2012–15 (Department of Health for Northern Ireland, 2012).

For Scotland there have been *The Same As You?* (Scottish Executive, 2000), *Keys to Life – Improving Quality of Life for People with Learning Disabilities* (Scottish Executive, 2013) and *Fairer Scotland for Disabled People* (Scottish Executive, 2016).

These are merely a selection of the ongoing initiatives which require leader and manager engagement.

According to *Fulfilling the Promises* (Welsh Assembly Government, 2001: 6) the aim of the *All Wales Strategy* was to 'enable people with learning disabilities to enjoy the full range of life opportunities and choices, to have positive identities and roles in their families and communities, to exercise choice and to develop independence, self-respect and self-fulfilment'.

Subsequent initiatives have aimed to address, despite differences in language, the same issues, how people with ID can be supported to live ordinary lives, access education and employment opportunities, reside in their own homes and have equal access to healthcare with similar outcomes to the general population, all the while experiencing equality of esteem, opportunity and access in life as a lead partner in the design and development of services. The importance of personalisation and co-production by people with ID and their representatives requires clinicians to embrace and apply new knowledge, skills and behaviours (attitudes) while employing a range of leadership styles. The demands for rapid reconfiguration and reform require an appreciation of and ability to apply the principles and practices of leadership and management in partnership, to deliver change consensually in an increasingly complex organisational environment.

Organisational structures delivering health, social care and education in the UK have changed significantly and become increasingly diverse. There are more differing and competing organisational forms inputting to the commissioning and provision of services designed and delivered to meet varied and sometimes competing social, professional, political, financial, legal, national, international and local standards. These include NHS Trusts, clinical commissioning groups, NHS England, Wales, Scotland and Northern Ireland, councils, regulators/professional bodies (Care Quality Commission, National Institute for Health and Care Excellence, General Medical Council, Professional Standards Authority for Health and Social Care, Health Education England, Royal Colleges), social enterprise organisations, charities, independent and private (for profit) health and social care providers, organisations and individuals representing service users.

It is essential that medical practitioners including psychiatrists working within the health and social care system appreciate their context and are aware of, accept and train to deliver as:

- clinicians, managers, leaders and advocates;
- communicators with skills to influence and educate;
- strategists and politicians in delivering change;
- systemic thinkers aware of the context in which they work at clinical, professional, multidisciplinary team, organisational, local health and social care, regional and national levels.

Richard Bach (1977) made an observation regarding the relationship between learning, doing and teaching which can be easily adapted to describe the interaction between clinical practice, management and leadership:

> Learning is finding out what you already know. Doing is demonstrating that you know it. Teaching is reminding others that they know just as well as you. You are all learners, doers, teachers. Richard Bach: *Illusions* (p. 46, in 1998 reprint)

This can be reinterpreted for clinical leadership and management purposes as follows:

> Clinical practice is the application of knowledge, skills and behaviours in common cause with an individual (patient) or population to address a health need.

Management is the process of controlling the resources to enable effective clinical practice with regard to a common cause.
Leadership is the means through which a group of people (organisation) is enabled to focus upon common cause and effect change.
You are all clinicians, managers, leaders. Paul Winterbottom (2019) Seminars in Intellectual Disability.

19.3 Context

The delivery of effective healthcare to people with ID and the leadership and management skills required are no different to that of a service supporting the general population; the same principles apply. The challenges lie in developing the partnerships that permit the *identification, design* and *delivery* of the reasonable adjustments that are required in order that the outcomes of the healthcare and social care interventions are equivalent to that experienced by the general population. If this is to be effective this requires skills in *communicating* and *influencing* in order that the need and resource implications, where relevant, are *recognised* and *prioritised*. These can vary in scope from awareness on the part of the practitioner of an individual's needs and this being sufficient, to the design and delivery of a parallel or separate specialist service with bespoke training and qualification.

As an example of context, currently services to people with ID remain in a public and political spotlight following reports regarding care provided at Winterbourne View and the independent review of deaths of people with a learning disability or mental health problem in contact with Southern Health NHSFT. The *Time for Change* report (Department of Health, 2014), *Transforming Care* (Department of Health, 2012) and the Better Care Fund are aimed at supporting the closure of hospital beds and preventing delayed discharge for people with ID who remain in hospitals.[1] In addition, there are still concerns about the premature deaths of people with ID as identified in the *Confidential Inquiry into Premature Deaths of People with Learning Disabilities (CIPOLD)* (Department of Health, 2013) and the contribution that unequal access to health, social and employment opportunities might make.

The NHS England business plan for 2016–17 identified the following key aims:

- improving health – closing the health and well-being gap;
- transforming care – closing the care and quality gap; and
- controlling costs and enabling change – closing the finance and efficiency gap.

And within them ten priority areas for action that include:

- upgrading the quality of care and access to mental health and dementia services;
- transforming care for people with learning disabilities;
- redesigning urgent and emergency care services;
- ensuring high quality and affordable specialised care; and
- new models of care to include, personalisation and choice, and integrated health and care.

---

[1] The Better Care Fund is a £3.8 billion budget, pooling health and social care funding, to support transformation and integration of health and social care services. More detail can be found at www.england.nhs.uk/ourwork/part-rel/ transformation-fund/bcf-plan [accessed 27 September 2018].

NHS Wales has developed a similar planning framework supporting the development of local health boards' and trusts' integrated plans up to 2016–17 that address similar issues through the collaboration of health boards and trusts.

Similarly NHS Scotland through NHS boards in conjunction with health and social care partnerships is developing local delivery plans that focus on quality, safety, integration, prevention, self-management, reduced hospital use and community support.

Northern Ireland is undertaking a similar task through Developing Better Health Services to support a modernisation plan for hospital and community and specialist services in conjunction with Transforming Your Care (2011), the Bamford Review and Action Plan (2012–15) (Department of Health for Northern Ireland, 2012) and the *Donaldson Report* (Department of Health for Northern Ireland, 2014).

In order to be effective as a clinical leader it is essential to have a clear understanding of the context in which you are working and how national, regional, local, political, financial and personal factors impact upon your opportunities to negotiate development.

19.4 Leadership and Management for Medical Practitioners

While not all doctors have formal management responsibilities associated with clinical management or the provision of training and education there are leadership responsibilities associated with the vast majority of job descriptions and job plans. It is perhaps helpful to consider leadership and management roles as a clinician in terms of:

- clinical (relating to the provision of safe and effective clinical care);
- clinical/multidisciplinary teams (relating to team processes and practice and the contribution of the doctor to the system);
- professional (contribution to Royal Colleges, BMA, etc.);
- educational (training and research);
- organisational (committee, service improvement, quality and development initiatives); and
- regional and national roles including policy and practice development.

Where job plans include specific managerial roles such as director of medical education, clinical director and medical director the responsibilities and scope of the role should be clearly identified within the job description and allocated time in the job plan. Any person undertaking these roles must ensure that they are in line with the practice of effective governance and that these responsibilities are addressed in appraisal, shared with the General Medical Council, their defence organisation and covered within their continuing professional development plans. There are of course a wide range of other leadership roles including responsible officer, Caldicott guardian, director of operations, chief executive or regional and professional organisational responsibilities that doctors undertake.

The General Medical Council has published a document entitled *Leadership and Management for all Doctors* (2012), which sets out the responsibilities of all doctors in this regard. In particular emphasising:

- responsibilities relating to employment issues;
- teaching and training;
- planning, using and managing resources;
- raising and acting on concerns; and
- helping to develop and improve services.

This document very helpfully identifies the additional responsibilities accruing to doctors with a leadership role in ensuring that there are systems and processes in place to support colleagues and provide assurance regarding the safety and quality of both the clinical services and the governance processes supporting them. All doctors should ensure that they are familiar with the instruction and advice provided and that they have taken this into account in their daily work as well as the assurance processes they use to demonstrate their adherence to good practice (personal development plan, continuing medical education, appraisal, supervision, mentoring and peer groups).

The following are examples of the expectations in the workplace:

- Engage with colleagues (includes non-medical and managerial colleagues) to maintain and improve the safety and quality of patient care.
- Contribute to discussions and decisions about improving the quality of services and outcomes.
- Raise and act on concerns about patient safety.
- Demonstrate effective team working and leadership.
- Promote a working environment free from unfair discrimination, bullying and harassment, bearing in mind that colleagues and patients come from diverse backgrounds.
- Contribute to teaching and training doctors and other healthcare professionals, including by acting as a positive role model.
- Use resources efficiently for the benefit of patients and the public.

Similarly the Royal College of Psychiatrists (2010a, 2010b) details within the core and specialist training curricula a series of areas for development identified under the headings knowledge, skills and attitudes demonstrated through behaviours, learning outcomes that describe leadership and management skills to be achieved in the course of training. These include understanding leadership styles, the role of the leader, the structure of NHS/social care organisation, the principles of change management and effective use of resource.

While the detailed content of both of the above documents will be subject to development the principle that these responsibilities are core to the doctors' role is unlikely to change.

19.5 Leadership and Management Resources

An exhaustive review of the various models developed to describe leadership and management styles and approaches cannot be delivered within this chapter. This section will focus upon the current approaches to leadership development within the NHS and provide some references for further reading and research.

Management may be considered the application of processes that are concerned with planning, budgeting, organising, staffing, controlling and problem-solving while leadership uses processes that involve establishing direction, aligning people, motivating and inspiring (Kotter, 1996).

The NHS Leadership Academy (2013a) has recognised the need for a shared approach to the description and development of leadership and management competencies which draws upon the meta-analysis of experience and research internationally both within healthcare and outside. This is intended to provide a national tiered approach and a common language to describe competencies and outcomes that support staff to engage in the development and assessment of skills. This approach acknowledges the difficulties that have been created by the simultaneous application of command and control, top-down (heroic) leadership models and contrasting distributed (shared) leadership models and the effect this can have on culture engagement and responsiveness. This work recognises the transactional (responsive, present orientated, working within the culture) and transformational (proactive, future orientated, developmental and creative) approaches.

The leadership model identifies three overarching elements:

- provision of and justification of a clear sense of purpose and contribution;
- motivation of individuals and teams to work effectively; and
- focus on improving performance.

This research has been developed to provide a model of healthcare leadership described through nine dimensions. Each of these is then further defined through observable leadership behaviours on a four-point scale from essential, through proficient, then strong to exemplary. These enable practitioners to assess themselves and through reflection identify how they can develop their practice.

NHS Leadership Academy (2013b) Model 9 Dimensions:

- inspiring shared purpose;
- leading with care;
- evaluating information;
- connecting our service;
- sharing the vision;
- engaging the team;
- holding to account;
- developing capability; and
- influencing for results.

19.6 Summary

I have attempted to provide a practical insight into the challenges and opportunities that present themselves to colleagues working in the field of ID when considering leadership and management roles. I have referenced the standards doctors are expected to uphold in relation to the General Medical Council and Royal College of Psychiatrists. I have briefly shared the context and current thinking about the application of research to leadership development in the NHS but with application across health and social care communities. For those who wish for further information the bibliography includes a number of recent helpful texts.

The Faculty of Medical Leadership and Management established in 2011 is a body supported by all UK medical royal colleges and faculties with the aim of providing a professional home for medical leadership at all stages of a medical career. For those contemplating further the opportunities for development of their knowledge and skills in leadership and management it is well worth considering the resources that they have developed.

My parting offering is a checklist (Box 19.1) and acronym (Box 19.2) to assist in future practical exploration of this subject which may be of use in analysing a leadership opportunity and considering the forces at work.

> **Box 19.1 Checklist**
>
> (1) **Role** What is my job description? What roles and responsibilities for leadership and management are identified within it? Are there identified resources associated with these roles and responsibilities?
> (2) **Resource** Do I have the knowledge, skills and behavioural (attitudes) qualities required and/or an approach to acquiring, developing and maintaining them such as continuing medical education, continuing professional development, job planning, appraisal, supervision and mentoring?
> (3) **Situation** Do I understand the organisational context in which I am working and providing a service? Who are the commissioners, stakeholders, competitors, partners, colleagues and regulators? What are their values and vision?
> (4) **Partners** Do my and partner organisations' priorities relate to this area. Are they aligned?
> (5) **Politics** Is the MP and/or councillor interested or is there a party political/policy position?
> (6) **Strategy** What is the NHS or social care, local, regional and national strategy in relation to this area?
> (7) **Evidence** What is the evidence base to support practice and development in this area?
> (8) **Indicators** Are there organisational, local, regional or national key performance indicators that are relevant to this service?
> (9) **Monies** What is the funding is it sufficient and secure?
> (10) **Employees** What is the human resource associated with this service? Are there any resourcing issues affecting developing or sustaining training and education?

> **Box 19.2**
>
> The checklist with a little creativity and imagination can be rearranged as follows for those who enjoy an acronym:
> - evidence
> - monies
> - partners & politics
> - indicators
> - role & resource
> - employees
> - strategy & situation
>
> While the creation of an empire is not perhaps the most appropriate use of leadership and management skills in the NHS it can provide a memorable template for doctors undertaking an analysis of an opportunity and the context.

References

Bach, R. (1977) *Illusions: The Adventures of a Reluctant Messiah*. Dell. [reprinted 1998]

Burnes, B. (2004) Kurt Lewin and the planned approach to change: A reappraisal. *Journal of Management Studies*, **41**(6), 977–1002.

Department of Health (1971) *Better Services for the Mentally Handicapped*. HMSO.

Department of Health (2009) *Valuing People Now: A New Three Year Strategy for People with Learning Disabilities*. Available at: http://webarchive.nationalarchives.gov.uk/20130105064234/http:/www.dh.gov.uk/prod_consum_dh/groups/dh_digitalassets/documents/digitalasset/dh_093375.pdf [accessed 19 September 2018].

Department of Health (2012) *Transforming Care: A National Response to Winterbourne View Hospital. Department of Health Review: Final Report*. Available at: www.gov.uk/government/uploads/system/uploads/attachment_data/file/213215/final-report.pdf [accessed 19 September 2018].

Department of Health (2013) *Confidential Inquiry into the Premature Deaths of People with Learning Disabilities (CIPOLD)*. University of Bristol.

Department of Health (2014) *Winterbourne View: Time for Change. Transforming the Commissioning for Services for People with Learning Disabilities and/or Autism*. Report by the Transforming Care and Commissioning Steering Group, chaired by Sir Stephen Bubb.

Department of Health for Northern Ireland (2012) *Bamford Action Plan 2012–15*.

Department of Health for Northern Ireland (2014) *The Right Time – the Right Place* [Donaldson Report]. Available at: www.health-ni.gov.uk/topics/health-policy/donaldson-report [accessed 19 September 2018].

Department of Work and Pensions (2013) *Fulfilling Potential – Making It Happen*. Available at: https://assets.publishing.service.gov.uk/government/uploads/system/uploads/attachment_data/file/320745/making-it-happen.pdf [accessed 19 September 2018].

Garelick, A. & Fagin, L. (2005) The doctor–manager relationship. *Advances in Psychiatric Treatment*, **11**, 241–52.

General Medical Council (2012) *Leadership and Management for All Doctors*. Available at: www.gmc-uk.org/guidance [accessed 19 September 2018].

King's Fund (2011) *The Future of Leadership and Management in the NHS: No More Heroes*.

King's Fund (2015) The practice of system leadership: Being comfortable with chaos.

Kotter, J. P. (1996) *Leading Change*. Harvard Business.

Massie, S. (2015) *Talent Management: Developing Leadership Not Just Leaders*. King's Fund.

NHS Improvement and Leadership Development Board (2016) *Developing People – Improving Care: A National Framework for Action on Improvement and Leadership Development in NHS-Funded Services*.

NHS Leadership Academy (2013a) *NHS Leadership Academy Healthcare Leadership Model: The Nine Dimensions of Leadership Behaviour*.

NHS Leadership Academy (2013b) *Towards a New Model of Leadership for the NHS*. Available at: www.leadershipacademy.nhs.uk [accessed 17 September 2018].

Royal College of Psychiatrists (2010a) *Core Training in Psychiatry Curriculum*. Available at: www.rcpsych.ac.uk/pdf/CORE_CURRICULUM_2010_Mar_2012_update.pdf [accessed 19 September 2018].

Royal College of Psychiatrists (2010b) *Specialists in the Psychiatry of Learning Disability Curriculum* (rev. May 2017).

Scottish Executive (2000) *The Same as You? A Review of Services for People with Learning Disabilities*. Available at: www.scotland.gov.uk/Resource/Doc/1095/0001661.pdf [accessed 28 September 2018].

Scottish Executive (2013) *The Keys to Life – Improving Quality of Life for People with Learning Disabilities*. Available at: www.gov.scot/Publications/2013/06/6964/1 [accessed 28 September 2018].

Scottish Government (2013) *The Keys to Life*.

Scottish Government (2016) *A Fairer Scotland for Disabled People*. Available at: www.gov.scot/Publications/2016/12/3778 [accessed 19 September 2018].

Valuing People (2001) *A New Strategy for Learning Disability for the 21st Century*. Ref Cm 5086. Available at: www.gov.uk/government/publications/valuing-people-a-new-strategy-for-learning-disability-for-the-21st-century [accessed 19 September 2018].

Welsh Assembly Government (2001) *Fulfilling the Promises – Proposals for a Framework for Services for People with Learning Disabilities*.

Welsh Assembly Government (2007) *Statement on Policy and Practice for Adults with a Learning Disability*.

Welsh Office (1983) *All Wales Strategy for the Development of Services for Mentally Handicapped People*.

Recommended Reading

Bach, R. (1983) *Illusions: The Adventures of a Reluctant Messiah*. Dell.

Bowman, W. E. (1956) *The Ascent of Rum Doodle*. Pimlico.

Faculty of Medical Leadership and Management: website: fmlm.ac.uk

Gopee, N. & Galloway, J. (2014) *Leadership and Management in Healthcare* (2nd edn). Sage.

Royal College of Psychiatrists (2016) *Management for Psychiatrists* (4th edn).

Walshe, K. & Smith, J. (2011) *Healthcare Management* (2nd edn). Open University.

Chapter 20

Clinical Research in Intellectual Disabilities
Ethical and Methodological Challenges

Niall O'Kane, Sujata Soni and Angela Hassiotis

We all need to have a strong belief in our field of study, a willingness in our research to embrace new investigative and analytical techniques through interdisciplinary collaborations and a commitment to high scientific and ethical standards
Professor Tony Holland (2009)

20.1 Introduction

High-quality clinical research forms one of the core tenets of evidence-based practice (Guyatt, 1992). Research leads to improvements in health treatments, patient outcomes as well as development of innovative and efficient services (National Institute for Health Research, 2016). Importantly, research provides us with the necessary evidence for whether existing interventions work or not in the way we think they should. Within the field of intellectual disability (ID), the scope in clinical research is vast, and spans across health and social care settings. Despite the large scope, clinical research is all too often neglected in this field (Robotham, 2011). One particular area, which has suffered, is that of conducting clinical trials.

Furthermore, the lack of robust clinical research exacerbates inequalities in healthcare that are already known to exist for people with ID as highlighted in reports by MENCAP (2007) and the Confidential Inquiry into Premature Deaths of People with Learning Disabilities (Heslop et al., 2013). Without properly evaluated interventions, it is less likely that we will succeed in reducing morbidity and achieving the much-needed parity in care for people with ID.

As a group of clinicians with varying levels of involvement in research, the chapter provides an opportunity to explore the development of research in the field of ID but also to compile practical advice on ethical issues and legal frameworks that can be used to promote the involvement of people with ID in research. We will describe recruitment barriers and other challenges in conducting research in this field and how such challenges may be overcome, including the examination of the role of active public engagement. Finally, we will comment on future directions of research in the field of ID.

20.2 Historical Overview of Ethics in Research

It is widely accepted that there are several guiding ethical principles relevant to the ethics of research involving human subjects: the principles of respect of persons, non-maleficence, beneficence and justice (the *Belmont Report*, 1979). While these principles continue to guide research practice, historically, they were often ignored or seriously breached. During the Second World War, individuals with ID were among the victims held in concentration camps subjected to harrowing, unlawful medical experimentation. The Nuremberg Trials of 1947 exposed the unlawful experimentation and led to the development of the first international code of ethics in medical research: the Nuremberg Code. The Nuremberg Code consists of ten principles, including informed consent and absence of coercion; properly formulated scientific experimentation; and research that benefits the participants.

Following this, the World Medical Association (WMA) issued the Declaration of Geneva in 1948, to serve as a modernised Hippocratic oath for all medical professionals. The WMA subsequently produced the Declaration of Helsinki in 1964 to reflect the principles of the Nuremberg Code with some amendments. The main change related to informed consent. Under the Nuremberg Code, this was defined as 'absolutely necessary' but subsequently changed to 'if at all possible' under the Declaration of Helsinki. This amendment allowed for provision of a legal guardian to act as 'consent by proxy'. The declaration additionally stipulated that research is only justified in a vulnerable group if relevant and responsive to their needs, and it is not possible for the research to be completed in non-vulnerable groups. The declaration also stated that this group of individuals should stand to benefit from the knowledge, practices or interventions that result from the research.

20.3 The Modernisation of Ethical Codes of Conduct Governing Medical Experimentation

Notwithstanding the advances in ethical codes of conduct following the Second World War, exploitative practice in research continued especially with medical experimentation. An example of this included the Willowbrook State School experiments in the USA (1955–70), when thousands of children with ID were deliberately infected with hepatitis as a means of finding treatment and prophylactic agents (Rothman & Rothman, 1984). The subsequent inquiry described how 'consent by proxy' was obtained from parents of the children but done so retrospectively, and families were not clearly informed of the experiments taking place.

As a consequence of this and several other controversial studies in the USA, the National Commission for the Protection of Human Subjects of Biomedical and Behavior Research was developed. This gave rise to the *Ethical Principles and Guidelines for the Protection of Human Subjects of Research: The Belmont Report* (1979). Similarly, in the UK, following several medical tragedies including the thalidomide birth-related defects (1960s), the legal requirement for an independent evaluation of medicinal products before marketing was enacted (McCully, 2011). Worldwide harmonisation of practical and ethical standards for the conduct of clinical trials only became established in 1996, under what is known as the International Conference on Harmonisation (ICH) of Technical Requirements for Registration of Pharmaceuticals for Human Use. In 1998, the Medical Research Council (MRC) updated their guidance in line with these standards.

While there were international requirements for clinical trials, there was no harmonised legislation within the European Union (EU) until 2004, when the Medicines for Human Use (Clinical Trials) Regulations were implemented into UK law. Oversight and conduct of clinical research were laid down within this EU directive; the Medicines and Healthcare Products Regulatory Agency (MHRA) was designated as the UK competent authority, responsible for overseeing development of new medicines under this directive. The directive formally defined that 'any study examining the safety or efficacy of a medicine, foodstuff or placebo in humans' is referred to as a 'Clinical Trial of an Investigational Medicinal Product' otherwise known as a CTIMP. The MHRA became responsible for ensuring that medicines and medical devices work, and are acceptably safe. It should be noted that non-CTIMPs refer to trials that do not involve an investigational medicinal product (IMP) as defined under the 2004 legislation.

Since the 2004 legislation, it has continued to evolve with subsequent directives issued, including the EU Clinical Trials Regulation, 2014. One requirement under the new regulation is that a single decision on clinical trials will be made by each member state involved. In the UK, this means a single approval for clinical trials to replace the current separate approvals given by the MHRA and NHS research ethics committees (see section 20.4).

20.4 Current Ethical Review Processes for Research in the UK

Within the UK, research proposals are reviewed by research ethics committees (RECs). Almost all research requires ethical review and approval (Health Research Authority, 2016a) and RECs seek to maintain the necessary ethical standards in research. Exceptions to this may include research involving previously collected, non-identifiable information for which ethical review has preceded the collection of data and which allows the use of the data for future projects subject to scientific review, e.g. use of large data sets of primary care or national surveys. RECs give their opinion about the proposed participant involvement and whether the research is ethical, including the quality of the study. RECs are subcategorised depending on the type of research involved. For example, there are specific RECs for clinical trials; for projects involving individuals lacking capacity; or individuals currently in prison. The UK has a range of bodies, which have roles in regulating different aspects of health research. The National Health Service (NHS) has a designated ethical approval process that brings together the assessment of governance and legal compliance, known as the Health Research Authority (HRA). The HRA acts as an independent arm's-length body to the RECs. In the UK, ethical approval occurs through a single submission channel known as the Integrated Research Application System (IRAS).

20.5 Current Frameworks for Consent in the UK

Research can be usefully categorised as intrusive or non-intrusive. Intrusive research involves direct contact with patients, for example, appraisals of clinical interventions or studies where interviews, observations or questionnaires are administered and studies where non-anonymised data is processed.[1] It is defined as any research, which would be unlawful if carried out on a person capable of giving consent, but without that consent. Non-intrusive research refers to that carried out in the absence of participant contact, for example, analysing anonymised data or samples. For any research involving contact with individuals, their consent must be sought.

The Mental Capacity Act (MCA) 2005 in England and Wales allows people who lack capacity to be lawfully included in intrusive research, except for CTIMPs, and applies to research undertaken in any setting, not just healthcare organisations or public bodies. The Act stipulates that certain criteria must be met before intrusive research can be carried out on, or in relation to, a person who lacks capacity. The relevant sections (sections 30–34)

---

[1] www.hra.nhs.uk/resources/research-legislation-and-governance/questions-and-answers-mental-capacity-act-2005 [accessed 20 September 2018].

are summarised in Box 20.1. In addition to the fundamental guiding principles for ethical research, the MCA includes advice on seeking consultees to contribute to decisions regarding participation in research of persons lacking capacity. It also makes provisions in case of loss of capacity of a consenting participant during the course of the research (section 30); in this case, there are options for the participant being withdrawn or remaining in the study; and for loss of capacity in participants entered into projects which were approved before the MCA came into force (section 34). Similar guidance is available in other countries of the UK as set out in the relevant capacity legislation.

(1) The research is in relation to an impairing condition (or treatment of the condition) affecting the participant who is unable to consent.

(2) The research could not be carried out with equal effectiveness in participants who have capacity to consent.

(3) Either:
  (a) The research offers potential benefit to the participant without imposing a disproportionate burden, or
  (b) The research provides knowledge of the causes, treatment or care of others with the same or similar condition.

If (a) does not apply, the following criteria must also be met:
  (c) The research must involve negligible risk to the participant.
  (d) The research must not interfere significantly with the participant's freedom of action or privacy.
  (e) The research is not unduly invasive or restrictive.

(4) Reasonable steps should be taken to seek advice from a *consultee* (section 32):
  – A consultee is a person who is engaged in caring for the individual lacking capacity or interested in their welfare and who is not acting in a professional capacity or receive remuneration for their caring role (personal consultee).
  – Where such a person cannot be identified, the researcher can nominate another person who is prepared to be consulted but has no connection with the research project (nominated consultee).
  – The role of the consultee is to give an opinion on whether the individual should participate in the research project and what their wishes or feelings would be regarding this. The consultee provides advice regarding this decision, which should be respected by the researchers; however, they do not consent on behalf of the individual.

(5) If a participant needs urgent treatment, appropriate arrangements are in place to seek agreement from a doctor who is not connected in the project where practicable. If not practicable, other arrangements are in place to decide on the inclusion of the participant.

(6) Additional safeguards (section 33):
  – Nothing must be done to which the participant appears to object unless it is to protect him/her from harm, reduce or prevent pain or discomfort.

- If the participant indicates he/she wishes to be withdrawn, this must be done without delay unless there would be a significant risk to his/her health.
- Any advance statement by the participant must be respected.
- In conducting the research, the interests of the participant must always be assumed to outweigh those of science and society.

Box 20.1 Approval criteria for research under MCA, ss. 30–33

[see HRA, 2106b, 2017: www.hra.nhs.uk/documents/7/standard-operating-procedures-version-7-2.pdf]

CTIMPs have an appropriately higher level of scrutiny due to their invasive nature and due to the potential risks involved in trialling medicines. They are governed by Clinical Trials Regulations rather than the MCA and require both clinical trial authorisation (CTA) from the MHRA and ethics committee approval.

The threshold for including people who lack capacity has to be set higher than that set out in the MCA provisions for non-clinical trials. Justification for including people who lack capacity in clinical trials must be clear: that is, the trial must relate directly to the participant's clinical condition; it must be essential that the trial be carried out in order to validate data from other trials involving consenting subjects; and there must be an expectation that the treatment being trialled will be of benefit to the participant, outweighing the risks or carrying no risks at all. RECs reviewing applications for CTIMPs involving people who lack capacity have a duty to seek expert advice before approving trials.

Where people lack capacity to consent in CTIMPs, a legal representative must be appointed to provide written informed consent, which legally represents the presumed will of the subject. A legal representative is defined as any person independent of the trial who by virtue of their relationship with the individual lacking capacity, is suitable, available and willing to act as their legal representative for the purposes of that trial. If no such person can be identified, a doctor primarily involved in the individual's care such as their GP or consultant or another person nominated by the relevant healthcare provider can act as the legal representative.

Deviations from trial protocols may occur in clinical trials (MHRA). While most of these do not result in harm to the trial participants or significantly affect the scientific value of their reported results, these cases need to be documented to allow appropriate actions to be taken within the context of good clinical practice (GCP). In addition, these deviations should be included and considered when the clinical study report is produced, as they may have an impact on the analysis of the data. However, not every deviation from the protocol needs to be reported to the MHRA as a serious breach. A serious breach is defined as a 'breach which is likely to effect to a significant degree – (a) the safety or physical or mental integrity of the subjects of the trial; or (b) the scientific value of the trial'. Examples may include serious adverse events such as a subject dosed with an IMP from the incorrect treatment arm, suspected unexpected serious adverse reactions such as subject death or other aspects to the clinical trial such as trial fraud (www.gov.uk/government/uploads/system/uploads/attachment_data/file/404588/GCP_serious_breaches_guide.pdf).

Clinical trials are considered the gold standard for evidencing treatment and interventions, yet they remain significantly underused in this field (Hassiotis et al., 2009). Tyrer (2007) has highlighted that much of the evidence for health interventions in this group draws from poor-quality, low-grade evidence studies. For example, most of the historical evidence to support the use of antipsychotic medication for challenging behaviour derives from non-experimental descriptive studies, comparative studies or case-control studies; or even evidence from expert committee reports, opinion and the clinical experience of respected authorities. There has since been an RCT by Tyrer et al. (2008) which showed that antipsychotics were no better than

> **Box 20.1 (cont)**
>
> placebo in the management of challenging behaviour, yet such treatments continue to be used in this population (Sheehan et al., 2015). RCTs in ID face an array of ethical, consent and practical issues (Hassiotis, 2009; Oliver-Africano et al., 2010). Poor levels of recruitment into these studies often mean that the reliability of findings is low and data collected requires careful interpretation.
>
> In addition to research directly involving participants, it is recognised that valuable work takes part in the NHS and in medical research that requires the use of identifiable patient information but where it is not always possible to seek consent. An example of this would be the use of national data sets which are collected from care records and which can subsequently be used to answer specific questions for research and service development. To overcome the difficulties in obtaining consent for using such data, section 251 of the NHS Act was introduced in 2006. It allows lawful disclosure of non-anonymised data where it was not practicable to obtain consent. This function is monitored by the Confidentiality Advisory Group (CAG) who are appointed by the HRA to provide advice on whether the processing of confidential patient information without consent should be approved or not (www.hra.nhs.uk/about-the-hra/our-committees/section-251). A Caldicott guardian is appointed by individual organisations to oversee the use of identifiable patient data and ensure that the individual's rights to confidentiality are protected.
>
> For non-intrusive research, the processing of non-identifiable patient data or anonymised tissue samples collected for other procedures is governed by other legislation such as the Data Protection Act (1998) and the Human Tissue Act (2004).

20.6 Barriers to Involvement of People with ID in Clinical Research

There are many ethical and practical barriers that affect people with ID taking part in RCTs and clinical research in general. Issues surrounding consent have at times hampered obtaining ethical approval for ID-related research projects (Goldsmith et al., 2015; Hassiotis et al., 2009). Many ethical committees have requested that researchers exclude participants who are unable to give consent (Iacono et al., 2006). Even in cases where consent by proxy can be achieved, if an adult patient lacking capacity for informed consent indicated that they were unwilling to participate in the study, they would not be included in that study (Oliver-Africano et al., 2010). RCTs in this area may also have issues relating to the concept of clinical equipoise. Clinical equipoise is defined as the assumption that there is not one 'better' intervention present (for either the control or experimental group) during the design of an RCT (Robotham et al., 2009). However, genuine uncertainty over the merits of the treatment being tested may arise. Oliver-Africano et al. (2010) described how the neuroleptics in the treatment of aggressive challenging behaviour for people with ID (NACHBID) trial revealed quite opposite views regarding clinical equipoise for antipsychotic medication for adults with ID and challenging behaviour. Thus, thought should be given to how such concepts may be presented to participants and their carers as well as the professionals who are tasked to recruit to the studies. Nonetheless, the concept of clinical equipoise has undoubtedly been influential as an ethical justification and scientific rationale for randomisation in RCTs (Gifford, 2007).

The access to participants, particularly through gatekeepers and stakeholders, such as former carers, family members and health professionals, can prove very challenging (Oliver et al., 2002). Nicholson et al. (2013) identified a number of participant factors (interview anxiety, difficulties in understanding the concept of research, worry about negative feedback). Gatekeepers may have misconceptions about what research may involve. Notably, individuals with greater impairments may be more likely to be perceived by gatekeepers as being at risk of vulnerability and exploitation (Iacono, 2006; McVilly et al., 2006). This may reduce the rate of individuals taking part where consent is given by proxy.

General research design factors may also affect recruitment such as inclusion and exclusion criteria which can often prevent individuals with ID from enrolling onto studies (Lewis, 2011, as cited in Shepherd, 2016). Within this population, communication difficulties can form significant barriers to participation and recruitment especially those with more severe ID. For example, individuals with ID may have difficulties in receptive and expressive language or memory as a result of cognitive impairment (Gilbert, 2004).

Oliver-Africano et al. (2010) have suggested, based on earlier qualitative studies, that the inexperience of participating clinicians can influence recruitment into RCTs. Clinicians have reported concerns about protecting vulnerable patients, and the impact on the doctor–patient relationship; the perceived lack of skill and confidence of clinicians to introduce a request for research participation; and priority of clinical practice versus research participation.

20.7 Overcoming Barriers to Recruitment and Participation in Research

There are many strategies which can be used to address practical barriers such as communication difficulties. For example, through using accessible information, pictures, DVDs or sign language or through considering factors such as the environment, timing and style in which information is given (Nind, 2008). For those who are likely to gain capacity with time, delaying the decision about participating in research should be considered. By enhancing communication, individuals with ID may be able to participate in research in more meaningful ways. When addressing communication issues researchers need to be mindful of acquiescence, suggestibility and using abstract concepts when, for example, collecting qualitative data from the person with ID concepts (Gilbert, 2004). Adequate training of researchers in adapting their communication style is strongly recommended due to the implications not only for engagement but also for ensuring reliable data collection (Goldsmith et al., 2015).

Nicholson et al. (2013) suggest overcoming some of the participant factors may be achievable by using a personal approach, meeting potential participants prior to recruitment and thinking about motivators to partake in research (including things that may enhance enjoyment and giving participants and carers something in return for their input such as financial rewards).

In terms of practical design issues, it is recognised that certain RCT designs may be more favourable over others. For example, Oliver-Africano et al. (2010) suggested that the method of cluster randomised trial should be used if appropriate. This method involves distributing participants to the different arms of a trial via 'social clusters' which can be a particular setting such as an outpatient clinic or hospital setting. This approach is said to allow for decreased contamination within these units, across intervention groups and is also more feasible in those situations when in ordinary practice the participants in a similar population group would all receive the same treatment. Robotham (2011) recommends that researchers include ongoing education on RCT design during trials, tailoring it to all stakeholders with emphasis on strong service user and care involvement. This could be a pivotal element in improving acceptability of and recruitment to RCTs.

A further innovation in the context of healthcare research is that of 'complex interventions'. Complex interventions are most commonly thought of as those which contain several interacting components, as well as complexity relating to implementing an intervention and determining its interaction with its context. Complex interventions commonly attempt to alter the functioning of systems which may respond in unpredictable ways. There are a number of key dimensions of complexity identified by the MRC framework including the skill requirements of those delivering the intervention, the number of groups targeted by the intervention, variability of outcomes, the degree of flexibility or tailoring of the intervention. Process evaluation is an integral part of a complex intervention aiming to develop an in-depth understanding of the functioning of an intervention by examining the implementation, mechanism of impact and the range of context factors (Craig et al., 2008).

The large body of social research suggests that inclusive approaches offer the prospect of empowerment to people with ID but great care has to be taken to avoid participation being tokenistic or outcomes being professionally driven (Kiernan, 1999; Walmsley, 2001). Inclusive approaches also face challenges such as balancing the voice of the researcher with that of an individual with ID and role clarification (Walmsley, 2001). Staley (2009) and Brett et al. (2010) reported that inclusive, emancipatory approaches such as patient and public involvement (PPI) in research have multiple influences and benefits, including the choice of research topics and direction of research, project design and methods, recruitment and data collection, analysis and dissemination. Furthermore, Staley (2009) concluded that public involvement could improve recruitment to all types of research (e.g. in qualitative research where participants are asked to share their views and experiences; or in clinical trials where it can help to improve trial design and ensure the use of relevant outcome measures). PPI is endorsed and funded by the National Institute for Health Research (NIHR). Evidence from NIHR Clinical Research Network (NIHR CRN) suggests that PPI can lead to treatments that better meet people's needs and are more likely to be put into practice. NIHR currently fund INVOLVE, a national advisory group bringing together expertise, insight and experience in the field of public involvement in research (INVOLVE, 2015. Figure 20.1 highlights how people with ID can be involved at the different stages of research using a PPI framework.

It should be noted that research involvement, participation and engagement are different activities although they are linked. Research involvement describes when members of the public are actively involved in the research. Examples can include identifying research priorities, people with ID as members of a project advisory or steering group and people with ID undertaking interviews with research participants. Participation refers to when people with ID take part in research studies, for example, participating in a focus group as part of the study or using people with ID recruited into the study to take part in the research. Engagement refers to where information and knowledge about research is provided and disseminated, such as providing knowledge about the research through open days or dissemination of study findings to research participants (INVOLVE, 2012).

Green (2016) suggests that while PPI promotes empowerment and some emancipatory approaches to research, there appears to be less evidence of a change in the power dynamic that manifests in social relations between the scientific research community and the public.

Choosing Study Topic: People with ID deciding what should be studied	**Research Methodology:** People with ID deciding what questions to ask and how	**Steering Committee:** >50% representation by people with ID	**Data Analysis:** Undertaken in a participatory manner

→ **Involving People with ID in Research** →

Funding: People with ID involved in writing funding forms	**Ethics:** People with ID attending meetings, easy read applications	**Data Collection:** Co-researchers undertaking interviews and running focus groups	**Dissemination:** Presenting at conferences and producing newsletters

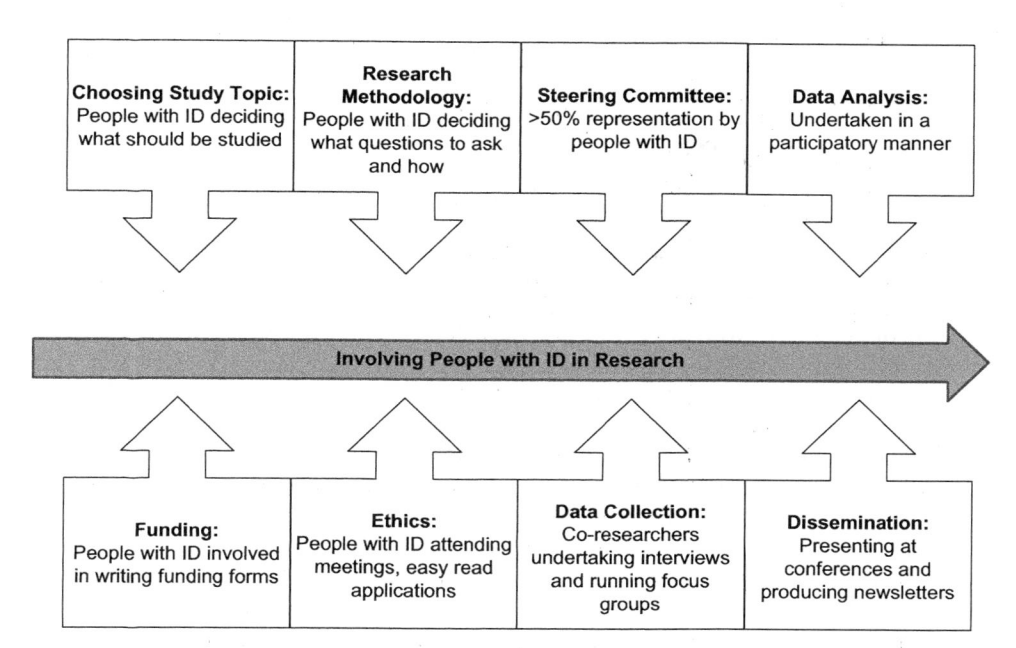

Figure 20.1 Example of people with ID: PPI flow chart (adapted with permission from Wilson et al., 2013, www.invo.org.uk/wp-content/uploads/2013/01/1.2-Wilson.pdf)

Green (2016) argues that as a result, the biomedical model remains dominant and largely unchallenged in research decision-making, and therefore issues similar to those from earlier inclusive research frameworks persist. For example, potentially tokenistic involvement of people with ID who may not feel sufficiently empowered to challenge researchers in their decision-making or choice of topic.

20.8 Conclusion

As clinicians, we have a responsibility to embrace clinical research practice. By doing so, we can help to develop high-quality evidence for interventions which may lead to improvements in the lives of people with ID, as well as informing services and policymakers. Despite the large scope to undertake research within the field of ID, it has been historically neglected and plagued by issues relating to ethics and consent as well as various practical barriers. Sadly, this means that individuals with ID continue to receive numerous interventions and services supported by limited, often inferior levels of evidence.

Nonetheless, we have seen much-needed advances in research frameworks, consent legislations (e.g. the MCA 2005) as well as concerted efforts to streamline ethical review and permission frameworks. Our understanding of barriers to participation and how to overcome these is improving. Such advances and improvements have allowed for much safer, more robust and ethically sound research practices. Progress is evidenced by the increasing funding of several multi-centred RCTs as well as other designs using national primary care data or population level surveys. Examples include the London Down Syndrome Consortium (LonDownS): which is an integrated study of cognition and risk of Alzheimer's disease in Down syndrome (Strydom et al., 2013); a trial of group-based cognitive-behavioural anger management for people with mild-to-moderate ID (Willner et al., 2013); clinical and cost effectiveness of manualised PBS staff training for managing challenging behaviour in adults with ID (Hassiotis et al., 2014).

20.9 Future Directions

NICE have suggested a number of research recommendations following recent release of guidelines for people with ID experiencing mental health problems (for further information, see NICE NG11 and NG54 research recommendations – see National Institute for Health and Care Excellence, 2015, 2016). Undoubtedly, people with profound and multiple learning disabilities (PMLD) face greater ethical and practical challenges with engagement in research compared to those with less severe ID; and therefore remain particularly at risk of poor evidence-based practice.

There is increasing interest in the use of technology, such as using the internet as an efficient way of providing mental health treatments and services. However, people with ID are likely to remain at risk of exclusion from using digital technology through lack of resources, skills and confidence (Robotham, 2016). More research in this area is required.

While research in genetics has implicated chromosomal copy-number variants (CNVs) in the aetiology of neurodevelopmental disorders, including ID, schizophrenia and autism spectrum disorders (ASDs), the majority of adults with idiopathic ID presenting to services have not been tested for CNVs (Wolfe et al., 2016). While clinicians' awareness of genetic disorders is increasing, further research in this area needs to be undertaken. Furthermore, research investigating biomarkers predicting response to both pharmacological and psychosocial interventions, otherwise known as precision medicine, is gaining popularity (Symons & Roberts, 2013).

Active public involvement in research remains vital for advances in clinical research in ID, particularly if we wish for new discoveries in this area to lead to better treatment options. Involving individuals with ID more centrally in research is not only empowering but also has the potential to identify changes in processes and systems that are required in order to make services accessible and appropriate to their users' needs (Hassiotis, 2015).

20.10 Summary

- The guiding ethical principles in research involving human subjects include the principles of respect of persons, non-maleficence, beneficence and justice.
- As clinicians, we have a responsibility to embrace clinical research as part of evidence-based practice.
- A multitude of ethical and logistical barriers have impeded research in this field.
- Advances in ethical frameworks and consent legislation have contributed to safer and robust research practice in this field although RCTs and clinical trials remain underused.
- Multi-centred RCTs are necessary for improving recruitment and evidencing psychological and pharmacological interventions in this population.
- PPI and inclusive approaches can empower individuals with ID to partake in research, and can help identify key future research priorities.
- People with greater degrees of ID remain at greater risk of exclusion from research, and thus subject to interventions which have limited evidence base.

- Future research directions should consider development of an evidence base for communication-based interventions in PMLD, the use of internet enabled technology for therapeutic inventions in people with ID and molecular genetics as part of identifying treatment options.
- New ethical and practical issues are likely to arise through new research discoveries.

References

Brett, J., Staniszewska, S. & Mockford, C. (2010) *The PIRICOM Study: A Systematic Review of the Conceptualisation, Measurement, Impact and Outcomes of Patient and Public Involvement in Health and Social Care Research*. United Kingdom Clinical Research Collaboration.

Craig, P., Dieppe, P., Macintyre, S. et al. (2008) Developing and evaluating complex interventions: new guidance. MRC.

Data Protection Act (1998) TSO.

Department of Health (2005a) *Mental Capacity Act: Code of Practice*. TSO.

Department of Health (2005b) *Research Governance Framework for Health and Social Care* (2nd ed). COI.

Department of Health, Research and Development Directorate England (2011) *Governance Arrangements for Research Ethics Committees: A Harmonised Edition*. HMSO.

Gifford, F. (2007) Pulling the plug on clinical equipoise: A critique of Miller and Weijer. *Kennedy Institute of Ethics Journal*, 17(3), 203–26.

Gilbert, T. (2004) Involving people with learning disabilities in research: Issues and possibilities. *Health and Social Care in Community*, 12(4), 298–308.

Goldsmith, L. & Skirton, H. (2015). Research involving people with a learning disability – Methodological challenges and ethical considerations. *Journal of Research in Nursing*, 20(6), 435–46.

MHRA (2018) *Guidance for the Notification of Serious Breaches of GCP or the Trial Protocol*. Available at: www.gov.uk/government/uploads/system/uploads/attachment_data/file/404588/GCP_serious_breaches_guide.pdf [accessed 22 December 2016].

Green, G. (2016) Power to the people: To what extent has public involvement in applied health research achieved this? *Research Involvement and Engagement*, 2, 28.

Guyatt, G. (1992) Evidence-based medicine: A new approach to teaching the practice of medicine. *JAMA*, 268(17), 2420–5.

Hassiotis, A. (2009) Research in mental health learning disabilities: Present challenges and future drivers. *Psychiatry*, 11, 457–60.

Hassiotis, A., Scior, K. & Hamid, A. (2015) Engaging service users in identifying priorities for research on intellectual disabilities. University College London. Available at: www.ucl.ac.uk/ciddr/documents/FinalReport21Jan2015.pdf [accessed 19 September 2018].

Hassiotis, A, Strydom, A., Crawford, M. et al. (2014) Clinical and cost effectiveness of staff training in Positive Behaviour Support (PBS) for treating challenging behaviour in adults with intellectual disability: A cluster randomised controlled trial. *BMC Psychiatry*, 14, 219.

Health Research Authority (2016a) Before you apply for approval. Available at: www.hra.nhs.uk/research-community/before-you-apply/determine-which-review-body-approvals-are-required [accessed 19 September 2018].

Health Research Authority (2016b) Questions and answers – Mental Capacity Act 2005. Available at: www.hra.nhs.uk/resources/research-legislation-and-governance/questions-and-answers-mental-capacity-act-2005 [accessed 22 December 2016].

Health Research Authority (2017) Standard operating procedures for research ethics committees. Available at: www.hra.nhs.uk/documents/7/standard-operating-procedures-version-7-2.pdf [accessed 22 March 2018].

Heslop, P., Blair, P., Fleming, P. et al (2013) *Confidential Inquiry into Premature Deaths of People with Learning Disabilities (CIPOLD): Final Report*. Bristol University. Available at: www.bristol.ac.uk/media-library/sites/cipold/migrated/documents/fullfinalreport.pdf [accessed 30 November 2016].

Holland, T. (2009) 'Editorial'. *Journal of Intellectual Disability Research*, 53(1), 1–2.

Human Tissue Act (2004) TSO.

Iacono, T. (2006) Ethical challenges and complexities of including people with intellectual disability as participants in research. *Journal of Intellectual and Developmental Disability*, 31, 173-9.

INVOLVE (2012) Briefing notes for researchers: Involving the public in NHS, public health and social care research. Eastleigh.

INVOLVE (2015) Public involvement in research: Values and principles framework. Eastleigh.

Kiernan, C. (1999) Participation in research by people with learning disability: Origins and issues. *British Journal of Learning Disabilities*, 27, 43-7.

McCully, S. (2011) *The UK Clinical Trials Regulations: An Introduction to the Regulations and Guidelines that Govern Clinical Trials in the UK*. Compliance Healthcheck Consulting UK. Available at: www.chcuk.co.uk/pdf/2011-09-01_UK_Clinical_Trials_Regulations-(Stuart_McCully)_Low_Res.pdf [accessed 21 December 2016].

McVilly, K. R. & Dalton, A. J. (2006) Commentary on Iacono (2006): Ethical challenges and complexities of including people with intellectual disability as participants in research. *Journal of Intellectual and Developmental Disability*, 31, 186-8.

MENCAP (2007) *Death by Indifference*. Available at: www.mencap.org.uk/sites/default/files/2016-06/DBIreport.pdf [accessed 22 December 2016].

National Commission for the Protection of Human Subjects of Biomedical and Behavioral Research (1979) *Ethical Principles and Guidelines for the Protection of Human Subjects of Research: The Belmont Report*. Office of the Secretary, DHEW.

National Institute for Health and Care Excellence (2015) *Challenging Behaviour and Learning Disabilities: Prevention and Interventions for People with Learning Disabilities Whose Behaviour Challenges (NG11)*.

National Institute for Health and Care Excellence (2016) *Mental Health Problems in People with Learning Disabilities: Prevention, Assessment and Management (NG54)*.

National Institute for Health Research [no date] Why research matters. Available at: www.nihr.ac.uk/patients-and-public/why-join-in/why-research-matters.htm [accessed 22 December 2016].

National Institute for Health Research (2016) Health Technology Assessment Programme: Improving communication for adults with profound and multiple learning disabilities (HTA no. 16/156). Available at: www.nets.nihr.ac.uk/__data/assets/pdf_file/0020/172460/16_156cb.pdf [accessed 22 December 2016].

National Research Association (2013) Does my project require review by a research ethics committee? Available at: www.hra.nhs.uk/documents/2013/09/does-my-project-require-rec-review.pdf [accessed 22 December 2016].

NHS Research Authority (2018) *Standard Operating Procedures for Research Ethics Committees*. UK Health Departments Research Ethics Service, vers. 7.3, September 2016. Available at: file:///C:/Users/owner/Downloads/RES_Standard_Operating_Procedures_Version_7.3_September_2018.pdf [accessed 20 September 2018].

Nicholson, L., Colyer, M. & Cooper, S. A. (2013) Recruitment to intellectual disability research: A qualitative study. *Journal of Intellectual Disability Research*, 57(7), 647-56.

Nind, M. (2008) Conducting qualitative research with people with learning, communication and other disabilities: Methodological challenges. ESRC National Centre for Research Methods Review Paper. Available at: http://eprints.ncrm.ac.uk/491 [accessed 22 December 2016].

Oliver, P. C., Piachaud, J., Done, J. et al. (2002) Difficulties in conducting a randomized controlled trial of health service interventions in intellectual disability: Implications for evidence-based practice. *Journal of Intellectual Disability Research*, 46, 340-5.

Oliver-Africano, P., Dickens, S., Ahmed, Z. et al. (2010) Overcoming the barriers experienced in conducting a medication trial in adults with aggressive challenging behaviour and intellectual disabilities. *Journal of Intellectual Disability Research*, 54, 17-25.

Regulation (EU) 536/2014 of the European Parliament and of the Council of 16 April 2014 on clinical trials on medicinal products for human use, and repealing Directive 2001/20/EC.

Robotham, D. & Hassiotis, A. (2009) Randomised controlled trials in learning disabilities: A review of participant experiences. *Advances in Mental Health and Learning Disabilities*, 3(1), 42-6.

Robotham, D., King, M. & Canagasabey, A. (2011) Social validity of randomised controlled trials in health services research and intellectual disabilities: A qualitative exploration of stakeholder view. *Trials*, **12**, 144.

Robotham, D., Satkunanathan, S., Doughty, L. et al. (2016) Do we still have a digital divide in mental health? A five-year survey follow-up. *Journal of Medical Internet Research*, **18**(11), e309.

Rothman, D. & Rothman, S. (1984) *The Willowbrook Wars*. HarperCollins, 265–6.

Sheehan, R., Hassiotis, A., Walters, K. et al. (2015) Mental illness, challenging behaviour, and psychotropic drug prescribing in people with intellectual disability: UK population based cohort study. *British Medical Journal*, **351**, h4326.

Shepherd, V. (2016) Research involving adults lacking capacity to consent: The impact of research regulation on 'evidence biased' medicine. *BMC Medical Ethics*, 7(1), 55. doi: 10.1186/s12910-016-0138-9

Staley, K. (2009) *Exploring Impact: Public Involvement in NHS, Public Health and Social Care Research*. Eastleigh.

Strydom, A. (2013) *The London Down Syndrome Consortium (LonDownS): An Integrated Study of Cognition and Risk for Alzheimer's Disease in Down Syndrome*. Available at: www.hra.nhs.uk/news/research-summaries/londowns-cohort/#sthash.PsNOEF54.dpuf [accessed 29 December 2016].

Symons, F. J. & Roberts, J. (2013) Biomarkers, behavior, and intellectual and developmental disabilities. *American Journal on Intellectual and Developmental Disabilities*, **118**, 413–15. doi:10.1352/1944-7558-118.6.413

Trials of War Criminals before the Nuremberg Military Tribunals under Control Council Law No. 10, Volume II (1949) pp. 181–2. US Government Printing Office.

Tyrer, P. (2007) Oral presentation of the NACHBID study at the academic programme of the Department of Mental Health Sciences, UCL, Bloomsbury Campus (10 October 2007).

Tyrer, P., Cooper, S.-A. & Hassiotis, A. (2014) Drug treatments in people with intellectual disability and challenging behaviour. *British Medical Journal*, **349**: g4323.

Tyrer, P., Oliver-Africano, P., Ahmed, Z. et al. (2008) Risperidone, haloperidol, and placebo in the treatment of aggressive challenging behaviour in patients with intellectual disability: A randomised controlled trial. *The Lancet*, **371**(9606), 57–63. doi: 10.1016/S0140-6736(08)60072-0

Tyrer, P., Oliver-Africano, P., Romeo, R. et al. (2009) Neuroleptics in the treatment of aggressive challenging behaviour for people with intellectual disabilities: A randomised controlled trial (NACHBID). *Health Technology Assessment*, **13**(21), iii–iv, ix–xi, 1–54.

Walmsley, J. (2001) Normalisation, emancipatory research and inclusive research in learning disability. *Disability & Society*, **16**(2), 187–205.

Willner, P., Rose, J., Jahoda, A. et al. (2013) Group-based cognitive-behavioural anger management for people with mild to moderate intellectual disabilities: Cluster randomised controlled trial. *British Journal of Psychiatry*, **203**, 288–96.

Wilson, P., Cowe, M. & Mathie, E. (2013) *Research with Patient and Public Involvement: A Realist Evaluation*. Available at: www.invo.org.uk/wp-content/uploads/2013/01/1.2-Wilson.pdf [accessed 22 March 2018].

Wolfe, K., Strydom, A. & Morrogh, D. (2016) Chromosomal microarray testing in adults with intellectual disability presenting with comorbid psychiatric disorders. *European Journal of Human Genetics*, **25**, 66–72.

World Medical Association (2008) *Declaration of Helsinki: Ethical Principles for Medical Research Involving Human Subjects*.

Further Reading

CTIMPs: EU legislation: www.hra.nhs.uk/resources/before-you-apply/types-of-study/clinical-trials-of-investigational-medicinal-products/clinical-trials-investigational-medicinal-products-ctimps-eu-legislation/#sthash.liQ59aYM.dpuf

C. Freeman & P. Tyrer (eds.) *Research Methods in Psychiatry* (3rd edn). RCPsych Publications, 2006.

HRA: www.hra.nhs.uk

Good clinical practice for clinical trials: www.gov.uk/guidance/good-clinical-practice-for-clinical-trials

National Institute for Health Research: www.nihr.ac.uk/Pages/default.aspx

Recommendations for research, National Institute for Health and Care Excellence. NG54 Mental health problems in people with learning disabilities: prevention, assessment and management: www.nice.org.uk/guidance/ng54/chapter/Recommendations-for-research

Recommendations for research, National Institute for Health and Care Excellence: *Challenging Behaviour and Learning Disabilities: Prevention and Interventions for People with Learning Disabilities Whose Behaviour Challenges (NG11)*: www.nice.org.uk/guidance/ng11/chapter/2-Research-recommendations

Research with Patient and Public Involvement: A Realist Evaluation. The RAPPORT study. Health Services and Delivery Research 3, 38: http://dx.doi.org/10.3310/hsdr03380

Research funding information, for example about new calls and deadline for applications can usually be obtained from the NIHR official site and from the sites of other bodies such as the MRC and the Wellcome Trust. We recommend establishing clinical–academic partnerships as early as possible if interested in research as both recruitment and methodological know-how are of importance. Other options include involvement with the work of Collaboration for Leadership in Applied Health Research and Care (www.clahrcprojects.co.uk) and academically ambitious trainees can seek further information about getting into academic training at www.nihr.ac.uk/funding-and-support/funding-for-training-and-career-development/training-programmes/integrated-academic-training-programme/integrated-academic-training/academic-clinical-fellowships

Chapter 21

Training in Intellectual Disability Psychiatry

Bernice Knight and Joanna Kingston

21.1 Introduction

Welcome to this chapter on training in intellectual disability (ID) psychiatry. Both of us are higher trainees in ID psychiatry reaching the end of our training, one in London and the other in Severn. In writing this chapter, we have imagined you are reading this either because you are intrigued to know a little more general information, or you have some specific questions about training. In order to cover the topics we think are relevant, we have set it out as questions with answers. One of the beauties of ID psychiatry is that you can shape your career depending on your own areas of special interest, as well as the needs of your local population. So if something you are particularly keen to know is missing, contact your local trainees or consultants, who are usually an enthusiastic and approachable group of people.

Specialist training in ID psychiatry predominantly focuses on working with adults with learning disabilities and we have written this chapter with that in mind. However, we recognise ID psychiatrists work in a wide variety of settings including in services for children with ID and forensic services. We are aware there is regional variation both in areas related to training and in the local service provision. We are also aware that training in ID psychiatry is rare globally, though we hope this chapter will be of interest to our international colleagues and give an insight into this training pathway in the UK.

21.2 Why Choose ID Psychiatry?

ID psychiatry offers quite a unique opportunity to integrate all your skills as a psychiatrist in order to work with a population who are some of the most vulnerable and poorly served in our society. Working across the adult lifespan from 18 years until the end of life, you have a continuity of care that is rare in other branches of medicine. For your patients and along with your team, you usually provide care that covers mental illness, neurodevelopmental disorders (autism and attention deficit hyperactivity disorder (ADHD)), dementia and behaviours that challenge, along with elements of forensic and neuropsychiatry. Epilepsy is common and may contribute to changes in behaviour and mental state, thus requiring an understanding of diagnosis and management and in some teams, ID psychiatrists are responsible for epilepsy management. Patients may also have medical conditions such as underlying genetic syndromes which can add further complexity to assessment and management. Furthermore, people with ID may not have language skills sufficient to inform us of their symptoms. As an ID psychiatrist, therefore, you have to be in tune with behaviour, be good at observation and have some working knowledge of common physical ailments as these may cause diagnostic overshadowing. You also have a role to ensure any physical health needs are appropriately assessed and managed through liaison into primary and secondary care.

> **Quote 21.1 Newly appointed consultant**
>
> I like that intellectual disability psychiatry is broad – anxiety, depression, bipolar, psychosis, dementia, personality disorders, autism – there is lots of core psychiatry stuff, which is not always the case in general adult psychiatry where care is divided into condition-specific service lines.

Psychotherapeutic skills continue to play a core role in your daily work, for example, when formulating ideas, communicating concepts of attachment and relationship, and in building therapeutic understanding and trust with patients. Many people with an ID have experienced a disproportionate number of losses, traumas and significant life events that have an impact on their psychological interaction with the world around them. Some psychiatrists choose to develop even more specialist skills in order to provide cognitive-behaviour therapy, systemic therapy, group therapy and long-term psychotherapy for people with ID. So, if you are worried that you won't continue using your therapeutic skills, then don't be: there are plenty of opportunities in the core work and more formally.

> **Quote 21.2 Newly appointed consultant**
>
> People with intellectual disability don't exist in isolation; they are always part of a system. This may be their family, supported living or day activities, and the presenting problem and its solution often will be partly related to issues in that system. So if you enjoy systemic thinking or the challenge of working with people, their carers and their networks, then ID psychiatry is great.

An attractive part of working in ID psychiatry is the true multidisciplinary working, where team members have maintained their professional specialty rather than working generically, which is not always the case in other psychiatric specialities. For example, a physiotherapist would advise on postural support for a patient and a speech and language therapist would provide expertise on communication strategies. This usually provides a sense of identity, translating into high morale. You may work alongside ID nurses, psychologists, occupational therapists, speech and language therapists, physiotherapists, specialist support workers, behavioural specialists, art therapists, music therapists and a range of other professionals. There is close collaboration with social care, and depending upon local services, teams may be integrated with social workers. Working across disciplines and organisations requires extensive collaboration and flexible communication skills.

In addition to the clinical work there are plenty of opportunities to have a portfolio career for those who would like more variety in their work life. A portfolio career is when an individual has multiple strands to their career rather than a single strand, either by having two or more part-time jobs at once, or a series of short-term jobs. As a relatively small specialty, there are options to interact with and work for the Royal College of Psychiatrists, medical schools, Parliament, commissioners, international organisations, academic departments, psychological institutions, forensic services and many more. All this means that if you want a career working with a unique but diverse group of patients, which utilises your general and specialist psychiatry knowledge, involves multidisciplinary team working, and provides ample opportunities for diversification, then ID psychiatry may be for you.

> **Quote 21.3** Newly appointed ST4 higher trainee
>
> The choice to specialise in ID psychiatry was one which crept up on me. I initially chose an ID psychiatry placement in core training because people told me 'everyone who does ID loves it'. I had neutral thoughts but I kept an open mind. The more time I spent in ID psychiatry, the more I truly appreciated the diversity and complexity of the clinical work, and I found the people working in ID were a universally friendly, supportive and dedicated bunch. There also seemed to be more time to spend with patients and for discussion in the multidisciplinary team. Particularly rewarding for me is close working with other colleagues in the ID team and also with professionals from schools, primary care and acute hospital settings; realising that we really can make a positive difference in the lives of our patients. I am now happily about to start my higher training in ID psychiatry and I don't regret my decision one bit – they don't call it the hidden gem of psychiatry for nothing!

21.3 What Is the Training Pathway?

ID psychiatry is a subspecialty of the broader medical specialty of psychiatry. To clear something up quickly, the terms intellectual disability (ID) and learning disability (LD) are currently used interchangeably in the UK but the more contemporary, internationally recognised concept is ID. Once the General Medical Council (GMC) formally recognise this name, the Royal College of Psychiatrists will change the specialty name from LD to ID. ID psychiatry is described by the Faculty of the Royal College of Psychiatrists in Box 21.1.

In the UK the current postgraduate training pathway to become a specialist in ID psychiatry takes a minimum of eight years. The pathway involves completing foundation training, core psychiatry training (or via broad-based training while this existed) and finally higher training in ID psychiatry (see Figure 21.1). Currently doctors have to competitively apply for posts at each of these stages through a process of national recruitment. All training

> **Box 21.1** Faculty of Intellectual Disability Psychiatry, Royal College of Psychiatrists
>
> People with learning disability are much more likely than the general population to experience mental health conditions, because they experience more biological and psychosocial risk factors. Specialist psychiatrists who work with people with learning disability offer treatment for severe mental illness, but also for a wide range of other mental health conditions such as autistic spectrum disorders and anxiety disorders. Because people with learning disability may have less internal resources to cope with mental distress, more minor disorders can have a severe effect, so services usually have a much lower threshold for referral than mainstream mental health services.
>
> More information can be found at: www.rcpsych.ac.uk/discoverpsychiatry/studentassociates/psychiatriccareerpaths/subspecialties/learningdisability.aspx [accessed 20 September 2018]

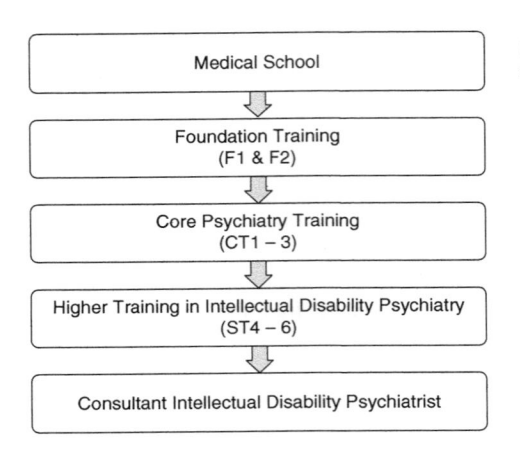

Figure 21.1 UK training pathway to become a consultant in ID psychiatry

```
Medical School
      ↓
Foundation Training
    (F1 & F2)
      ↓
Core Psychiatry Training
      (CT1 – 3)
      ↓
Higher Training in Intellectual Disability Psychiatry
              (ST4 – 6)
      ↓
Consultant Intellectual Disability Psychiatrist
```

programmes are coordinated regionally and how this is organised differs in the different regions of the UK. For example, in England this is through four local education and training boards (LETBs). Previously, training was organised in deaneries and a legacy of this geographical division still exists, through the existence of postgraduate deans and their offices.

After completing their medical degree, the doctor will undertake foundation training (F1 and F2) where they will rotate around a number of specialities predominantly based in acute hospitals. Depending upon the range of rotations these may include general practice and psychiatry. It is not a requirement to have done a foundation post in psychiatry to apply for core psychiatry training. For example, of the two authors of this chapter only one undertook psychiatry placements during foundation training. If you don't have a post in psychiatry, it is possible to gain experience through undertaking 'taster days' where you spend a day in the speciality.

Core psychiatry training (CT1–3) involves three years of training, rotating (usually every six months) around a variety of psychiatry posts. This will include posts in General Adult and Old Age Psychiatry in addition to other specialities. Trainees will gain experience in both hospital and community environments. Usually trainees undertake one neurodevelopmental post (either ID or child and adolescent psychiatry) and at times this has been a requirement by the Royal College of Psychiatrists. During this training period trainees will work to undertake the examinations for membership of the Royal College of Psychiatrists, which is a requirement for applying for higher training.

Higher training in psychiatry (ST4–6) is divided into six specialities and trainees have to decide which speciality they want to work in as a consultant, in order to obtain the necessary certificate of completion of training. Currently the options are: general adult, old age, child and adolescent, forensic, psychotherapy and ID psychiatry. The training programme for all specialities is currently three years full-time equivalent. Many trainees will work less than full-time for some or all of their training, usually because of caring or parenting responsibilities. Sometimes there are options for dual training (e.g. general adult and old age) and these require a longer length of training (typically four or five years depending upon the speciality combinations). Currently there are two relevant dual training programmes approved by the GMC: ID psychiatry and forensic psychiatry, and ID psychiatry and child and adolescent psychiatry. All higher trainees have one day per week away from their normal clinical duties for 'special interest' sessions to gain additional experience in both clinical and non-clinical areas.

ID psychiatry higher training is the same as other major subspecialities. Trainees must undertake a minimum of three years full-time equivalent and obtain the necessary competencies to progress at each stage. Posts are often for twelve months but there may be some six-month post options. Although all trainees will need to gain a broad range of experience in ID psychiatry, the options available for posts will vary from region to region, largely dependent on the services in that region.[1]

21.4 What Is the ID Psychiatry Curriculum?

The curriculum for higher training in ID psychiatry is specified by the Royal College of Psychiatrists. It is reviewed by the Faculty of Intellectual Disability Psychiatry via relevant committees and is updated at regular intervals; the last update was in August 2016. Over the course of the training programme, trainees need to display evidence they have achieved competency in all these areas. As the curriculum is updated every few years it is important to follow the most up-to-date version. The current curriculum is divided into intended learning outcomes (ILOs) (Royal College of Psychiatrists, 2010). These are summarised and listed in Table 21.1.

According to the curriculum, the Royal College of Psychiatrists (2013) currently expects at least two years of higher training to be spent within designated ID psychiatry posts, which should comprise:

- acute treatment and management of people with learning disabilities and their mental and behavioural problems within inpatient settings;
- working in multidisciplinary community teams; and
- seeing patients and their carers in a variety of outpatient and community settings.

One year can be within ID psychiatry services for children. The third year can comprise either a specialist post or further community-based experience as above, perhaps with an emphasis on:

- neuropsychiatry;
- neurodevelopmental disorders;
- brain injury;
- experience within designated ID psychiatry posts in forensic psychiatry; and
- experience within designated posts in relevant psychiatric specialty: e.g. general adult psychiatry or one of its subspecialties.

An integrated academic career pathway is available through posts funded by the National Institute of Health Research (NIHR). Usually they are advertised by an academic institution at core trainee level (academic clinical fellow) and applied for by the individual at higher training level. Other fellowship or research funding may be available through charities and universities. Opportunities change regularly so we have not been more specific here.[2]

---

[1] Further information can be found on the Royal College of Psychiatrists website at: www.rcpsych.ac.uk/workinpsychiatry/faculties/intellectualdisability.aspx [accessed 18 September 2018].
[2] More information can be found at: www.nihr.ac.uk/funding-and-support/funding-for-training-and-career-development/fellowship-programme.htm, or by searching online.

Table 21.1 A competency-based curriculum for higher training in ID psychiatry

	ILO 1	Specialist assessment of patients and document-relevant history and examination in culturally diverse patients
	ILO 4	Risk assessment of harm to self and others including intervention and involuntary treatment
	ILO 5	Conduct therapeutic interviews; demonstrate a range of therapies and integrate with other interventions
	ILO 7	Specialist assessment and treatment of those with chronic and severe mental disorders
	ILO 8	Research methodology and critical appraisal of research literature
	ILO 10	Develop ability to conduct and complete audit in clinical practice
	ILO 11	To develop an understanding of the implementation of clinical governance
	ILO 13	Demonstrate effective communication with patients, relatives and colleagues, and therapeutic alliances
	ILO 14	Demonstrate ability to work effectively with colleagues, including team working
	ILO 15	Develop appropriate leadership skills
	ILO 16	Demonstrate the knowledge, skills and behaviours to manage time and problems effectively
	ILO 17	Develop ability to teach, assess and appraise
	ILO 19	Ensure that you act in a professional manner at all times; ensure lifelong learning and reflective practice

(source: Royal College of Psychiatrists, 2010). ILO = Intended Learning Objective

21.5 What Is It Like as a New Trainee in ID Psychiatry?

Starting training in ID psychiatry can be both an exciting and daunting time. ST4–6 training equates to what was previously referred to as specialist registrar (SpR). Doctors will be familiar with the role of the medical registrar in the acute hospital and this is someone whom most of us have looked up to, seeing them as a senior doctor responsible for looking after the acute medical patients. However, unlike the medical registrar, for most people starting higher training in ID psychiatry they will only have at most six months' experience of working in ID psychiatry and so it can feel like joining a new specialty with lots to learn. Such feelings are not uncommon and trainers will be familiar with this. It is important for trainees to seek supervision and support when needed.

We are now able to reflect on our own experiences of this time and so here are some suggestions of things we wish we had known:

- There are two national conferences each year organised by the Faculty of Intellectual Disability, in spring and autumn. These are good opportunities to hear the latest updates in the field and meet colleagues from around the country. Bursaries may be available to apply for from the ID faculty if you have used all your study budget.

- An annual trainees' conference is organised by trainees for trainees, which is a great place to meet, network and socialise with your cohort. It is also a great opportunity for anyone who wants to organise the conference in their area.
- Supervisors are usually very willing to discuss career and domestic issues with you, so don't be afraid to ask for advice or support.
- Opportunities are plentiful in higher training, be as creative and ambitious as you wish, because it's a time for exploration and development.
- Training goes really quickly, so start doing things early.
- Towards the start of your training, it may be helpful to identify areas of the curriculum you will need to cover in special interest sessions (i.e. outside your usual training post, for example, in a specialist clinic). This will vary depending on local services. You can then incorporate this into planning special interest sessions over the three years.
- Use all your study budget each year, as you can't carry it over to another year. There are lots of courses, for example, in autism, ADHD, epilepsy and psychotherapy you will want to attend over the three years.
- Life outside of medicine is really important, so don't forget to nourish yourself as well as the trainee.

21.6 How Do I Progress through Training?

The overarching aim of higher training is to achieve a certificate of completion of training (CCT) in order to practise as a consultant psychiatrist for adults with ID. Trainees should gain sufficient clinical competence in order to diagnose and manage routine through to complex presentations for their patients. They are required to blend their knowledge of general adult psychiatry with the specialist knowledge required to understand the similarities and differences in adults with varying degrees of ID. Alongside clinical expertise, it is crucial to develop effective multidisciplinary working, advanced communication skills and an ability to manage ambiguity. Trainees are likely to further develop resilience and a deeper understanding of themselves, so that by the end of training doctors should have gained the confidence to take on a role as clinical leader within an ID service. Of course the learning does not stop there, but a trainee should be equipped to take on the new challenge of being a consultant by the end of their higher training.

In England trainees have three formal layers of supervision to support their learning. Ideally, these are different people but sometimes one person will provide more than one role and there may be variation in different regions of the UK:

(1) Clinical supervisor: changes with each placement to oversee the daily clinical work by monitoring competency development and providing structured feedback through electronic appraisal documents.
(2) Educational supervisor: may remain the same over the course of training and typically offers mentoring about three times each year, to help guide career development and progress towards CCT.
(3) Training programme director (TPD): has responsibility for monitoring progress of all trainees on the programme by undertaking formal reviews of clinical progress (usually annually) and reports back to Health Education England.

Trainees are required to undertake formal appraisal in order to progress through the three years of training (ST4–6). Usually this is done on an annual basis through the annual review of competence progression (ARCP). This can be a stressful and time-consuming process but when done well by the supervisors and trainee, it offers a fulfilling and developmental opportunity. As the ARCP maps to the curriculum learning objectives (see above) the process should help to drive curriculum-focused learning. You can read the *Gold Guide* produced by the Conference of Postgraduate Medical Deans for more information (COPMeD, 2016).

Many trainees will experience significant life events during their training or have physical or mental health problems of their own. Life crises do not pay attention to whether you are in a training programme or not, and being a psychiatrist is a demanding job. Informal support through your friends and family, and your trainee network, may be a place to start for help and advice. However, there are many other avenues of support available to trainees. This includes discussing with your clinical/educational supervisors and TPD, your GP and trust occupational health department, the LETB/deanery professional support unit or the NHS Practitioner Health Programme (NHS, 2017). If you need some time out of training or need to reduce some of your work commitments, there are a number of options available through the above routes. Sometimes your TPD may suggest extending your training to compensate for any time out but this is specific to the individual and their circumstance. It is generally best to address the problem early rather than wait for it to reach crisis point, as supervisors can't help you, if they don't know what is happening. It is very common for trainees to have some personal difficulties during their training, so don't think it is unusual or that it will be difficult to make things easier for you.

21.7 What Are the Training Opportunities in Higher Training?

The opportunities that are available to you are broadly divided into national and regional. National opportunities are open to everyone, regardless of where they train, and they are often advertised through the Faculty of Intellectual Disability Psychiatry at the Royal College of Psychiatrists. Regional opportunities depend on the services, consultants and special interest sessions available in your area. However, there is nothing to say you can't take advantage of things going on further afield in agreement with your supervisors.

Broader clinical experience outside of the traditional day job can be achieved through special interest sessions and on-call work. As explained above, every higher trainee has about one day per week (full-time equivalent) to undertake special interest sessions in an area of their interest or where development is needed. Examples of regional opportunities are: autism services, psychotherapy long cases, deaf services, epilepsy clinics and neuropsychiatry clinics. National opportunities currently include a position as a parliamentary researcher in the House of Lords or as a trainee representative for the Royal College of Psychiatrists. On-call working provides a lot of trainees with emergency psychiatry experience including crisis management and use of the Mental Health Act.

The Royal College of Psychiatrists offers prizes for posters, presentations, essays and international work throughout the year, so keep an eye out for deadlines. Audit and quality improvement projects should be available locally through your teams or through special interest sessions and they make good submissions for prizes when done well. Research can be done through collaboration with your local academic or research department, a taught programme such as a certificate or MSc, or through an academic career path like the NIHR or university-led scheme.

Table 21.2 Examples of opportunities available in higher training

	Psychotherapy	Research	Teaching	Management
Job-specific	Clinical psychotherapy post	Clinical lecturer NIHR ACF	Teaching fellow	Darzi fellow FMLM fellow
Qualification	BACP qualifications	MSc PhD	PG cert	MBA NHS Leadership programme
Informal	Special interest sessions	Departmental research	Teaching sessions for medical students	Quality improvement projects
	Joint working with psychologists	Personal research	Foundation and core trainees	Audits
	Specific experience within post	Reviews	Local academic programmes	Management projects within your organisation
		Book chapters	MDT teaching	Local leadership and management programmes

Out-of-programme experiences are also available through an application to your LETB/deanery after discussion with your TPD. Trainees have used this time to undertake international work, complete a PhD, work as a teaching or clinical fellow or other specialist skill development. As long as you have a robust plan and a clear timescale, trainers are usually very supportive of you broadening your expertise. Table 21.2 gives some further ideas of opportunities available depending on the degree to which you want to concentrate on it.

21.8 How Do I Prepare to Be a Consultant?

In the final year of training the focus is likely to turn to preparing to be a consultant. The modern consultant role is often a combination of clinician, manager and educator. A lot of the decisions regarding your first consultant job will depend on what is advertised at the time. In the final year of training there may be the opportunity to undertake an 'acting up' consultant post for up to three months, which is a good opportunity to gain insight into working as a consultant. It is worth spending some time considering what post is most likely to suit your skill set. You may wish to balance what is most important to you, taking into account whether you thrive during inpatient or outpatient positions, and considering the relative importance of location, team formations and access to subspecialities. Preparation may also include addressing training gaps, interview preparation and CV writing. Most newly appointed consultants we have spoken to recommend gaining mentoring and advice from colleagues you trust, and, if possible, visiting any job before the interview to make sure you are compatible.

Thank you for reading and we wish you all the very best with your future career, in whatever specialty you choose.

References

COPMeD (2016) *The Gold Guide: A Reference Guide for Postgraduate Specialty Training in the UK* (6th edn). Conference of Postgraduate Medical Deans. Available at: www.copmed.org.uk/publications/the-gold-guide [accessed 21 September 2018].

NHS (2017) *NHS Practitioner Health Programme: Supporting the Health of Health Professionals*. Available at: http://php.nhs.uk [accessed 21 September 2018].

Royal College of Psychiatrists (2010) *A Competency Based Curriculum for Specialist Training in Psychiatry: Specialists in the Psychiatry of Learning Disability*. GMC-approved February 2010 – revised August 2016. Available at: www.rcpsych.ac.uk/pdf/Psychiatry_of_Learning_Disability_Curriculum_August_2016.pdf [accessed 21 September 2018].

Royal College of Psychiatrists (2013) *A Competency Based Curriculum for Specialist Core Training in Psychiatry: Core Training in Psychiatry CT1–CT3*. GMC-approved July 2013 – revised August 2016. Available at: www.rcpsych.ac.uk/pdf/Core_Psychiatry_Curriculum_August_2016.pdf [accessed 21 September 2018].

Index

A-Z Reference Book of Syndromes and Inherited Disorders (Gilbert), 28
ability to testify, 61–62
Absolute Discharge, 152
Accessible Cause-Outcome Representation and Notation System (ACORNS), 130
Accessible Information Standard, 48
Accreditation for Inpatient Mental Health Services (AIMS), 209
Acute Care Hospitals, 196
Acute Hospital Trusts, 199
adaptive behaviour
  challenging behaviour and, 175
  defined, 1–2, 3
  dementia and, 95, 138
  influence of, 2
  introduction to, 1–2, 3
  tools for assessing, 90, 95, 139
Adaptive Behaviour Dementia Questionnaire (ABDQ), 139
adults with intellectual disability
  accurate diagnosis, 127–128
  aetiology, 130–131
  assessment, 128–129
  epidemiology, 125–127
  interventions, 131
  introduction to, 125
  prognosis, 132
  psychiatric symptoms and classification, 129–130
aetiology of intellectual disability, 5–6
affective disorder, 7, 31, 58, 132, 204, 215
age at death, 107
age-related cognitive impairment, 95
Alzheimer's disease, 6, 29, 67
Alzheimer's Society, 166

American Association on Intellectual and Developmental Disabilities' manual (AAIDD), 2, 6
American Psychiatric Association, 2, 55
Angelman syndrome (AS), 17, 18, 30
anger management, 165, 172–174
Annual Review of Competence Progression (ARCP), 251–252
Antecedent, Behaviour and Consequence (ABC) charts, 169–170
antidementia drugs, 140
antidepressant medication, 141, 179
antiepileptic medication, 142
antipsychotic medication, 140–141, 179
antisocial behaviour, 28
anxiety/anxiety disorders
  assessment of, 120
  autism and, 59, 122
  in children, 122–123
  Glasgow Anxiety Scale, 208
  incidence of, 132, 204
  medication for, 122–123, 220
  psychological interventions for, 172
  social anxiety, 31, 32–33, 123
APP gene and dementia, 137
Applied Behaviour Analysis conceptual framework, 171
Asperger, Hans, 53
Asperger syndrome, 53
assessment. See also biopsychosocial approach to assessment; instruments of screening
  adults with intellectual disability, 128–129
  anxiety/anxiety disorders, 120

attention deficit and hyperactivity disorder, 120
behaviour with epilepsy, 74
biopsychosocial approach to, 86, 89–96
cognitive skills assessment, 90
depression, 120, 139
developmental history assessment, 90
difficulty accessing, 104
engaging with carers, 89
engaging with physical health colleagues, 87–89
epilepsy, 72, 74, 91
forensic psychiatric patients, 154–155
improvements to, 85–89
learning disability, 175
least restrictive principle in, 86–87
motor skills assessment, 90
normalisation in, 86–87
person centred approach to, 86
reasonable adjustments in, 86
respiratory conditions assessment, 93
vision assessment, 94
Association of Director of Social Care (ADASS), 209
attention deficit and hyperactivity disorder (ADHD)
  assessment of, 120
  autism, 58
  Cornelia de Lange syndrome, 31
  fragile X syndrome, 33
  lack of screening tool, 121
  mental health legislation, 215–216
  sex aneuploidy, 34
Atypical Autism, 53
atypical mood disorders, 123
atypical psychosis, 31
auditory memory, 47

255

Index

autism spectrum
  disorders (ASD)
  ability to testify, 61–62
  aetiology of, 56–57
  anxiety and, 122
  child-specific concerns, 116,
    120–121
  comorbidity, 29, 58–60
  Cornelia de Lange
    syndrome, 31
  decision making and mental
    capacity, 62
  differential diagnosis, 168
  epidemiology of, 57–60
  evolving concepts, 53–54
  foetal valproate
    syndrome, 31
  fragile X syndrome, 33
  genetic risk factors, 13
  identification and screening,
    54–56
  instruments for, 55
  interviews, 56
  introduction to, 7
  management of, 60–61
  mental health legislation,
    215–216
  offending behaviour, 61
  prevalence of, 57–58
  questionnaires, 55
  summary of, 62
autosomal dominant
  disorders, 16
avoidant learning style, 29

Bach, Richard, 223
barriers to involvement in
  clinical research, 236–237
basal ganglia, 49
behavioural phenotypes
  Angelman syndrome, 30
  Cornelia de Lange
    syndrome, 31
  defined, 28
  Down syndrome, 29
  foetal alcohol syndrome,
    31–32
  foetal valproate
    syndrome, 31
  fragile X syndrome,
    32–33
  hypothyroidism, 35, 36–38*t*
  introduction to, 28–29, 130
  Lesch-Nyhan syndrome, 33
  phenylketonuria, 35, 36–38*t*
  physical health, 29

Prader-Willi syndrome,
  30–31
Rett syndrome, 33
sex aneuploidy, 33–34
Smith-Magenis
  syndrome, 34
summary of, 39
tuberous sclerosis complex,
  34–35
William syndrome, 35
Belmont Report on Ethical
  Principles and Guidelines
  for the Protection of
  Human Subjects of
  Research, 232
bezoars concerns, 92
biomarkers in genetics, 240
biopsychosocial approach to
  assessment
  age-related cognitive
    impairment, 95
  cardiac conditions, 93
  description of cognitive/
    motor skills, 90
  developmental history, 90
  eating and choking
    symptoms, 92
  endocrine system, 93
  epilepsy, 91
  gastrointestinal system,
    91–92
  health promotion/living, 95
  healthcare management,
    95–96
  hearing and vision, 94
  in hospital setting, 96–97
  introduction to, 86, 89
  life events, 90
  medications, 94
  mental illness symptoms, 94
  musculoskeletal system, 93
  overview of, 89–96
  pain, 91
  physical/mental health
    issues, 95
  psychiatric review of, 96
  respiratory conditions, 93
  usual behaviour, 90–91
bipolar disorder and autism,
  59–60
borderline intellectual
  functioning, 3, 153
borderline learning
  disability, 153
Bradley Report, 150
Brief Psychotic Disorder, 59

British Psychological Society,
  138, 142, 161
Broca's area of the brain, 49
Building the Right
  Support, 152

capacity legislation, 218–220,
  235–236
cardiac conditions
  assessment, 93
Care and Treatment Review
  (CTR), 207
Care Quality Commission, 199
carers and dementia, 143
catatonia and autism, 59–60
Catholic identity, 195
cause of death. *See also*
  mortality
  age-related, 102, 103
  choking, 92
  intellectual disability and,
    7–8, 105
  overview of, 108
Cause of Death certificate, 105
cause-specific mortality,
  108, 109
celiac disease, 92
Center for Disease Control
  and Prevention
  (CDC), 57
central coherence, 56
cerebral palsy, 33, 67, 92, 93,
  103, 109, 153
Certificate of Completion of
  Training (CCT), 251
challenging behaviour and
  pharmacology
  conceptual framework for
    understanding, 180
  formulation informed
    intervention plans,
    180–183, 182*f*
  good prescribing practices,
    183–185, 184*f*, 186–187*t*,
    187*f*
  harm to others, 185
  harm to self, 185
  introduction to, 179
  summary of, 185
challenging behaviour and
  psychotherapy
  achieving/maintaining
    change, 174
  anger management, 165,
    172–174
  case study, 160

differential diagnosis and diagnostic overshadowing, 166–168
differential reinforcement, 172t
functional analysis, 168–170
interventions, 170
introduction to, 165–166
measuring outcomes, 174–175
Positive Behaviour Support, 170–171
summary of, 175
Child and Adolescent Mental Health Services (CAMHS), 115, 119
child-environment transactions, 130
childhood Obsessive Compulsive Disorder, 57
Childhood Schizophrenia, 53
children with intellectual disability
anxiety, 122–123
atypical mood disorders, 123
autism and, 116, 120–121
common problems, 120–123
depression, 121
epilepsy and, 121
family issues, 117–118
introduction to, 115–116
multidisciplinary teams, 119–120
psychosis, 123
school issues, 118–119
self-talk, 123
sleep disorders, 120
summary of, 124
Tourette's syndrome, 121
transitioning from school, 119
choking symptoms, 92
Clinical Commissioning Groups, 209
clinical criterion of intellectual disability, 1
Clinical Global Impression Scale (CGI), 208
Clinical Practice Research Database, 107, 109
clinical research/trials
barriers to involvement, 236–237
consent for inclusive research, 235–236

ethical codes for medical experimentation, 232–233
ethical review process, 233
future directions, 240
historical overview of ethics, 231–232
introduction to, 231
overcoming barriers to involvement, 237, 239f
summary, 239–241
Clinical Trial Authorisation (CTA), 235
Clinical Trial of an Investigational Medicinal Product (CTIMP), 233, 235
clobazam medication, 77
close-knit peer support, 88
clumsiness and autism, 58
Cochrane Collaboration reviews, 140
cognitive behaviour therapy (CBT), 121, 131, 165, 170, 172
cognitive skills assessment, 90
cognitive treatment, 154
Commissioning for Quality and Innovation (CQUINs), 209
communicable disease, 1
communicating skills in leadership and management, 224
communication with intellectual disability
auditory memory, 47
during clinical appointment, 51–52t
easy read information, 48
expressive language use, 44–47
inclusive/total communication, 47
introduction to, 42
language difficulties, 43,
language neurology, 48–49
management of disorders, 60
motor system for speech, 49–50, 50t
psychotherapy and, 159
real objects in, 46, 47t
receptive language, 47
signing systems, 45
speech difficulties, 42, 43t
speech neurology, 49
spoken output, 44

symbols, pictures and photographs, 45–46, 46t
written language, 44
community care, 199t, 200t, 201
community disposal of forensic patients, 152
Community Forensic Intellectual Disability teams, 152
comorbidity, 29, 58–60, 61, 141
complex interventions, 238
concomitant neurodevelopmental disorders, 128
Confidential Inquiry into Premature Deaths of People with Learning Disabilities (CIPOLD), 104, 107, 110t, 111, 224
Confidentiality Advisory Group (CAG), 236
consent for inclusive research, 235–236
consent-to-treatment procedures, 183
constipation concerns, 92
copy-number variants (CNVs), 214–221, 240
Cornelia de Lange syndrome (CdLS), 31
Court Diversion Schemes, 150
court reports for forensic patients, 154
Cri-du-chat syndrome, 16
criminal justice system (CJS), 147, 148, 149–151
Criminal Procedure rule (2005), 150
Cygnet program, 117
cytogenetic abnormalities, 13–16
cytogenetic technique, 13
cytokines, 130

Danish Civil Registration System, 5
Data Protection Act, 236
Database of Genomic Variants (DGV), 19
de novo mutations (DNMs), 13, 21
Death by Indifference (Mencap report), 103, 104
Death by Indifference campaign, 199

Deciphering Developmental Disorders (DDD) study, 21
decision-making capacity, 62, 172, 219
delivery skills in leadership and management, 224
delusions, 181
dementia in Alzheimer's disease (DAD), 136, 140, 143–144
Dementia Questionnaire for people with Learning Disabilities (DLD), 139
Dementia Scale for Down's syndrome (DSDS), 139
Dementia Screening Questionnaire for Individuals with ID (DSQIID), 139
dementia with intellectual disabilities
 antidementia drugs, 140
 antipsychotic medication, 140–141
 carers and, 143
 co-morbidity treatments, 141–142
 diagnosis and evaluation, 137–139
 direct tests, 139
 environmental factors, 143
 epidemiological issues, 136–137
 informant questionnaires, 139
 introduction to, 132
 mortality and, 109
 non-pharmacological interventions/treatment, 142–143, 144
 pharmacological interventions/treatment, 140–142
 psychological approaches to, 142–143
 summary of, 143–144
 treatments, 139–143
dementia with Lewy Bodies, 137
depression
 Alzheimer's and, 29
 antidepressant medication, 141, 179, 220
 assessment of, 120, 139
 autism, 59

in children, 121
 cognitive behavioural therapy for, 131
 comorbidity, 141
 Cornelia de Lange syndrome, 31
 low self-esteem with, 130
 mood disorders, 59
 psychological interventions for, 172
 sex aneuploidy, 34
Deprivation of Liberty Safeguards (2007), 198–199, 217
design skills in leadership and management, 224
developmental delay (DD), 12, 19
developmental disorders, 149
developmental history assessment, 90
diagnosis and evaluation. *See also* assessment
 adults with intellectual disability, 127–128
 dementia with intellectual disabilities, 137–139
 epilepsy, 70t
 importance of, 181–182
 intellectual disability, 2–4
Diagnostic and Statistical Manual of Mental Disorders (DSM 5)
 autism spectrum disorders, 55
 intellectual disabilities, 126
 introduction to, 2
 mental handicap, defined, 197
 mental retardation, 200
Diagnostic Criteria for Psychiatric Disorders for Use with Adults with Learning Disabilities/ Mental Retardation (DC-LD), 129–130
Diagnostic Manual-Intellectual Disability 2 (DM-ID2), 129–130
diagnostic overshadowing, 127, 166–168
Dialectical Behaviour Therapy, 154
diet and epilepsy, 77
differential diagnosis
 autism spectrum disorders, 168

behavioural disorders, 166–168
epilepsy, 71t, 167
differential reinforcement, 172t
disability service providers, 97
Disability Services Commission of Western Australia, 7
Disorders of Intellectual Development (DID), service history
 community care and, 199t, 200t, 201
 incarceration of, 194–196
 introduction to, 12–13, 191
 legislation and policy documents, 200–201
 pre-specialist care, 191–193
 specialist care, 193–194
DNA (deoxyribonucleic acid), 12
DNA microarrays, 19
Down, Langdon, 193
Down Syndrome
 Alzheimer's disease and, 6, 29
 behavioural phenotypes, 29
 celiac disease, 92
 dementia and, 136
 epilepsy in, 67
 genetic risks, 16
 psychotherapy and, 161
 self-talk, 123
 speech difficulties, 42
 vision impairment impact, 84
dravet syndrome, 68–69
dual criterion of intellectual disability, 1

early vocabulary development, 44
easy read information, 48
Education, Health and Care Plan (EHCP), 119
education with intellectual disability, 60, 143
electroconvulsive therapy (ECT), 215
electroencephalogram (EEG), 167
emotional support, 143
employment with intellectual disability, 60
endocrine system assessment, 93

England, inpatient care,
    206–207
English Autism Act (2009), 199
English Mental Capacity Act
    (2005), 198
English Poor Law (1834), 193
environmental factors and
    intellectual disabilities,
    131, 143
epidemiological community
    surveys, 4
epilepsy
  in adults, 130
  aetiology of, 66–67
  antiepileptic medication, 142
  assessment of risk, 72
  autism and, 58
  behaviour assessment, 74
  behavioural phenotype
    and, 29
  biopsychosocial approach to
    assessment, 91
  in children, 121
  Cornelia de Lange
    syndrome, 31
  diagnosis of, 70t
  diet and, 77
  differential diagnosis of,
    71t, 167
  dravet syndrome, 68–69
  epidemiology of, 65, 66t
  improving care and
    outcomes, 78
  introduction to, 65
  lennox-gastaut syndrome, 68
  mental health and, 69–70
  morbidity and mortality,
    69, 109
  non-pharmacological
    interventions, 77–78
  outcome measures, 73–74
  pharmacological
    interventions, 74–77, 76t
  phenotypes, 67
  psychiatric management
    of, 245
  seizure types, 67–68
  summary of, 75f, 78
  surgery for, 77
  treatment, 72–73
  vagus nerve stimulation, 78
Equality Act (2010), 111
equality legislation, 217–218
ethical codes for medical
    experimentation, 232–233
eugenics, 147, 194

European Convention on
    Human Rights, 213, 214,
    216–217
event recording, 169
evidence-based health/
    medicine, 72, 102, 170,
    181, 231
executive function, 56
exome sequencing, 21–22, 23
expressive language use, 44–47

family issues, 117–118
Farr, William, 102
fatuus naturalis, 191
feeble-minded persons,
    191, 195
fitness to plead, 151
foetal alcohol syndrome (FAS),
    31–32
foetal valproate syndrome, 31
forensic psychiatric patients
  background on, 147–148
  community disposal, 152
  court reports, 154
  criminal justice system, 147,
    148, 149–151
  fitness to plead, 151
  inpatient services, 152–153
  Mental Health Act, 149,
    150, 151
  offending by, 148–149
  prevalence of, 148
  risk assessment, 154–155
  summary of, 155
  treatment, 154
forensic rehabilitation
    needs, 205
formulation informed
    intervention plans,
    180–183, 182f
fragile X mental retardation
    protein (FMRP), 32
fragile X syndrome (FXS), 17,
    23, 32–33
frontotemporal dementia
    (FTD), 137
functional analysis of
    behavioural disorders,
    168–170

gastrointestinal system
    assessment, 91–92
gatekeepers, 237
General Medical Council
    (GMC), 184, 225, 247
genetic pleiotropy, 13

genetic testing, 22–23
genetics/genetic risk factors
  autism spectrum disorders, 13
  biomarkers, 240
  copy number variations,
    18–21
  Cri-du-chat syndrome, 16
  cytogenetic abnormalities,
    13–16
  Down Syndrome, 16
  epilepsy, 72
  exome sequencing, 21–22, 23
  future directions, 23
  genetic testing, 22–23
  introduction, 14, 6, 12–13
  psychiatric disorders, 130
  sex chromosome
    aneuploidies, 16
  single-gene disorders, 16–18
  summary of, 23–24
  whole-genome
    sequencing, 22
Glasgow Anxiety Scale, 208
Glasgow epilepsy outcome
    measure (geos), 74
Global Burden of Disease
    study, 4
Goddard, Henry, 147
Good Medical Practice,
    213, 235
good prescribing practices, 183,
    183–185, 184f, 186–187t,
    187f
Griffiths Report (1988), 198
Guardianship Order, 152

hallucinations, 59, 123,
    181
harm to others, 180, 185
harm to self. *See* self-harm/
    self-injury
health inequalities, 6–7
health literacy of carers, 85
Health of the Nation Scale-
    Learning Disability
    (HoNoS-LD), 208
health promotion/living
    assessment, 95
Health Research Authority
    (HRA), 233
healthcare management
    assessment, 95–96
hearing assessment, 94
hearing loss, 42
heterogeneity between genetic
    abnormalities, 67

Index

H.pylori concerns, 92
Human Genome Initiative, 21
Human Genome Project (HGP), 21–23
Human Rights Act, 214, 217
Human Tissue Act, 236
hyperactivity, 29, 32
hypothyroidism, 35, 36–38*t*
hypoxanthine guanine phosphoribosyltransferase (HPRT), 33

identification skills in leadership and management, 224
identity and psychotherapy, 159–160
Idiot and Imbecile Institution, 193
idiots, defined, 191–193, 195
Idiots Act (1886), 193
imbeciles, defined, 195
Improving Access to Psychological Therapies (IAPT), 160
impulsivity in fragile X syndrome, 32
in-hospital mortality and morbidity, 84
incarceration history, 194–196
incidence studies of intellectual disability, 4–5
inclusive/total communication, 47
individuation process, 160
Industrial Revolution, 204
industrialisation, 192
infantile spasms, 67
inflammatory cytokines, 130
influencing skills in leadership and management, 224
innocents, defined, 192
inpatient care
  care and treatment reviews, 207
  challenges for, 209
  England, 206–207
  for forensic patients, 152–153
  future planning, 209
  generic *vs.* specialist services, 204–206
  introduction to, 204
  need for, 205
  Northern Ireland, 208
  outcome measures, 208
  quality issues, 208–209
  reduction in use of specialist beds, 206–208
  Scotland, 207
  treatment issues, 208
  Wales, 208
insomnia and hypnotics, 141
Institution for Idiotic and Imbecile Children, 193
Institution for Imbecile Children, 193
institutional discrimination, 103
instruments of screening
  autism spectrum disorders, 55, 57
  dementia in Alzheimer's disease, 138
  dementia with intellectual disorders, 139
  epilepsy, 74
  risk assessments, 154–155
intellectual criterion of intellectual disability, 1
Intellectual Development Disorder (IDD), 3
intellectual disability. *See also* adults with intellectual disability; children with intellectual disability
  aetiology, 5–6
  introduction to, 1
  morbidity, 6–7
  mortality, 7–8
  perspectives of, 1–2
  prevalence and incidence, 4–5
  profound and multiple intellectual disability, 46
  summary of, 8
  terminology, classification and diagnosis, 2–4
Intellectual Disability (ID) Psychiatry training. *See* training in Intellectual Disability (ID) Psychiatry
intelligence quotient (IQ), 30
intelligence quotient (IQ) tests, 1, 106
inter-personal problems, 173
International Association for the Scientific Study of Intellectual and Developmental Disabilities (IASSIDD), 3
International Classification of Diseases (ICD-10), 2, 55, 126, 197, 200
International Classification of Functioning, Disability and Health (ICF), 2
International Conference on Harmonisation (ICH), 232
International Standard Cytogenomic Array (ISCA) Consortium, 19
interval recording, 169
interventions. *See also* pharmacological interventions/treatment; treatment
  adults with intellectual disability, 131
  anxiety/anxiety disorders, 172
  complex interventions, 238
  dementia with intellectual disabilities, 142–143, 144
  epilepsy, 74–78, 76*t*
  formulation informed intervention plans, 180–183, 182*f*
  Outcome Measures for Challenging Behaviour Interventions, 175
  psychological intervention with intellectual disability, 60
  understanding challenging behaviour, 180
interviews for autism spectrum disorders, 56
Investigational Medicinal Product (IMP), 233
INVOLVE advisory group, 238

Kanner, Leo, 53, 54
Klinefelter syndrome, 33–34

labelling concerns, 159
lacosamide medication, 77
lamotrigine medication, 75
language difficulties, 44, 43
language neurology, 48–49
leadership and management
  background, 222–224
  context for, 224–225
  introduction to, 222
  for medical practitioners, 225–226

Index

resources for, 226–227
summary of, 228
Learning Disabilities Mortality Review (LeDeR) Programme, 105, 112
learning disability
  profound and multiple learning disabilities, 240
learning disability (LD)
  assessment scales, 175
  assessment team, 152
  behavioural problems with, 167, 171
  challenging behaviour, 165
  communication standards, 51*t*, 52
  defined, 153, 198
  as diagnosis, 198
  health care providers for, 200
  inpatient care, 205–206, 207
  Mental Health Act and, 151
  mild learning disability, 160, 161
  social services for, 198
  specialists in children's homes, 118
  support for, 223, 224
  therapeutic approach to, 173
  training pathways, 247–249
Learning Disability Programme, 207
least restrictive principle in healthcare assessment, 86–87
legal provisions and restrictive practices
  capacity legislation, 218–220, 235–236
  equality legislation, 217–218
  European Convention on Human Rights, 213, 216–217
  introduction to, 213–214
  mental health, 214–216
  therapeutic restriction, 220–221
lennox-gastaut syndrome, 68
Lesch-Nyhan syndrome, 33
levetiracetam medication, 77
life events, 90, 131
life expectancy, 84, 107
life stages and psychotherapy, 159–160
Local Delivery Plans, 225
Local Education and Training Boards (LETBs), –248

London Down Syndrome Consortium (LonDownS), 239–240
lower motor neuron (LMN) pathways, 50
Lunacy Act (1845), 193

mainstream services with psychotherapy, 160–161
management and leadership. *See* leadership and management
Mansell Report, 166
Massachusetts Sanitary Commission, 102
Mazars report, 104–105
medical experimentation, 232–233
Medical Research Council (MRC), 232, 238
medication
  antidementia drugs, 140
  antidepressants, 141, 179
  antiepileptics, 142
  antipsychotics, 140–141, 179
  anxiety/anxiety disorders, 122–123, 220
  assessments for, 94
  biopsychosocial approach to assessment, 94
  clobazam, 77
  evidence-based health/medicine, 72, 102, 170, 181, 231
  lacosamide, 77
  lamotrigine, 75
  levetiracetam, 77
  perampanel, 77
  start low go slow policy with, 73
  topiramate, 75–77
Medicines and Healthcare Products Regulatory Agency (MHRA), 232, 235
Medicines for Human Use (Clinical Trials) Regulations, 232
melatonin, 120
Mendelian disorders, 16–18
Mental Capacity Act (2005), 138, 217, 219, 235–236
Mental Care Hospitals, 196
Mental Deficiency Act (1913), 147, 194, 196
mental handicap, defined, 197–198

mental handicap hospitals, 197
Mental Health Act (1959), 196
Mental Health Act (1983), 149, 150, 151, 198, 204, 217
mental health/illness
  biopsychosocial approach to assessment, 94
  epilepsy and, 69–70
  introduction to, 7
  legislation for, 214–216
  physical health and, 83–85
Mental Health Treatment Requirement option (MHTR), 152
mental retardation. *See* intellectual disability
mental subnormality, 196
mentally defective, 193, 194, 195
mentally deficient, 195–196
Metropolitan Asylums Board, 193
Michael, Jonathan, 104
mild learning disability, 160, 161
Modified Overt Aggression Scale, 166, 208
mood disorders, 59
moral imbeciles, 195
morbidity
  comorbidity and, 29, 58–60, 61, 141
  epilepsy, 69, 109
  in-hospital, 84
  intellectual disability, 6–7
mortality. *See also* cause of death
  age at death, 107
  cause of death, 108
  cause-specific mortality, 108–110
  emergence as key issue, 103–105
  in-hospital, 84
  introduction to, 7–8, 102
  life expectancy, 107
  potentially unavoidable deaths, 109–110
  reducing premature deaths, 110–111, 112*t*
  standardised mortality rates, 107
  standardized mortality ratio, 106*t*–107–108
  summary of, 111–112
  surveillance component, 105–107

Motivation Assessment Scale (MAS), 170
motor skills assessment, 90
motor system for speech, 49–50, 50t
multidisciplinary team (MDT), 119–120, 139, 144, 174, 215, 246
musculoskeletal system assessment, 93

National Commission for the Protection of Human Subjects of Biomedical and Behaviour Research, 232
National Health Service (NHS), 204, 233
National Institute for Health and Care Excellence (NICE), 128, 170–171, 179, 184
National Institute of Health Research (NIHR), 238, 249
National Patient Safety Agency (NPSA), 103
National Task Group on Intellectual Disabilities and Dementia Practices (NTG), 137–138, 143
negative social determinants of health, 84
neonatal hypotonia, 30
neuroleptics in the treatment of aggressive challenging behaviour for people with intellectual disabilities (NACHBID), 236
neurological disturbance behaviour, 220
New Poor Law Commissioners, 193
next generation sequencing (NGS), 13
NHS Leadership Academy, 226
NIHR Clinical Research Network (NIHR CRN), 238
non-pharmacological intervention for dementia, 142–143, 144
non-synonymous exonic mutations, 21
normalisation in healthcare assessment, 86–87, 197
Northern Ireland, inpatient care, 208
nucleic acid microarrays, 19
Nuremberg Trials, 231–232
nutritional concerns, 92

obsessions, 181
obsessive compulsive disorder (OCD), 29, 31, 57, 59
offending behaviour, 61
Office for National Statistics death certification data, 109
operant conditioning, 168–169
Outcome Measures for Challenging Behaviour Interventions, 175
outward aggression, 180
over-values ideas, 181
oxidative stress, 130

pain assessment, 91
palliative care status, 84
parasitic infections, 92
PASSAD checklist, 168
Pathological Demand Avoidance (PDA), 54
Patient and Public Involvement (PPI), 238
peer review of casework, 88
penetrance, defined, 12
People with Disorders of Intellectual Development, 191
perampanel medication, 77
perinatal risk factors in intellectual disability, 6
person-centred care, 86, 171, 206
Person Centred Planning, 119
personality disorder with autism, 58
pharmacological interventions/ treatment, 140, 74–77, 76t *See also* challenging behaviour and pharmacology; interventions; medication
phenylalanine hydroxylase *(PAH)* gene, 17
phenylketonuria (PKU), 17, 35, 36–38t
photographs, in communication, 45–46, 46t
physical abuse, 117

physical health
behavioural phenotypes, 29
biopsychosocial approach to assessment, 86, 89–96
in hospital setting, 96–97
improvements to healthcare assessments, 85–89
introduction to, 6–7, 83
mental health and, 83–85
multidisciplinary approach to, 88
summary of, 97–98
pictures, in communication, 45–46, 46t
Police and Criminal Evidence Act (PACE) (1984), 149
polymerase chain reaction (PCR), 16
polypharmacy, 129
portfolio career, 246–247
Positive Behaviour Support (PBS), 143, 144, 170–171
potentially unavoidable deaths, 109–110
Prader-Willi Syndrome (PWS), 17, 18, 30–31
Pragmatic Language Impairment, 53
pre-existing disabilities, 128
pre-existing physical disorders, 128
pre-specialist care, 191–193
precentral gyrus, 49
premature deaths, reduction factors, 110–111, 112t
prenatal risk factors for intellectual disability, 6
prevalence studies of intellectual disability, 4–5
prioritised resources in leadership and management, 224
problem behaviours, 127
profound and multiple intellectual disability (PMID), 46
profound and multiple learning disabilities (PMLD), 240
pseudo-hallucinations, 181
psychiatric disorders, 19–20
psychiatric review of assessment, 96
psychiatrist role, 181
psychological mindedness, 218
psychopathic personalities, 196

psychosis in adults, 129
psychosis in children, 123
psychotherapy. *See also* challenging behaviour and psychotherapy
 challenging behaviour, 160
 choosing modality, 161, 162*t*
 communication and, 159
 context for, 158–159
 dementia with intellectual disabilities, 142–143
 developing skills in, 161–163, 246
 intervention with intellectual disability, 60
 introduction to, 158
 labelling and stigma concerns, 159
 life stages and identity, 159–160
 mainstream *vs.* specialist services, 160–161
 summary of, 163

quality issues with inpatient care, 208–209
questionnaires for autism spectrum disorders, 55

random controlled trials (RCTs), 77, 235–238, 239, 240
real objects in communication, 46, 47*t*
reasonable adjustments in healthcare assessment, 86
receptive language communication, 47
recognized resources in leadership and management, 224
Reed, Andrew, 193
Regional Clinical Genetics Services, 22
Research Autism, 60
Research Ethics Committees (RECs), 233, 235
respiratory conditions assessment, 93
respiratory diseases and mortality, 109
restricted, repetitive patterns of behaviour, interests or activities (RRBI), 54–55, 59
restrictive practices. *See* legal provisions and restrictive practices

Rhett syndrome, 17, 18, 23, 33
risk assessment, 154–155. *See also* genetics/genetic risk factors
Rochester Epidemiology Project, 5
role-playing therapy, 174
Royal College of Psychiatrists, 119, 138, 161, 197, 205, 247, 248
Royal College of Speech and Language Therapists, 51*t*, 52
Royal Commission on the Care and Control of the Feeble Minded, 194

Schizoid Personality Disorder, 53
schizophrenia
 autism and, 59
 Childhood Schizophrenia, 53
 genetic risk factors, 13, 19–20
 16p11.2 deletion syndrome, 21
 22q11.2 deletion syndrome, 20
school issues, 118–119
Scotland, inpatient care, 207
Scotland's Census, 126
Scottish Intercollegiate Guideline Network (SIGN), 208
seizures, 142, 167
Selective Serotonin Reuptake Inhibitors (SSRI) antidepressants, 123, 144
self-fulfilling prophecy, 28
self-harm/self-injury, 168, 169, 180, 185
self-talk, 32, 123
Semantic Pragmatic Disorder, 53
sensory deficits, 29
severe subnormality, 196
sex aneuploidy, 33–34
sex chromosome aneuploidies, 16
sexual abuse, 117, 159
sexual offenses, 149
signing systems, 45
single-gene disorders, 16–18
single nucleotide polymorphism (SNP) microarrays, 19

single nucleotide variants (SNVs), 13
16p11.2 deletion syndrome, 20–21
sleep disorders, 120
Smith-Magenis syndrome, 34
social anxiety, 31, 32–33, 123
Social Communication Disorder (SCD), 53
social contextual processes, 180
social criterion of intellectual disability, 1
social factors in psychiatric disorders, 131
social learning theory, 172
socio-economic disadvantage, 6
sodium valproate, 31
somatic mosaicisms, 23
Sparrowhawk, Connor, 104–105
spastic paralysis, 50
specialist care, 160–161, 193–194
specialist registrar (SpR), 250
speech and language therapists, 120
speech difficulties, 42, 43*t*
speech neurology, 49
spoken output, 44
stakeholders, 237
standardized mortality ratio (SMR), 107–108
STAR form, 170
start low go slow policy with medication, 73
stigma concerns, 159
stimulation-orientated treatments, 142–143
stop over-medication of people with an intellectual disability (STOMP), 179
subnormality, 196, 198
substance misuse disorders, 149
sudden unexplained death in epilepsy (SUDEP), 69
Support Needs model of disability, 2
Suspected Unexpected Serious Adverse Reactions (SUSARs), 235
symbols, in communication, 45, 46

syndrome-specific behaviours, 168

Thalidomide birth related defects, 232
Theory of Mind, 56
therapeutic restrictions, 220–221
time sampling, 169
tonic-clonic seizures, 67–68
tonic seizures, 68
topiramate medication, 75–77
Tourette's syndrome, 121, 168
training for people with autism, 60
training in Intellectual Disability (ID) Psychiatry
  curriculum studies, 249, 250t
  higher training opportunities, 252–253, 253t
  introduction to, 245
  new trainee experiences, 250–251
  pathway to, 247–249, 248f
  preparation as consultant, 253
  progressing through training, 251–252
  reasons to choose, 247
training programme director (TPD), 251, 252
Transforming Care programme, 153, 199
transition cliff, 4
transitioning from school, 119
treatment. *See also* challenging behaviour and psychotherapy; interventions; psychotherapy
  cognitive treatment, 154
  consent-to-treatment procedures, 183
  dementia with intellectual disabilities, 139–143, 144
  epilepsy, 72–73
  forensic psychiatric patients, 154
  inpatient care, 207, 208
  stimulation-orientated treatments, 142–143
trinucleotide repeat expansion, 32
Triple P (Positive Parenting Programme), 117
Trisomy X, 34
tuberous sclerosis complex (TSC), 34–35, 67
Turner syndrome, 33–34
22q11.2 deletion syndrome, 20

UBE3A gene, 30
ubiquitin-protein ligase E3A (*UBE3A*), 18
UK Office for National Statistics, 102
United Kingdom Supreme Court, 221
University of California Santa Cruz (UCSC) genome browser, 21
upper motor neuron (UMN) pathways, 50

usual behaviour assessment, 90–91

vagus nerve stimulation, 78
Valuing People, 205, 222
Valuing People Now, 205, 222
verbal aggression, 149
vision assessment, 94
vision impairment and Down Syndrome, 84
vulnerability factors for challenging behaviour, 180

Wales, inpatient care, 208
Wernicke's area of the brain, 49
whole-genome sequencing (WGS), 22, 23
William syndrome (WS), 35
Wing, Lorna, 53, 54
Winterbourne View investigation, 175
Witness Intermediary Scheme, 154
World Health Organization, 2, 105
World Medical Association (WMA), 232
World Psychiatric Association (WPA), 3
written language communication, 44

X chromosome, 12

Y chromosome, 12